MEDICAL LIBRARY SERVICE

Uterine Cancer

CURRENT CLINICAL ONCOLOGY

Maurie Markman, MD, SERIES EDITOR

For other titles published in this series, go to
http://www.springer.com/series/7631

UTERINE CANCER

Screening, Diagnosis, and Treatment

Edited by

FRANCO MUGGIA, MD

New York University, School of Medicine,
Division Medical Oncology, New York, NY

ESTHER OLIVA, MD

Massachusetts General Hospital,
Department of Pathology, Boston, MA

Humana Press

Editors
Franco Muggia
New York University
School of Medicine
Division Medical Oncology
550 First Avenue, BCD 556
New York, NY 10016
USA
franco.muggia@nyumc.org

Esther Oliva
Massachusetts General Hospital
Department of Pathology
55 Fruit St.
Boston, MA 02114
USA
eoliva@partners.org

ISBN 978-1-58829-736-5   e-ISBN 978-1-60327-044-1
DOI 10.1007/978-1-60327-044-1
Springer Dordrecht Heidelberg London New York

Library of Congress Control Number: 2008939889

Printed on acid-free paper

Springer is part of Springer Science+Business Media (www.springer.com)

Preface

For the Editors, the task of writing a Preface is most satisfying. It represents the completion of the book and a moment of reflection on whether the whole is more than the sum of all the parts. And also, one must reflect on how this book is likely to be utilized in this era of rapid communications.

The Editors first met in May 2003 at a stimulating Italian symposium on endometrial cancer (organizers Drs. Luigi Frigerio, Roberto Grassi and Andrea Lissoni, with participation of the deans of Italian Gynecologic Oncology, Ugo Bianchi and Constantino Mangioni) that took place at Bergamo and Caravaggio. The impressive gains in biology and clinical trials were further discussed by the two editors and others that are co-authors in this venture on this side of the Atlantic at a 2004 Educational Session at the American Society of Clinical Oncology (ASCO). The pace of progress in various aspects of management of uterine cancer was noteworthy, not only was tumor biology fueling novel hypotheses such as questioning the mesenchymal origin of carcinosarcomas, but knowledge of molecular pathways was beginning to be applied as prognostic and as predictive factors portending benefit from systemic therapies. Surgical staging and sensitive imaging provided the underpinning for refining our treatment algorithms. Finally, a role for chemotherapy had finally become established, principally through phase III studies comparing chemotherapy to radiation in mostly locally advanced stages III and IV that had undergone resection.

Inevitably, this task brought back thoughts of prior efforts going into books covering endometrial cancer. In 1987, an international symposium resulted in publication of a multiauthored book. To this day, it remains a valuable reference to the advent of pharmacology and hormone receptor work in the evaluation of hormonal therapy relevant to endometrial cancer. However, in the intervening 20 years biomedical science has moved far beyond focusing systemic therapy on the first of 'targeted therapies'. We are indebted to all contributors, mostly selected on first-hand knowledge of their expertise and often based on interactions within our institutions or in cooperative groups and scientific societies. We know we added some additional work to their already busy daily lives, but hope they will be pleased with the results.

Covering the subject in a comprehensive manner is a challenge for the Editors. On the one hand, one needs to discourage encyclopedic reviews in order to focus on what is new – the prime motivation for highlighting various aspects of uterine cancer. On the other hand, if one of the functions will be to become a handy reference on which to build the near future of therapeutics, all aspects of the foundations as well as of advancing science need to be included. In finally surveying the components that make up this new venture, we are hopeful that we have come close to our goals to emphasize new aspects while providing useful reference material.

January 2, 2009   Franco Muggia and Esther Oliva
                                                                                         Editors

Contents

Contributors

Lea Baer, MD, Department of Radiation Oncology, NYU Cancer Institute, NYU Medical Center, New York NY

Patricia M. Baker, MD, Department of Pathology, Health Sciences Centre, University of Manitoba, Winnipeg, Canada

Richard R. Barakat, MD, FACS, Gynecology Service, Department of Surgery, Memorial Sloan-Kettering Cancer Center, New York, NY

Stephanie V. Blank, MD, Department of Obstetrics and Gynecology, NYU Medical Center, New York, NY

Karine Chung, MD, MSCE, Departments of Preventive Medicine and Obstetrics and Gynecology, USC/Norris Comprehensive Cancer Center, Keck School of Medicine, University of Southern California, Los Angeles, CA

John Curtin, MD, MBA, Department of Obstetrics and Gynecology, NYU Medical Center, New York, NY

Paola Dal Cin, PhD, Pathology Department, Brigham and Women's Hospital, Boston, MA

Marcela G. del Carmen, MD, MPH, Vincent Obstetrics and Gynecology Service, Division of Gynecologic Oncology, Massachusetts General Hospital, Boston, MA

Linda R. Duska, MD, Division of Gynecologic Oncology, Department of Obstetrics and Gynecology, University of Virginia, VA

Gini F. Fleming, MD, Section of Hematology/Oncology, Department of Medicine, University of Chicago Medical Center, Chicago, IL

Silvia Formenti, MD, Department of Radiation Oncology, NYU Cancer Institute, NYU Medical Center, New York, NY

Barbara Goff, MD, Department of Obstetrics and Gynecology, University of Washington, Seattle, WA

Leslie I. Gold, PhD, Departments of Medicine and Pathology, NYU Medical Center, New York, NY

Annekathryn Goodman, MD, Division of Gynecologic Oncology, Gillette Center for Women's Cancers, Massachusetts General Hospital, Boston, MA

Martee L. Hensley, MD, Gynecologic Medical Oncology Service, Department of Medicine, Memorial Sloan-Kettering Cancer Center, New York, NY

Neil S. Horowitz, MD, Vincent Obstetrics and Gynecology Service, Division of Gynecologic Oncology, Massachusetts General Hospital, Boston, MA

Carolyn Krasner, MD, Department of Medical Oncology, Gillette Center for Women's Cancers, Massachusetts General Hospital, Boston, MA

Susanna I. Lee, MD, PhD, Department of Radiology, Massachusetts General Hospital, Boston, MA

Franco Muggia, MD, Division of Medical Oncology, NYU Cancer Institute, NYU Medical Center, New York, NY

Halla Nimeiri, MD, Section of Hematology/Oncology, Department of Medicine, University of Chicago Medical Center, Chicago, IL

Esther Oliva, MD, Department of Pathology, Massachusetts General Hospital, Boston, MA

Jose Palacios, MD, Pathology Department, Hospital del Rocio, Seville, Spain

Celeste L. Pearce, PhD, Departments of Preventive Medicine and Obstetrics and Gynecology, USC/Norris Comprehensive Cancer Center, Keck School of Medicine, University of Southern California, Los Angeles, CA

Malcolm C. Pike, PhD, Departments of Preventive Medicine and Obstetrics and Gynecology, USC/Norris Comprehensive Cancer Center, Keck School of Medicine, University of Southern California, Los Angeles, CA

Matthew A. Powell, MD, Division of Gynecologic Oncology, Department of Obstetrics and Gynecology, Washington University School of Medicine, St. Louis, MO

Mansi A. Saksena, MD, Department of Radiology, Massachusetts General Hospital, Boston, MA

Yukio Sonoda, MD, Gynecology Service, Department of Surgery, Memorial Sloan-Kettering Cancer Center, New York, NY

Robert A. Soslow, MD, Department of Pathology, Memorial Sloan-Kettering Cancer Center, New York, NY

Nicholas P. Taylor, Division of Gynecologic Oncology, Department of Obstetrics and Gynecology, Washington University School of Medicine, St. Louis, MO

A. Gabriella Wernicke, MD, Department of Radiation Oncology, Weill Cornell School of Medicine, New York, NY

Anna H. Wu, PhD, MPH, Departments of Preventive Medicine and Obstetrics and Gynecology, USC/Norris Comprehensive Cancer Center, Keck School of Medicine, University of Southern California, Los Angeles, CA

The Essential Epidemiology of Cancer of the Endometrium

Celeste L. Pearce, Karine Chung, Anna H. Wu, and Malcolm C. Pike

Abstract The central epidemiologic features of cancer of the endometrium are the much increased risk associated with obesity, evident both in premenopausal and postmenopausal women, the decreased risk with increasing parity and increasing duration of use of oral contraceptives (OCs), the increased risk with menopausal estrogen therapy (ET), and the sharp slowing down in the rate of increase in endometrial cancer incidence with age around the time of menopause. Sequential menopausal estrogen–progestin therapy (EPT) with the progestin given for 10–12 days per 28-day cycle is still associated with an increased risk, although of a much smaller magnitude than that associated with ET. Continuous-combined EPT is not associated with any increased risk and may be associated with a decreased risk. These phenomena are readily explained by a simple "unopposed estrogen hypothesis," by which estrogen "unopposed" by a progestin increases risk. The basis for this hypothesis is that estrogen unopposed by a progestin increases cell division rates in the endometrium. Considering the relationship between endometrial cell proliferation during the menstrual cycle and the diminishing effect of ET with increasing body mass index (kg/m^2), it is possible to show that there is a relatively low ceiling of biologically available estradiol (E$_2$), ~10.1 pg/ml, beyond which no further increase in endometrial cancer risk occurs. On the basis of this information, one would predict that reducing the standard dose of ET by as much as one half will produce little or no reduction in the risk of ET.

Keywords Endometrial cancer • Body mass index • Weight • Estrogen • Estrogen therapy

C.L. Pearce, K. Chung, A.H. Wu, and M.C. Pike (✉)
Departments of Preventive Medicine and Obstetrics and Gynecology, USC/Norris Comprehensive Cancer Center, Keck School of Medicine, University of Southern California, Los Angeles, CA
e-mail: mcpike@usc.edu

F. Muggia and E. Oliva (eds.), *Uterine Cancer*, Current Clinical Oncology,
DOI: 10.1007/978-1-60327-044-1_1,
© Humana Press, a Part of Springer Science+Business Media, LLC 2009

Introduction

The risk of endometrial cancer increases markedly with increasing body mass index (BMI; kg/m^2) and use of estrogen therapy (ET), while increasing parity and use of oral contraceptives (OCs) decrease risk significantly. The qualitative effects of these factors can be explained by a simple "unopposed estrogen hypothesis" for endometrial cancer (44). This hypothesis maintains that endometrial cancer risk is increased by exposure of the endometrium to estrogen "unopposed" by progesterone or a synthetic progestin, and that the increased risk is essentially caused by the increased mitotic activity of the endometrium induced by such exposure. Increased mitotic activity as a general risk factor is supported by a considerable amount of evidence; essentially, for a given tissue, the mitotic rate plays a central role in determining the rates at which the underlying carcinogenic processes, such as mutation, proliferation, and cell death, will occur in some stem cell compartment (6, 39). This simple "unopposed estrogen hypothesis" predicts that, for a given parity, the ages at which births occur will have little effect; however, epidemiologic studies show that there is significantly greater protection the later the ages at which births occur.

In order to obtain a comprehensive understanding of all these epidemiologic observations, it is first necessary to gain understanding of the relationship between unopposed estrogen "dose" and endometrial cell proliferation.

Estrogen Dose and Endometrial Cell Mitotic Rate

Estradiol (E$_2$) is the predominant intracellular estrogen in the endometrium and estrogens stimulate mitosis in endometrial cells (52). Progestins dramatically reduce mitotic activity by reducing the concentration of estrogen receptors, by increasing the metabolism of E$_2$ to the less active estrone (E$_1$), and by stimulating differentiation of endometrial cells to a secretory state (19).

The Menstrual Cycle

Figure 1 shows the plasma concentrations of E$_2$ and progesterone (P$_4$) and the mitotic rate of the glandular endometrial cells during the menstrual cycle (14, 17, 48). The mitotic rate rises rapidly from a very low level during menses to reach a near maximal level early on in the cycle around day 5. The rate stays roughly constant for ~14 days, until around day 19, after which it drops again to a very low level when P$_4$ increases. The maximal mitotic rate is induced by the relatively low early follicular plasma E$_2$ concentration of ~50 pg/ml; later increases in E$_2$ levels do not appear to induce any further increase in mitotic rate. Thus, there appears to be an upper limit to the effective plasma concentration of E$_2$ no greater than ~50 pg/ml.

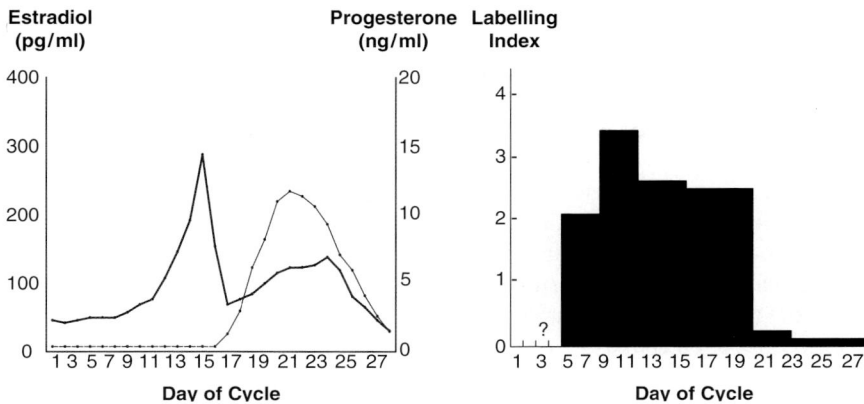

Fig. 1 Plasma concentrations of estradiol and progesterone and endometrial mitotic rate by day of cycle.

The existence of a low ceiling of E_2 effect has important implications. In particular, this limit implies that, in premenopausal women, changes in E_2 will have little effect. Increases in E_2 concentration above normal will not increase endometrial cell division, while decreases in E_2 may, at most, only decrease mitotic activity for the few days of the cycle during which E_2 is normally close to the basal ~50 pg/ml level. However, in postmenopausal women, E_2 plasma levels are well below the ~50 pg/ml ceiling; thus increases in E_2 may, therefore, increase the endometrial mitotic rate until the upper limit for E_2 effect is reached.

Bioavailable E_2

Plasma E_2 is bound with high affinity to sex hormone-binding globulin (SHBG) and SHBG-bound E_2 is not bioavailable (31). SHBG levels decrease significantly with increasing BMI (kg/m^2), so that, for example, SHBG levels decrease ~46% with a BMI change from 20 to 30 kg/m^2, and the proportion of E_2 that is bioavailable increases from ~49% at a BMI of 20 kg/m^2 to ~64% at a BMI of 30 kg/m^2. [The above figures were calculated using the mass action approach of Södergard et al. (46) with the estimated association constants as given by Dunn et al. (10) – which were used by the Endogenous Hormones and Breast Cancer Collaborative Group (11) – and with the E_2 and SHBG values given by the same group (12).] Estimating the average BMI of the women contributing to Fig. 1 at 25 kg/m^2, the ~50 pg/ml ceiling of effective E_2 translates into a upper limit of bioavailable E_2 of ~28.4 pg/ml. This is not, of course, the ceiling but an upper bound of the ceiling. We see below that we can refine this estimate by considering the effects of menopausal ET on endometrial cancer risk.

Body Mass Index

Increasing body mass index (BMI) is strongly associated with a greatly increasing risk of endometrial cancer, the risk approximately doubling between a BMI of 23 kg/m^2 and a BMI of 30 kg/m^2 (16). This is evident both in premenopausal (19) and postmenopausal women (51). At premenopausal ages, increasing BMI, especially obesity, is associated with an increase in anovulatory cycles (18), in which in the absence of P$_4$, the endometrium is stimulated throughout the cycle. During the postmenopausal period, increasing BMI is associated with higher levels of E$_2$ from conversion of androgens to estrogens, as well as lower levels of SHBG, so that the estrogen is more bioactive (43, 45). It should be noted that the added risk associated with increasing BMI will, of course, increase as the duration of "exposure" to the added BMI increases, as is seen with ET use.

Menopausal Hormone Therapy

Menopausal Estrogen Therapy

The dose of menopausal ET most commonly used in the USA, that is, conjugated estrogens (CE) at 0.625 mg/day, results in endometrial cell proliferation approximating that found during the follicular phase of the menstrual cycle (23). Thus, it is not surprising that menopausal ET substantially increases a woman's risk of developing endometrial cancer, which is strongly dependent on the duration of use. In our study, an increased risk of ~16.8% per year of use was found (37) and similar risks have been reported in other studies (3, 9, 34) (*see* Table 1 and Fig. 2).

However, the increased risk from ET use is strongly dependent on BMI. The increased risk per year of use of ~16.8% is an average of 19.3% for women with a BMI of <30 kg/m^2 and of 7.7% for women with a BMI of $\geq$ 30 kg/m^2 in our study (37). This BMI effect was also seen in the Multiethnic Cohort Study, where there was a slight decreased risk in women with a BMI of $\geq$ 30 kg/m^2 (33). Similar results were reported by Brinton and coworkers (5) with a relative risk of 3.8 for women with a BMI of <28 kg/m^2 and 1.05 for women with a BMI of $\geq$ 28 kg/m^2. Finally, the Million Women Study Collaborators report (28) also found that ET use was associated with no increase in risk in women with a BMI of $\geq$ 30 kg/m^2. We conservatively estimate that there is no increased risk from ET use in women with a BMI $\geq$ 32 kg/m^2. Plasma E$_2$ is $\geq$ 15.7 pg/ml in a 32 kg/m^2 woman (12), and it can be concluded that the ceiling of effective non-SHBG-bound plasma E$_2$ is ~10.1 pg/ml (calculated as described above).

All effective doses of ET are likely to result in plasma estrogen levels above this effective ceiling level. This can be seen most easily by considering the plasma estrogen levels achieved by the 50 µg E$_2$ transdermal patch, which achieves roughly the same effects as a CE dose of 0.625 mg/day. A 50 µg E$_2$ patch increases steady

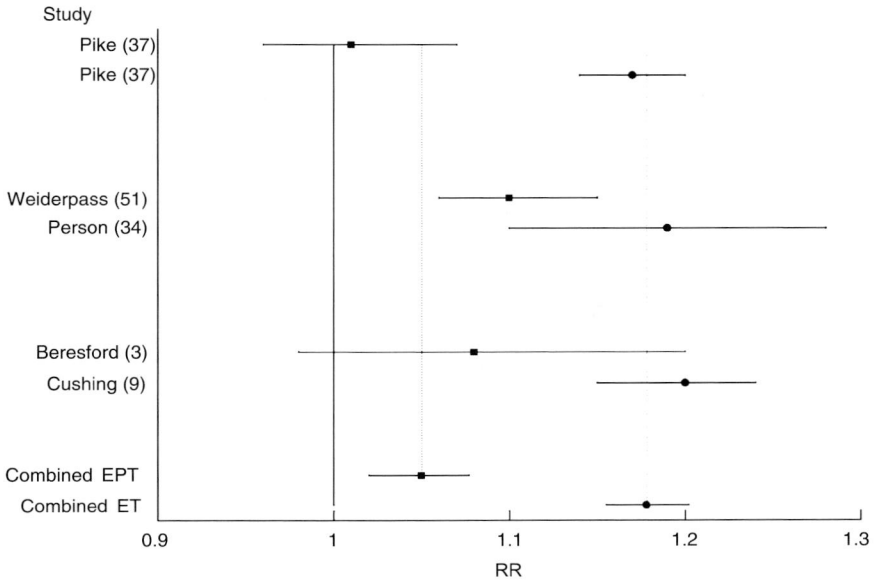

Fig. 2 Relative risks of endometrial cancer per year of estrogen therapy use (*ET*) and sequential estrogen–progestin therapy use (*EPT*) (*P* given for 10–12 days per 28-day cycle).

Table 1. RRs of endometrial cancer per year of ET and sequential EPT use (*P* given for 10–12 days per 28-day cycle)

Study area	References	Therapy	RR (95% CI)
Los Angeles	(37)	ET	1.17 (1.14–1.20)
	(37)	EPT	1.01 (0.98–1.05)
Sweden	(34)	ET	1.19 (1.10–1.28)
	(51)	EPT	1.10 (1.06–1.15)
Washington State	(9)	ET	1.20 (1.15–1.24)
	(3)	EPT	1.08 (0.98–1.20)
Combined		ET	1.18 (1.16–1.20)
		EPT	1.05 (1.02–1.08)

RR relative risks, ET estrogen therapy, EPT estrogen-progestin therapy

state plasma E_2 levels by ~30 pg/ml (38, 41, 42) and has little effect on SHBG (29, 40), so that non-SHBG-bound E_2 will increase from ~4.0 to ~18.4 pg/ml in a 20 kg/m^2 woman (calculated as described above). Thus, the steady state plasma non-SHBG-bound E_2 level of all women on a 50 μg E_2 patch is well above the ceiling level of ~10.1 pg/ml. Even with only half the dose, that is, a 25 μg E_2 patch, the non-SHBG-bound E_2 will be ~13.6 pg/ml in a 20 kg/m^2 woman, still above the ceiling. Thus, different doses of ET should have similar effects, as it has been observed (9).

Menopausal Estrogen–Progestin Therapy

To reduce the increased endometrial cancer risk from menopausal ET, progestins were added to ET [estrogen–progestin therapy (EPT)] between 5 and 15 days (usually 7 or 10 days) per month in a sequential fashion (sequential EPT). Sequential EPT causes regular bleeding in many women and is associated with other negative side effects; as a result, continuous-combined therapy regimens were developed in which the estrogen and progestin are always taken together (continuous-combined EPT).

Endometrial cell proliferation associated with CE at 0.625 mg/day is completely blocked by oral medroxyprogesterone acetate (MPA) at 5 or more mg/day (26). This finding and the observation that the level of progesterone is above 5 ng/ml in the normal menstrual cycle during seven days (15) persuaded many prescribers that 7 days of progestin was sufficient to abolish any risk. However, Flowers et al. (15) found that such short progestin use only caused 40 to 50% of the functional layer of the endometrium to desquamate and did not completely remove the risk of hyperplasia (32). As a result, 10 or more days of progestin therapy became standard practice (23). It should be pointed out that, as can be seen in Fig. 3, endometrial cancer incidence is increasing rapidly in the premenopausal period, even where obesity is uncommon, so that the notion that mimicking the progestin phase of the menstrual cycle would provide adequate protection was always suspect.

As expected, our endometrial cancer case-control study (37) showed that women who received sequential EPT with MPA at ≥ 5 mg/day given for ~7 days per month still had a markedly elevated risk of ~13% per year of such EPT use and this result has been found consistently.

Key and Pike (22) argued that if endometrial cell proliferation in the basalis layer was the key to increased risk from ET, there would still be an increased risk from sequential EPT even with 10 days of progestin use. This is because there would still be unopposed estrogen for around 15 days per treatment cycle since sequential EPT was usually given for 25 days per 28-day cycle (37). Subsequent studies have reported similar results with a meta-analysis estimate of a relative risk per year of use of 1.05 (95% CI 1.02–1.08) (Fig. 2).

Continuous-combined EPT should reduce the risk of endometrial cancer as it would be expected that the progestin component would block endogenous estrogen in addition of blocking the action of estrogen in the EPT. However, the extent of this action is not completely clear with the relatively low dose of MPA (2.5 mg/day) used in the USA with continuous-combined EPT. The Women's Health Initiative randomized trial of continuous-combined EPT found a decreased risk of endometrial cancer with a relative risk of 0.81 (95% CI 0.48–1.36; based on 27 and 31 cases of endometrial cancer) during 5.6 years of use (2). Similar results were observed in the much smaller HERS II randomized trial (21), and in a number of epidemiological studies (20, 28, 50). However, other studies have failed to show a decreased risk (30, 37). Nonetheless, although the question of a decreased risk of endometrial cancer associated with continous EPT remains to be settled, notably for the situation with low-dose progestin, it is clear that there is no increased risk with continuous-combined EPT.

Fig. 3 Age-specific incidence rates for endometrial cancer in the Birmingham region of the UK, 1968–1972 (49)

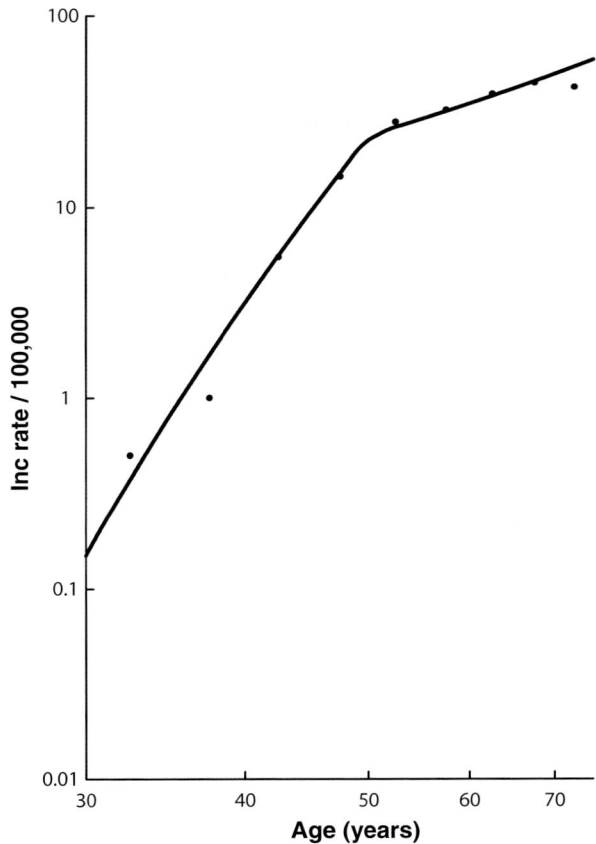

Menopause

Figure 3 shows the age-specific incidence rates for endometrial cancer in the Birmingham Region of the UK from 1968 to 1972 (49). It shows that the rate of increase in the incidence of endometrial cancer slows down around age 50. This older data is used in order to avoid distorsion due to high hysterectomy rates, high obesity rates, and widespread use of OCs and menopausal hormone therapy in the USA, all of which profoundly affect the incidence of endometrial cancer.

This age–incidence curve shown is for a time period (and location) when obesity was uncommon. Under such circumstances, the effective total 28-day estrogen dose to the endometrium will be much decreased at menopause (22). However, with increasing average BMI, the slowing down of the rate of increase in incidence of endometrial cancer at menopause will decrease, until a situation is reached where there will be no decrease in this rate (BMI of ~28 kg/m^2), and at higher average BMI, there may well be a slight increase in the rate of increase at menopause as shown in several studies (33, 37).

Parity

Endometrial cancer risk decreases significantly with increasing parity, and there is a greater reduction in risk with the first birth than with subsequent births (30–40% reduction in risk with the first birth compared to an ~15% reduction with each subsequent birth) (1, 4, 24, 25, 35). There is also evidence that births at older ages are more protective. In particular, a number of studies have reported that a late age at last birth was associated with significant reduction in risk independent of parity (1, 24, 25). However, this finding has not been corroborated in other studies (27, 35). McPherson et al. (27) showed that older age at last pregnancy appeared to be protective until it was controlled for gravidity, but the authors did not give the adjusted (controlled) results. We found that compared to a nulliparous woman, the risk of endometrial cancer was reduced by 51% in a woman with a last birth after age 35 and that additional births (before the last) reduced the risk further by an average of an additional 15% per birth. A last birth before age 25 was associated with only a 12% reduced risk of endometrial cancer. However, ages at all births were highly correlated and we were unable to prove that this age-at-birth effect was particularly so for last births (35).

In a detailed analysis from Norway, Albrektsen et al. (1) found that the protective effect of age at last birth was most pronounced in the period immediately after the birth and declined gradually thereafter. The authors concluded that the effect of age at last birth disappeared after adjustment for time since last birth, supporting the hypothesis that the reduction in risk for endometrial cancer is related to a mechanical shed of malignant or premalignant cells at each delivery.

Oral Contraceptives

The use of OC is associated with a significant reduction in endometrial cancer risk. Early studies of young premenopausal women estimated that risk is reduced by ~10% per year of use (7, 19). However, the reduction in risk declines with increasing age and a more representative figure is closer to 7% per year of use. OCs are a mixture of an estrogen (ethinyl-E_2) and a progestin. Their composition is such that they are progestin dominant for the endometrium, so that endometrial proliferation is confined effectively to the days on which OC is not taken. On the assumption that endometrial proliferation will be proportional to the number of days of unopposed estrogen, the observed reduction in risk with OC use is very close to that predicted by our mathematical model of incidence based on the simple unopposed estrogen hypothesis (36). Contrary to what has been observed with the protective effect of parity, where the extent of protection is much greater the later the age at the birth, no such effect has been reported with regards to the protective effect seen with OC use.

Chemoprevention

The use of OC remains an effective approach to chemoprevention of endometrial cancer. In recently published studies, this protective effect was seen to be very long term although of lesser magnitude than originally observed in younger women.

The substantial reduction in risk of endometrial cancer seen with late ages at births and possibly with time since last birth suggests that endometrial sloughing may have a substantial protective effect. If endometrial cells of the functionalis layer are susceptible to cancer, which would be consistent with the observation that early stage tumors often appear to arise in this layer, it would provide an explanation for the greater protective effect of late ages at births. Such endometrial sloughing would also provide an explanation for the observations made 15 years ago that CE at 0.625 mg/day did not produce endometrial hyperplasia if 10 mg/day of MPA was given for 14 days every 3 months (13, 53). Hyperplasia did occur in a trial in which E_2 valerate was given at 2 mg/day for 68 days, followed by norethisterone at 1 mg/day for 10 days, and finally E_2 valerate at 1 mg/day for 6 days (8). The only real difference in these regimens is the duration of progestin administration. Norethisterone at a dose of 1 mg is generally equated to MPA at 10 mg, so the dose of progestin does not appear to be the issue (47), and the dose of estrogen should not be relevant as both doses are in excess of the estimated ceiling of estrogen effect. It may be necessary to give the progestin for longer than 10 days to achieve the desired effect. Whether blocking endometrial hyperplasia will completely prevent any increase in endometrial cancer is an open question.

Further detailed studies of the endometrium – at or soon after delivery, at the end of the sloughing period while taking OCs, at the end of varying numbers of days of taking MPA at various doses, and at the end of the sloughing period – should lead to a deeper understanding of the basis of the protective effect of births and how we might hope to mimic their protective effect.

Conclusions

- Proliferation of the endometrium is dependent on estrogen unopposed by a progestin.
- Maximum profliferation is achieved at a relatively low level of bioavailable estradiol.
- Basal estrogen levels in the postmenopausal age group are dependent on body mass index (BMI).
- Bioavailable estradiol levels are also dependent on BMI.
- The above facts explain many epidemiologic observations concerning the risk of developing endometrial cancer in relation to age, obesity, and type of exogenous hormonal use.

References

1. Albrektsen G, Heuch I, Tretli S, Kvale G. Is the risk of cancer of the corpus uteri reduced by a recent pregnancy? A prospective study of 765,756 Norwegian women. Int J Cancer 1995;61:485–490.
2. Anderson GL, Judd HL, Kaunitz AM, et al. Effects of estrogen plus progestin on gynecologic cancers and associated diagnostic procedures. JAMA 2003;290:1739–1748.
3. Beresford SA, Weiss NS, Voigt LF, McKnight B. Risk of endometrial cancer in relation to use of oestrogen combined cyclic progestagen therapy in postmenopausal women. Lancet 1997;349:458–461.
4. Brinton LA, Berman ML, Mortel R, et al. Reproductive, menstrual, and medical risk factors for endometrial cancer: results from a case-control study. Am J Obstet Gynecol 1992;167:1317–1325.
5. Brinton LA, Hoover RN. Estrogen replacement therapy and endometrial cancer risk: Unresolved issues. The Endometrial Cancer Collaborative Group. Obstet Gynecol 1993;81:265–271.
6. Cairns J. Somatic stem cells and the kinetics of mutagenesis and carcinogenesis. Proc Natl Acad Sci 2002;99:10567–10570.
7. Cancer and Steroid Hormone Study. Combination oral contraceptive use and the risk of endometrial cancer. The Cancer and Steroid Hormone Study of the Centers for Disease Control and the National Institute of Child Health and Human Development. JAMA 1987;257:796–800.
8. Cerin A, Heldaas K, Moeller B. Adverse endometrial effects of long-cycle estrogen and progestogen replacement therapy. N Engl J Med 1996;334:668–669.
9. Cushing KL, Weiss NS, Voigt LF, McKnight B, Beresford SA. Risk of endometrial cancer in relation to use of low-dose, unopposed estrogens. Obstet Gynecol 1998;91:35–39.
10. Dunn JF, Nisula BC, Rodbard D. Transport of steroid hormones: binding of 21 endogenous steroids to both testosterone-binding globulin and corticosteroid-binding globulin in human plasma. J Clin Endocrinol Metab 1981;53:58–68.
11. Endogenous Hormones and Breast Cancer Collaborative Group. Free estradiol and breast cancer risk in postmenopausal women: comparison of measured and calculated values. Cancer Epidemiol Biomark Prev 2003;12:1457–1461.
12. Endogenous Hormones and Breast Cancer Collaborative Group. Body mass index, serum sex hormones, and breast cancer risk in postmenopausal women. J Natl Cancer Inst 2003;95:1218–1226.
13. Ettinger B, Selby J, Citron JT, Vangessel A, Ettinger VM, Hendrickson MR. Cyclic hormone replacement therapy using quarterly progestin. Obstet Gynecol 1994;83:693–700.
14. Ferenczy A, Bertrand G, Gelfand MM. Proliferation kinetics of human endometrium during the menstrual cycle. Am J Obstet Gynecol 1979;133:859–867.
15. Flowers CE, Wilborn WH, Hyde BM. Mechanisms of uterine bleeding in postmenopausal patients receiving estrogen alone or with a progestin. Obstet Gynecol 1983;61:135–143.
16. Friedenreich C, Cust A, Lahmann PH, et al. Anthropometric factors and risk of endometrial cancer: the European prospective investigation into cancer and nutrition. Cancer Causes Control 2007;18:399–413.
17. Goebelsmann U, Mishell DR. The menstrual cycle. In: *Reproductive Endocrinology Infertility and Contraception*, pp 67–89. Mishell DR, Davajan V (Eds). F.A. Davis Company: Philadelphia. 1979.
18. Hartz AJ, Barboriak PN, Wong A, Katayama KP, Rimm AA. The association of obesity with infertility and related menstrual abnormalities in women. Int J Obesity 1979;3:57–73.
19. Henderson BE, Casagrande JT, Pike MC, Mack T, Rosario I, Duke A. The epidemiology of endometrial cancer in young women. Br J Cancer 1983;47:749–756.
20. Hill DA, Weiss NS, Beresford SA, et al. Continuous combined hormone replacement therapy and risk of endometrial cancer. Am J Obstet Gynecol 2000;183:1456–1461.
21. Hulley S, Furberg C, Barrett-Connor E, et al. Noncardiovascular disease outcomes during 6.8 years of hormone therapy: Heart and Estrogen/Progestin Replacement Study Follow-up (HERS II). JAMA 2002;288:58–66.

22. Key TJ, Pike MC. The dose-effect relationship between 'unopposed' oestrogens and endometrial mitotic rate: its central role in explaining and predicting endometrial cancer risk. Br J Cancer 1988;57:205–212.

23. King RJ, Whitehead MI. Progestin action in relation to the prevention of endometrial abnormalities. In: *Medical Management of Endometriosis*, pp 67–77. Raynaud JP, Ojasoo T, Martini L (Eds). Raven Press: NewYork. 1984.

24. Kvale G, Heuch IG. Reproductive factors and risk of cancer of the uterine corpus: a prospective study. *Cancer Res* 1988;48:6217–6221.

25. Lambe M, Wuu J, Weiderpass E, Hsieh CC. Childbearing at older age and endometrial cancer risk (Sweden). Cancer Causes Control 1999;10:43–49.

26. Lane G, Siddle NC, Ryder TA, Pryse-Davies J, King RJB, Whitehead MI. Is Provera the ideal progestogen for addition to postmenopausal estrogen therapy? Fertil Steril 1986;45:345–352.

27. McPherson CP, Sellers TA, Potter JD, Bostick RM, Folsom AR. Reproductive factors and risk of endometrial cancer. The Iowa Women's Health Study. Am J Epidemiol 1996;143:1195–1202.

28. Million Women Study Collaborators. Endometrial cancer and hormone-replacement therapy in the Million Women Study. Lancet 2005;365:1543–1551.

29. Nachtigall LE, Raju U, Banerjee S, Wan L, Levitz M. Serum estradiol profiles in post-menopausal women undergoing three common estrogen replacement therapies: associations with sex hormone-binding globulin, estradiol, and estrone levels. Menopause 2000;7:243–250.

30. Newcomb PA, Trentham-Dietz A. Patterns of postmenopausal progestin use with estrogen in relation to endometrial cancer (United States). Cancer Causes Control 2003;14:195–201.

31. Pardridge WM. Serum bioavailability of sex steroid hormone. Clin Endocrinol Metab 1986;15:259–278.

32. Paterson ME, Wade-Evans T, Sturdee DW, Thom MH, Studd JW. Endometrial disease after treatment with oestrogens and progestogens at the climacteric. BMJ 1980;22:822–824.

33. Pearce CL, Setiawan W, Chung K, Wu AH, Pike MC. Endometrial cancer risk as it relates to ages at births and to the joint effects of BMI and use of menopausal estrogen therapy and age at menopause. In preparation.

34. Persson I, Weiderpass E, Bergkvist L, Bergström R, Schairer C. Risks of breast and endometrial cancer after estrogen and estrogen-progestin replacement. Cancer Causes Control 1999;10:253–260.

35. Pettersson B, Adami HO, Bergström R, Johansson EDB. Menstruation span – a time-limited risk factor for endometrial carcinoma. Acta Obstet Gynecol Scand 1986;65:247–255.

36. Pike MC. Age-related factors in cancers of the breast, ovary, and endometrium. J Chron Dis 1987;40:59S–69S.

37. Pike MC, Peters RK, Cozen W, et al. Estrogen-progestin replacement therapy and endometrial cancer. J Natl Cancer Inst 1997;89:1110–1116.

38. Powers MS, Schennkel L, Darley PE, Good WR, Balestra JC, Place VA. Pharmacokinetics and pharmacodynamics of transdermal dosage forms of 17-β estradiol: comparison with conventional oral estrogens used for hormone replacement. Am J Obstet Gynecol 1985;152:1099–1106.

39. Preston-Martin S, Pike MC, Ross RK, Jones PA, Henderson BE. Increased cell division as a cause of human cancer. Cancer Res 1990;50:7415–7421.

40. Ropponen A, Aittomaki K, Vihma V, Tikkanen MJ, Ylikorkala O. Effects of oral estradiol administration on levels of sex hormone-binding globulin in postmenopausal women with and without a history of intrahepatic cholestasis of pregnancy. J Clin Endocrinol Metab 2005;90:3431–3434.

41. Schiff I, Sela HK, Cramer D, Tulchinsky D, Ryan KJ. Endometrial hyperplasia in women on cyclic or continuous estrogen regimens. Fertil Steril 1982;37:79–82.

42. Selby PL, Peacock M. Dose dependent response of symptoms, pituitary, and bone to transdermal estrogen in postmenopausal women. BMJ 1986;293:1337–1339.

43. Siiteri PK, MacDonald PC. In: Handbook of physiology, pp 615–629, Sect. 7 Part I,2. American Physiological Society: Washington, DC. 1973.

44. Siiteri PK. Steroid hormones and endometrial cancer. Cancer Res 1978;38:4360–4366.
45. Siiteri PK, Hammond GL, Nisker JA. Increased availability of serum estrogens in breast cancer: a new hypothesis. In: *Banbury Report: Hormones and Breast Cancer*, pp 87–106. Pike MC, Siiteri PK, Welsch CW (Eds). Cold Spring Harbor. 1981.
46. Södergard R, Backstrom T, Shanbhag V, Carstensen H. Calculation of free and bound fractions of testosterone and estradiol-17β to human plasma proteins at body temperature. J Steroid Biochem 1982;16:801–810.
47. Stanczyk FZ. Pharmacokinetics and potency of progestins used for hormone replacement therapy and contraception. Rev Endocrin Metab Disord 2002;3:211–224.
48. Thorneycroft LH, Mishell DR, Stone SC, Kharma KM, Nakamura RM. The relation of serum 17-hydroxyprogesterone and estradiol-17-beta levels during the human menstrual cycle. Am J Obstet Gynecol 1971;111:947–951.
49. Waterhouse J, Muir C, Correa P, Powell J (Eds). *Cancer Incidence in Five Continents*. IARC Sci Publ No. 15: Lyon (France). 1976.
50. Weiderpass E, Adami H-O, Baron JA, et al. Risk of endometrial cancer following estrogen replacement with and without progestins. J Natl Cancer Inst 1999;91:1131–1137.
51. Weiderpass E, Persson I, Adami H-O, Magnusson C, Lindgren A, Baron JA. Body size in different periods of life, diabetes mellitus, hypertension, and risk of postmenopausal endometrial cancer (Sweden). Cancer Causes Control 2000;11:185–192.
52. Whitehead MI, Townsend PT, Pryse-Davies J, Ryder TA, King RJB. Effects of estrogens and progestins on the biochemistry and morphology of the postmenopausal endometrium. N Engl J Med 1981;305:1599–1605.
53. Williams DB, Voigt BJ, Yao SF, Schoenfeld MJ, Judd HL. Assessment of less than monthly progestin therapy in postmenopausal women given estrogen replacement. Obstet Gynecol 1994;84:787–793.

Endometrial Cancer: Screening, Diagnosis, and Surgical Staging

Annekathryn Goodman and Barbara Goff

Abstract Through case studies, the authors point out environmental and hereditary factors that contribute to increased risk of developing endometrial cancer and how to apply screening modalities in pre- and postmenopausal women. Attention is drawn to certain anatomic abnormalities that prevent vaginal bleeding – the most common symptom related to cancer. Diagnostic tests that are available to pursue various aspects of the diagnosis in a sequential fashion are described, culminating in the endometrial biopsy. Recommendations for screening and diagnosis in the asymptomatic as well as the symptomatic patients are summarized. Surgical staging represents the final event in the diagnostic workup. Instances when such staging can be modified to deal with various comorbidities are delineated.

Keywords Endometrial cancer • Heredity • Screening • Endometrial biopsy • Surgical staging

Screening

Case Report 1

A 32-year-old thin, nulliparous woman presented with menorrhagia. The bleeding was unresponsive to birth control pill use. She had no other medical conditions. There was no family history of malignancies. She underwent a rollerball endometrial ablation. She did not have an endometrial biopsy done prior to this procedure. Three months later a hysterectomy was performed because of persistent bleeding.

A. Goodman(✉) and B. Goff
Division of Gynecologic Oncology, Gillette Center for Women's Cancers,
Massachusetts General Hospital, Boston, MA
e-mail: agoodman@partners.org

F. Muggia and E. Oliva (eds.), *Uterine Cancer*, Current Clinical Oncology,
DOI: 10.1007/978-1-60327-044-1_2,
© Humana Press, a Part of Springer Science + Business Media, LLC 2009

Her pathology showed a deeply invasive grade 2 endometrioid endometrial adeno-carcinoma with metastases to a para-aortic lymph node.

While endometrial cancer is the most common malignancy of the female genital tract with 41,200 new cases and 7,350 deaths in 2006 (1), routine screening is not recommended. The rationale for the lack of massive screening is that symptoms develop at an early stage and the female genital tract allows easy access to the uterus for diagnostic evaluation. Therefore, the focus has been on efficient evaluation in the setting of symptoms.

There are certain groups of women who have an increased risk for the development of endometrial cancer. Evaluation of the endometrial cavity should be considered and a higher index of suspicion for the development of endometrial cancer should be entertained even in the absence of symptoms for these women. Table 1 summarizes the groups of women who are at increased risk for the development of endometrial cancer. Whether screening should be performed in asymptomatic women is controversial.

Any factor that increases the exposure to unopposed estrogen increases the risk of endometrial cancer (2). Premenopauasal women who have had chronic anovulation will develop a build up of the endometrial lining (3). Women with polycystic ovarian syndrome will present with years of anovulation since their teenage years (4). Other causes of anovulation include thyroid disease, hyperprolactinemia, and certain exogenous drugs such as antipsychotics (5). Estrogen secreting ovarian tumors such as granulosa cell tumors and thecomas can lead to stimulation and the build up of the endometrial lining (6).

Table 1. Factors associated with increased risk of developing endometrial cancer

Premenopausal women
Endogenous estrogen exposure:
Anovulatory cycles
Polycystic ovarian syndrome
Morbid obesity
Estrogen secreting tumors
Hereditary syndromes:
Hereditary nonpolyposis colorectal cancer
BRCA1 mutation
Postmenopausal women
Endogenous estrogen exposure:
Morbid obesity
Estrogen secreting tumors
Cirrhosis of the liver
Exogenous estrogen exposure:
Exogenous estrogens without progestins
Tamoxifen use
Pelvic radiation
Hereditary syndromes:
Hereditary nonpolyposis colorectal cancer
BRCA1 mutation

Morbid obesity is a risk factor at all ages as these women have higher endogenous estrogens due to the aromatization of androgens to estradiol and the conversion of androstendione to estrone in peripheral adipose tissue (7). Use of exogenous estrogen without the balance of progesterone is associated with endometrial cancer (8). Women with liver disease who cannot adequately metabolize their endogenous or exogenous estrogens are also at risk for the development of endometrial malignancies (9).

Tamoxifen increases the risk of endometrial cancer two- to threefold (10). Tamoxifen effect on the endometrial lining is not seen before 2 years of use (11). However, the absolute risk of developing endometrial cancer while taking tamoxifen is 1.2/1,000 per year or only 6/1,000 after 5 years (12). Currently, the American College of Obstetrician Gynecologists (ACOG) does not recommend screening in asymptomatic women taking tamoxifen (13).

Women with breast or colon cancer may have a higher genetic risk of gynecologic malignancies. A careful family history will help guide the decision to evaluate the endometrium. Hereditary nonpolyposis colon cancer (HNPCC), an autosomal dominant syndrome, confers a 40–60% risk of endometrial cancer (14). Women with known HNPCC who are undergoing surgery for colorectal cancer should be counseled about the potential benefits of total abdominal hysterectomy and bilateral salpingo-oophorectomy (TAH–BSO) at the time of colorectal surgery (15). BRCA1 gene mutation, in addition to the well-known increased risk of ovarian cancer, has been associated with an increased endometrial cancer risk (16).

Pelvic radiation for other malignancies such as cervical or rectal cancer will increase the risk of uterine corpus cancers. The most common postradiation pelvic malignancy is adenocarcinoma of the endometrium (17).

Even in the absence of personal or family risk factors of endometrial cancer, all women with abnormal bleeding need to be evaluated for malignancy. Any vaginal bleeding in postmenopausal women regardless of the quantity needs to be evaluated. The risk of endometrial cancer in a 50-year-old woman with postmenopausal bleeding is 9%, 16% for a woman in her sixties, 28% for a woman in her seventies, and 60% for a woman in her eighties (18). Irregular bleeding in premenopausal women needs to be thoughtfully worked up. While hormonal irregularities, complication of pregnancy, and pelvic infection are other causes of premenopausal bleeding, the possibility of malignancy must be taken seriously. Twenty-five percent of all endometrial cancers occur in premenopausal women and 5% are found in women <40 years old (19).

Table 2 lists certain anatomical changes that may prevent the development of the warning sign of vaginal bleeding or impair the examiner's ability to fully evaluate the pelvic tract. Women who have developed cervical stenosis because of postmenopausal atrophy, or previous cervical procedures such as cryotherapy or cervical cone biopsies will not have an open cervical canal. On physical inspection, the examiner will see that a cutip or cytobrush cannot pass through the cervical os. Some women develop agglutination of the upper vagina secondary to atrophy, radiation, or infection. Certain congenital duplications of the lower genital tract such as a vaginal septum can also close of the uterus and not allow blood to exit the

Table 2. Anatomic abnormalities that prevent vaginal bleeding

Abnormality	Causes
Agglutinated Vagina	Postmenopausal atrophy
	Radiation
	Sequelae of infection (Toxic shock syndrome, Stevens-Johnson syndrome)
	Use of intravaginal Efudex cream
Cervical stenosis	Sequelae of therapy for cervical intraepithelial neoplasia (cryotherapy, cone biopsy, LEEP)
Vaginal septum	Congenital
Intrauterine synechia	Asherman's syndrome
	Endometrial ablation

LEEP loop electrosurgical excision procedure.

vagina. Women who have had an endometrial ablation may develop a malignancy deep to the scar of ablation, which is not amenable to detection by biopsy. For all these women, it is important to evaluate the upper genital tract especially if they also have other risk factors discussed above.

Comment on Case Report 1

The 32-year-old woman had no known risk factors for endometrial cancer. However, she had abnormal bleeding that was not fully evaluated before trying the therapeutic intervention of ablating her endometrial lining. It is extremely important to perform an endometrial biopsy when bleeding is unexplained. Only 10% of all gynecologic cancers are associated with a known genetic risk. Endometrial cancers that are not associated with hyperestrogenism seem to have a more aggressive behavior.

Diagnostic Tests

Case Report 2

A 49-year-old woman presented with mid cycle spotting. She had had several abnormal pap smears showing atypical glandular cells over the last 5 years. Colposcopy and cervical biopsies had been normal. An endometrial biopsy showed a grade 2 endometrioid adenocarcinoma. She underwent a total abdominal hysterectomy (TAH), bilateral salpingo oophorectomy (BSO), and pelvic node biopsies. Her final pathology showed a polypoid carcinoma of the endometrium with superficial myometrial invasion. All staging biopsies were negative for tumor.

Evaluation of the uterus occurs with physical examination, visual inspection, cytologic and histologic evaluation, and radiologic imaging. Table 3 summarizes the different diagnostic tests that are available to study the uterus.

Physical examination includes visual inspection of the external genitalia. In the setting of abnormal bleeding, it is important to rule out the possibility of an extrauterine lesion. The vulva, periurethral region, and anus are examined. The vagina and cervix are evaluated. The cervix is assessed for stenosis, friability, and gross lesions. The vagina should also be palpated circumferentially to make sure that there are no nodules that may have been missed on visual examination. The uterus is palpated on bimanual examination. It should be evaluated for size, tenderness, and irregularities of shape. A rectovaginal examination allows the examiner to evaluate the cul-de-sac, the back wall of the uterus, and the adnexal structures.

While Papanicolau smears were developed for screening of lower genital tract neoplasia, an occasional asymptomatic woman with endometrial carcinoma will

Table 3. Diagnostic tests for uterine corpus disease

Office procedures	Type of information
Physical examination	Origin of bleeding Cervical stenosis Uterine size, pelvic mass
Pap smear	Cytologic abnormalities of cervix, vagina Occasional information about upper tract disease
Endometrial biopsy	Endometrial lining
Hysteroscopy	Endometrial lining
Radiological procedures	**Type of information**
Transvaginal ultrasound	Endometrial stripe Uterine size Adnexal size, presence of cysts, masses
Sonohysterogram	Endometrial stripe Presence of submucosal fibroids, polyps, endometrial cavity masses
Pelvic MRI	Myometrial abnormalities Endometrial cavity Adnexal structures Invasion into parametria, vagina, bladder Pelvic nodal disease
Abdominopelvic CT scan	Ascites Pelvic and para-aortic adenopathies Intraparenchymal organ abnormalities Peritoneal and omental disease
Operative procedures	**Type of information**
Examination under anesthesia	Same as physical examination
Dilation and curettage	Endometrial lining
Hysteroscopy	Endometrial lining
Hysterectomy	Full pathologic analysis of the uterus

present with abnormal cytology. Cervical cytology is not a reliable screening test for endometrial cancer. However, endometrial cells seen on cervical cytology in women over 40 years of age can signify endometrial disease (20).

The risk of malignancy is increased twofold when atypical endometrial cells are seen on cervical cytology compared with benign appearing cells (21). In patients with endometrial cancer, suspicious cells on cervical cytology are associated with higher grade and more advanced stage disease (22). Some studies have not confirmed a higher risk of endometrial pathology in asymptomatic women with normal endometrial cells noted by cervical cytology screening (23).

Any abnormal uterine bleeding needs to be evaluated by endometrial biopsy. The accuracy of an office biopsy will be depending on the size of the endometrial lesion, the examiner's skills, the anatomy of the patient, and patient comfort. Small lesions, cervical stenosis with the inability to get deeply into the endometrial cavity, and distorting submucosal fibroids can all reduce the yield on office biopsies. Premedication with a nonsteroidal anti-inflammatory and the use of a paracervical block can help facilitate an office evaluation. An office hysteroscope can also increase the yield for diagnosing abnormalities. Many different types of office biopsy devices are thought to be effective diagnostic techniques (24). Table 4 lists some of the commercial devices that are available for outpatient endometrial biopsies.

If it is not possible to obtain an adequate sampling in the office because of patient distress, anatomic factors, or a discrepancy between normal office biopsy results and an abnormal imaging study (see below), a day surgical procedure should be scheduled. Under anesthesia, vaginal adhesions can be gently opened up. If cervical stenosis is a problem, an ultrasound can help safely guide the operator into the uterine cavity and avoid uterine perforation. Hysteroscopy combined with curettage of the endometrial cavity is recommended to avoid missing small lesions.

Imaging studies can be a helpful adjunct in the evaluation of endometrial pathology. In asymptomatic women, the addition of a transvaginal ultrasound can help determine the need for an endometrial biopsy. The stripe width varies with the menstrual cycle in premenopausal women. After the menopause, an endometrial stripe thickness >5 mm is usually considered abnormal (28). Tamoxifen can increase the incidence of a falsely thickened endometrial stripe because of tamoxifen-induced subendometrial edema (29). In addition, about 30% of women taking tamoxifen will develop endometrial polyps (30). A sonohysterogram can be helpful. Sterile saline is instilled into the endometrial cavity and then a transvaginal ultrasound is performed. The saline will reveal subtle irregularities such as small

Table 4. Commercial devices for endometrial biopsy

Device	Accuracy for diagnosis of endometrial cancer (%)	References
Novak curet	67–97	(25)
Pipelle (Unimar)	79–94	(26)
Vabra aspirator	80–98	(27)

Table 5. Endometrial cancer: recommendations for screening and diagnosis

Asymptomatic patient
No risk factors and normal physical examination: routine yearly follow-up Risk factors of estrogen excess: transvaginal ultrasound Tamoxifen use for >2 years: annual sonohysterogram Genetic risk factors: annual endometrial biopsy Abnormal physical examination: transvaginal ultrasound
Symptomatic patient
Office endometrial biopsy and transvaginal ultrasound Dilation and curettage if unable to perform office biopsy or abnormal ultrasound

polyps and it will reduce the error in measuring the stripe thickness. Some authorities recommend proceeding directly to a sonohysterogram in the evaluation of women on tamoxifen (31).

A pelvic MRI is useful preoperatively to help determine depth of myometrial invasion in a known invasive cancer (32). It is about 70% accurate in predicting myometrial invasion. A CT scan can also help to evaluate the lymph node chains and check for upper abdominal disease. Neither of imaging tests is indicated in screening for, and the diagnosis of endometrial cancer. In general, CT scan is recommended preoperatively in women with papillary serous or clear cell histologies. Table 5 summarizes screening and diagnostic recommendations.

Comment on Case Report 2

This patient had repetitively abnormal glandular cells on cervical cytology. She also had unexplained midcycle bleeding. When her cervical evaluation with colposcopy returned with negative results, she should have undergone an endometrial biopsy. An ultrasound may have been helpful to pick up the large polypoid lesion within her endometrial cavity.

Surgical Staging

Case Report 3

A 35-year-old G3P3 woman with menorraghia undergoes a total vaginal hysterectomy. The final pathology reveals a grade 3 endometrioid adenocarcinoma of the endometrium with inner one-third myometrial invasion. She is taken back to surgery and undergoes a laparoscopic BSO, pelvic and para-aortic lymph node dissection,

and pelvic washings. All staging biopsies are negative for cancer. She has a stage
Ib grade 3 endometrial cancer diagnosis.

The staging of a cancer serves three main purposes. An internationally agreed upon numeric classification of extent of disease allows the collection of statistics and worldwide interpretation of treatment outcome and survival. A stage assignment for a particular cancer gives information about prognosis. Third, with the knowledge of stage, a particular treatment regimen that is based on solid collective experience can be recommended. A stage is assigned for the cancer at initial presentation and this stage assignment never changes. For instance, a woman who develops lung metastases after an initial diagnosis of stage IIb endometrial cancer does not have stage IV disease. Her cancer is described as Stage IIb with lung metastases.

Since 1988, endometrial cancer has been staged surgically (33). For endometrioid carcinomas a degree of differentiation is also documented. A grade 1 tumor has ≤ 5% solid growth pattern of the glandular component. A grade 2 tumor has 6–50% solid growth pattern. Grade 3 tumors have > 50% solid component. Endometriod type endometrial cancer spreads in a predictable manner (34). It first occurs by direct invasion into the myometrium. Spread can also progress into the cervix and then the vagina. Tumor cells can also migrate transtubally with implantation on the ovaries, uterine serosa, or with free-floating cells in the peritoneum. Involvement of lymphovascular spaces can lead to lymphatic spread. Tumor then can involve the organs of the upper abdomen, the inguinal lymph nodes, or extraabdominal sites. Endometrial cancer can also spread hematogenously to involve the lungs. Surgical staging reflects this predictable behavior (*see* Table 6). While the rare subtypes have less predictable behavior, they are included in the FIGO endometrial cancer staging system. Clear cell and serous histologies commonly spread by transtubal route and follow the peritoneal fluid circulation in a manner similar to epithelial ovarian cancers (35). This spread frequently occurs while the primary cancer is small and noninvasive of the myometrium.

Table 6. Surgical staging of endometrial cancer

Stage	Site of tumor involvement	Substages
I	Uterine corpus	Ia: no myometrial invasion
		Ib: invasion of < one half of the myometrium
		Ic: invasion ≥ one half of the myometrium
II	Uterine cervix	IIa: endocervical gland involvement
		IIb: cervical stromal invasion
III	Pelvic Structures	IIIa: positive peritoneal cytology, serosal involvement or adnexal metastases
		IIIb: vaginal metastases
		IIIc: pelvic or para-aortic nodes
IV	Upper abdomen, extra-abdominal disease invasion outside the true pelvis	IVa: bladder or bowel invasion
		IVb: distant metastases including inguinal and intra-abdominal nodes

Operative Techniques for Staging

Laparotomy

The surgical approach chosen for removal of the uterus, tubes, and ovaries will be based on many factors. If a patient has had multiple prior surgeries, a history of peritonitis, diverticulitis, or abdominal radiation, an open approach may be judicious. A preoperative bowel preparation is an important addition to preoperative planning. The choice of the incision can be based on patient's body habitus, previous abdominal scars, and what surgery is planned. The classic incision for abdominal exploration is the low vertical incision, which can be extended as needed into the upper abdomen. Some surgeons prefer a slight paramedian approach to avoid compromising the structural integrity of the umbilicus. A low transverse incision is reasonable for grade 1 cancers where one is not planning to sample the high para-aortic nodal chains. This incision can be modified by the muscle cutting Maylard incision if more exposure is necessary. It is important not to compromise the blood supply to the skin by making a parallel incision to an old incision. As the skin and subcutaneous tissue is supplied by the superficial epigastric vessels that come in from a lateral position, a skin bridge between two incisions can develop necrosis. It is also important to understand the surgical techniques that have been performed previously when a woman has undergone a myofascial flap for breast reconstruction after breast cancer surgery. Commonly a mesh is placed after a TRAM flap. It is helpful to obtain advice about where to place the new fascial incision from the plastic surgeon who has done the previous surgery. This will reduce the risk of postoperative hernias.

Pelvic cytology is first collected by rinsing the pelvis with sterile saline and aspirating the fluid back. The abdomen is then carefully explored. After the uterus and both adnexa are removed, a decision about further staging is made. For grade 2 and 3 cancers, pelvic and para-aortic lymph node dissection should be performed. For grade 1 cancers, the uterus is sent to pathology for evaluation of the depth of invasion and then determine the need for lymph node dissection. Macroscopic examination of the fresh specimen correctly predicted depth of invasion in 87% of grade 1, 65% of grade 2, and 30% of grade 3 tumors (36). Lymph node dissection should be performed for deeply invasive grade 1 tumors.

Some investigators recommend staging all patients with endometrial cancer if technically feasible (37). Otherwise, potential pitfalls, seen in 15–20% of patients include: final pathology report with a higher grade than the preoperative endometrial biopsy and lack of accuracy in assesing depth of invasion for grade 2–3 tumors. Several studies have suggested a potential therapeutic benefit from lymphadenectomy as compared to lymph nodes sampling or no lymph node dissection (38).

Laparoscopy

A laparoscopically assisted vaginal hysterectomy with appropriate staging is an acceptable alternative to a laparotomy as long as the same information can be obtained (39). Uterine morcellation should not be performed because of the theoretical risk of seeding and spread of viable cancer cells.

Vaginal Approach

For patients who have multiple comorbidities, a simple vaginal hysterectomy without comprehensive surgical staging should be considered. The purpose of this surgery is to remove the uterus and stop bleeding. This surgery can be performed under spinal anesthesia. Vaginal hysterectomy with BSO is also appropriate for women with grade 1 minimally invasive tumors. It is not always technically possible to remove the ovaries through the transvaginal approach. As synchronous primary cancers of endometrium and ovary are found in 5–10% of women it is important to remove the ovaries if technically possible and medically safe to do so (40).

Comment on Case Report 3

The gynecologic oncology group demonstrated that 22% of women with clinical stage I disease had extrauterine spread (34). The patient had undergone a vaginal hysterectomy because of menorraghia without an endometrial biopsy. With the discovery of a grade 3 cancer, it was crucial that she had undergone a second surgery to evaluate her ovaries and nodal status. With the diagnosis of a stage Ib endometrial cancer, she did not need postoperative whole pelvic radiation. She was at higher risk for vaginal recurrence and vaginal brachytherapy was recommended.

Conclusions

- An endometrial biopsy is the key diagnostic test for abnormal vaginal bleeding.
- Any positive findings on biopsy should be pursued further beyond physical examination and cytologic evaluation, selecting from a number of radiologic and operative procedures (see also Chapter 3).
- With a diagnosis of invasive endometrial cancer, the operative approach beyond hysterectomy should include thorough surgical staging.

References

1. Jemal A, Siegel R, Ward E, Murray T, Xu J, Smigal C, Thun MJ. Cancer Statistics 2006. CA Cancer J Clin 2006; 56:106–130.
2. Hale GE, Hughes CL, Cline JM. Endometrial cancer: hormonal factors, the perimenopausal "window at risk", and isoflavones. J Clin Endocrinol Metab 2002; 87:3.
3. Coulam CB, Anneger JF, Kranz JS. Chronic anovulation syndrome and associated neoplasia. Obstet Gynecol 1983; 61:403.
4. Azziz R, Woods KS, Reyna R, et al. The prevalence and features of the polycystic ovary syndrome in an unselected population. J Clin Endocrinol Metab 2004; 89:2745.
5. Schlechte J, Sherman B, Halmi N, et al. Prolactin-secreting pituitary tumors in amenorrheic women: a comparative study. Endocr Rev 1980; 1:295.
6. Outwater EK, Wagner BJ, Mannion C, et al. Sex cord-stromal and steroid cell tumors of the ovary. Radiographics 1998; 18:1523.
7. Siiteri PK. Adipose tissue as a source of hormones. Am J Clin Nutr 1987; 45:277.
8. Persson I, Adami H-O, Bergkvist L, et al. Risk of endometrial cancer after treatment with estrogens alone or in conjunction with progestogens: results of a prospective study. BMJ 1989; 298:147.
9. Zumoff B, Fishman J, Gallagher TF, Hellman L. Estradiol metabolism in cirrhosis. J Clin Invest 1968; 47(1):20–25.
10. Cohen I. Endometrial pathologies associated with postmenopausal tamoxifen treatment. Gynecol Oncol 2004; 94:256.
11. Suh-Burgmann EJ, Goodman A. Surveillance for endometrial cancer in women receiving tamoxifen. Ann Intern Med 1999; 131:127–135.
12. Fisher B, Constantino JP, Redmond CK, Fisher ER, Wickerham DL, Cronin WM. Endometrial cancer in tamoxifen treated breast cancer patients: findings from the National Surgical Adjuvant Breast and Bowel Project (NSABP) B-14. J Natl Cancer Inst 1994; 86:527–537.
13. ACOG Commitee Opinior Number 232 April 2000-Tomoxifen and Endometrial Cancer.
14. Ollikainen M, Abdel-Rahman WM, Moisio AL, et al. Molecular analysis of familial endometrial carcinoma: a manifestation of hereditary nonpolyposis colorectal cancer or a separate syndrome? J Clin Oncol 2005; 23:4609.
15. Schmeler KM, Lynch HT, Chen L-M, et al. Prophylactic surgery to reduce the risk of gynecologic cancers in the Lynch Syndrome. N Eng J Med 2006; 354:261–269.
16. Levine DA, Lin O, Barakat RR, et al. Risk of endometrial carcinoma associated with BRCA mutation. Gynecol Oncol 2001; 80:395.
17. Kleinerman RA, Boice JD, Storm HH, et al. Second primary cancer after treatment for cervical cancer. Cancer 1995; 76:442–452.
18. Anderson B. Diagnosis of endometrial cancer. Clin Obstet Gynecol 1986; 13:739–750.
19. Pellerin GP, Finan MA. Endometrial cancer in women 45 years of age or younger: a clinicopathological analysis. Am J Obstet Gynecol 2005; 193:1640.
20. Cherkis RC, Patten SF, Jr, Andrews TJ, et al. Significance of normal endometrial cells detected by cervical cytology. Obstet Gynecol 1988; 71:242.
21. Cherkis RC, Patten SF, Jr, Dickinson JC, et al. Significance of atypical endometrial cells detected by cervical cytology. Obstet Gynecol 1987; 69:786.
22. DuBeshter B, Warshal DP, Angel C, et al. Endometrial carcinoma: the relevance of cervical cytology. Obstet Gynecol 1991; 77:458.
23. Chang A, Sandweiss L, Bose S. Cytologically benign endometrial cells in the papanicolaou smears of postmenopausal women. Gynecol Oncol 2001; 80:37.
24. Clark TJ, Mann CH, Shah N, Khan KS, Song F, Gupta JK. Accuracy of outpatient endometrial biopsy in the diagnosis of endometrial cancer: a systematic quantitative review. BJOG: An Int J Obstet & Gynaecol 2002; 109:313

25. Karlsson B, Granberg S, Wikland M, et al. Transvaginal ultrasonography of the endometrium in women with postmenopausal bleeding – a Nordic multicenter study. Am J Obstet Gynecol 1995; 172:1488.
26. Decensi A, Fontana V, Bruno S, Gustavino C, Gatteschi B, Costa A. Effect of tamoxifen on endometrial proliferation. J Clin Oncol 1996; 14:434–440.
27. Love CDB, Muir BB, Scrimgeour JB, et al. Investigation of endometrial abnormalities in asymptomatic women treated with tamoxifen and an evaluation of the role of endometrial screening. J Clin Oncol 1999; 17:2050.
28. Schwartz LB, Snyder J, Horan C, Porges RF, Nachtigall LE, Goldstein SR. The use of trans-vaginal ultrasound and saline infusion sonohysterography for the evaluation of asymptomatic postmenopausal breast cancer patients on tamoxifen. Ultrasound Obstet Gynecol 1998; 11:48–53.
29. Manfredi R, Gui B, Maresca G, Fanfaui F, Bonomo L. Endometrial cancer: magnetic reso-nance imaging. Abdom Imaging 2005; 30:626–636.
30. Novak E. A suction-curet apparatus endometrial biopsy. JAMA 1935; 104:1497–1498.
31. Behnamfar F, Khamehchian T, Mazoochi T, Fahiminejad T. Diagnostic value of endometrial sampling with pipelle suction curettage for identifying endometrial lesions in patients with abnormal uterine bleeding. J Res Med Sci 2004; 3:21–23.
32. Goldberg GL, Tsalacopoulos G, Davey DA. A comparison of endometrial sampling with the Accurette and Vabra aspirator and uterine curettage. S Afr Med J 1982; 61:114–116.
33. International Federation of Gynecology and Obstetrics. Annual report on the results of treat-ment in gynecologic cancer. Int J Gynecol Obstet 1989; 28:189–190.
34. Creasman WT, Morrow CP, Bundy BN, Homesley HD, Graham JE, Heller PB. Surgical pathologic spread patterns of endometrial cancer. Cancer 1987; 60:2035–2041.
35. Aquino-Parsons C, Lim P, Wong F, Mildenberger M. Papillary serous and clear cell carcinoma limited to endometrial curettings in FIGO stage Ia and Ib endometrial adenocarcinoma: treat-ment implications. Gynecol Oncol 1998; 71:83–86.
36. Goff BA, Rice LW. Assessment of depth of myometrial invasion in endometrial adenocarci-noma. Gynecol Oncol 1990; 38:46–48.
37. ACOG Partice bulleten, number 65, August 2005. Management of Endometrial Cancer.
38. Kilgore LC, Partridge EE, Alvarez RD, Austin JM, Shingleton HM, Noojian F, III, et al. Adenocarcinoma of the endometrium: survival comparisons of patients with and without pelvic node sampling. Gynecol Oncol 1995; 56:29–33.
39. Fowler JM. Laparoscopic staging of endometrial cancer. Clin Obstet Gynecol 1996; 39:669.
40. Soliman PT, Slomovitz BM, Broaddus RR, et al. Synchronous primary cancers of the endometrium and ovary: a single institution review of 84 cases. Gynecol Oncol 2004; 94:456.

Imaging in the Diagnosis and Treatment of Endometrial Cancer

Mansi A. Saksena and Susanna I. Lee

Abstract   Ultrasound, sonohysterography (SHG), magnetic resonance imaging, computed tomography (CT), and positron emission tomography (PET) are tools available for diagnosis and for post-treatment surveillance. The transvaginal ultrasound has a well-defined role in women presenting with postmenopausal bleeding. Magnetic resonance imaging (MRI) provides the most accurate modality for preoperative staging in patients with early disease; CT and PET are helpful in the detection of distant metastases; sonohysterography is a less-invasive alternative to hysteroscopy.

Keywords   Endometrial imaging • Ultrasound • MRI • Sonohysterography • CT/PET

Introduction

Imaging is employed in many steps during the diagnosis and treatment of endometrial cancer. Evaluation of abnormal uterine bleeding, preoperative tumor characterization and staging, and post-treatment surveillance all require imaging. This chapter provides an overview of various imaging modalities used in the evaluation of endometrial cancer, highlighting the strengths and limitations of the various applications.

Ultrasound

Ultrasound has long been known as an effective tool in the evaluation of women with postmenopausal bleeding (1–4). Although transabdominal ultrasound can be used to detect endometrial pathology, limited spatial resolution, patient body

M.A. Saksena and S.I. Lee(✉)
Department of Radiology, Massachusetts General Hospital, Boston, MA
e-mail: slee0@partners.org

F. Muggia and E. Oliva (eds.), *Uterine Cancer*, Current Clinical Oncology,
DOI: 10.1007/978-1-60327-044-1_3,
© Humana Press, a Part of Springer Science+Business Media, LLC 2009

habitus, uterine retroflexion, and coexisting conditions such as leiomyomas can make transabdominal endometrial evaluation challenging. The improved resolution afforded by high-frequency transvaginal ultrasound probe has led to the establishment of transvaginal ultrasound (TVUS) as the initial noninvasive study of choice in evaluating women presenting with postmenopausal bleeding. TVUS demonstrates better image quality than transabdominal ultrasound in 72% of patients (5) and performs significantly better in evaluating the endometrium in the retroverted uterus (6).

Cancer Detection

In a postmenopausal patient with abnormal vaginal bleeding, the primary role of TVUS is to identify women who need further evaluation for cancer in the form of endometrial biopsy. Endometrial appearance on TVUS is evaluated by thickness and morphology. Normal postmenopausal endometrium is < 5 mm in thickness and is homogenous in thickness and echotexture (Fig. 1a). Because TVUS demonstrates very high specificity and negative predictive value (7) for cancer comparable with other more invasive techniques (8–10) (Table 1), it identifies women who are highly unlikely to have endometrial cancer. Thus, a normal TVUS study can be used to triage patients to diagnostic algorithms that are effective in detecting benign causes of postmenopausal bleeding, for example endometrial polyps or submucosal fibroids.

Endometrial Thickness

Endometrial thickness measurement is an integral part of a TVUS endometrial evaluation. Numerous studies have attempted to establish a size threshold, below which endometrial pathology can be excluded with measurements ranging from 4 to 7 mm (6, 7, 11). A large meta-analysis including 35 studies with 5,892 women demonstrated that, using a 5 mm threshold to define endometrial thickening, 96% of women with endometrial cancer had an abnormal TVUS result, whereas 92% of women with any endometrial disease such as cancer, polyp, or hyperplasia had an abnormal TVUS. This threshold of 5 mm is particularly accurate in excluding endometrial disease in symptomatic women on tamoxifen (Table 1). In postmenopausal women with vaginal bleeding, a 10% pretest probability of endometrial cancer was reduced to a 1% posttest probability after a normal TVUS (7). Thus, TVUS is a powerful tool for identifying patients with postmenopausal bleeding who are highly unlikely to have endometrial pathology.

While a threshold of ≤5 mm endometrial thickness is highly sensitive for detecting endometrial cancer, it is not very specific. Seventy percent of women with postmenopausal bleeding and endometrial thickness >5 mm demonstrate benign

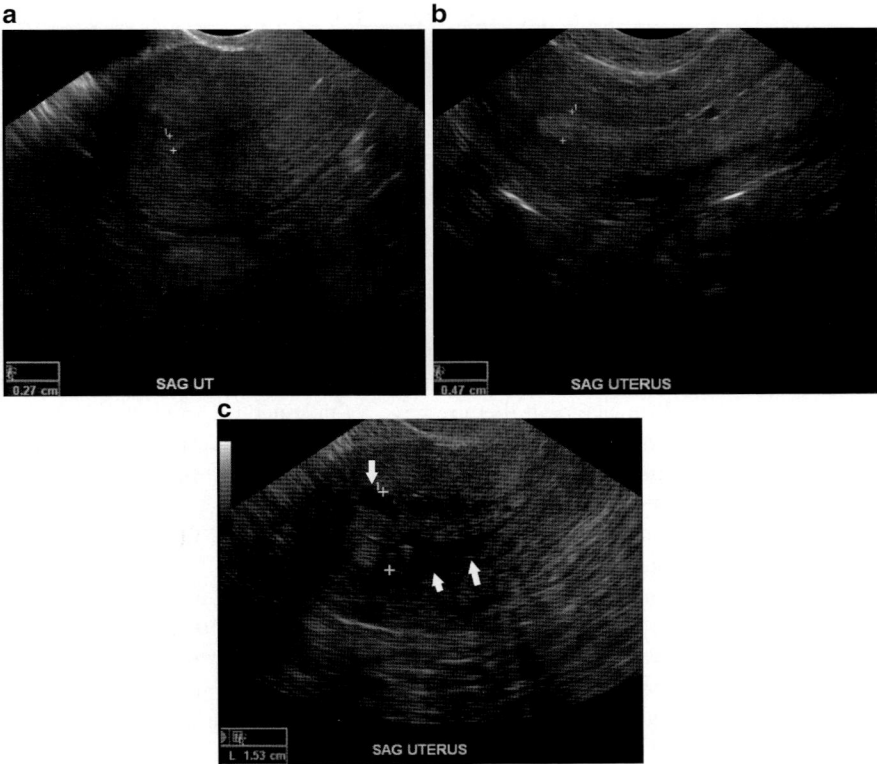

Fig. 1 Transvaginal ultrasound of normal postmenopausal endometrium. Endometrial thickness of a patient not on hormone replacement therapy (**a**), on hormone replacement therapy (**b**), and on tamoxifen (**c**) are measured on sagittal images of the uterus. Note that the patient on hormone replacement therapy displays a slightly thickened endometrium. The patient on tamoxifen demonstrates subendometrial cysts (arrows) and apparent thickening of the endometrium.

Table 1. Diagnostic modalities for endometrial cancer detection

Modality	Sensitivity (%)	Specificity (%)	PPV[a] (%)	NPV[b] (%)
Transvaginal ultrasound (TVUS) not on hormone replacement therapy (7)	96	99	57	99
TVUS on hormone replacement therapy (7)	96	77	31	99
Nonfocal biopsy (8)	87	99	82	99
Hysteroscopy (9)	86	99	72	99
Sonohysterography (10)	89	46	16	97

[a]Positive predictive value
[b]Negative predictive value

Table 2. Common causes of postmenopausal bleeding (13)

Polyps	30%
Submucosal fibroids	30%
Endometrial atrophy	8%
Hyperplasia	4–8%
Endometrial carcinoma	10%

pathology (12). Multiple etiologies for postmenopausal bleeding have been reported (13) (Table 2), some of which result in a thickened endometrium. Postmenopausal women on hormonal replacement therapy have a thickened endometrium at base-line than those who are not on hormone replacement. Patients on sequential hormo-nal therapy demonstrate greater endometrial thickness than in those on continuous hormonal replacement (14) (Fig. 1b). Patients on tamoxifen with cystic suben-dometrial atrophy can also demonstrate apparent abnormal thickening of the endometrium (15) (Fig. 1c).

Note that normal endometrial thickness does not exclude endometrial cancer as a cause for postmenopausal bleeding. A study of women with postmenopausal bleeding not on tamoxifen showed that half the patients with endometrial cancer had an endometrial thickness between 3 and 4 mm (12). Thus, even in patients with normal endometrial thickness, persistent or recurrent bleeding should be further evaluated to definitively identify the cause of the symptoms.

Endometrial Morphology

In addition to endometrial thickness, TVUS assesses endometrial morphology, which can be classified as either focal or diffuse. Diffuse endometrial thickening is often due to hyperplasia or carcinoma and a nonfocal biopsy will usually be ade-quate to establish a histologic diagnosis (Fig. 2a). Focal thickening is usually due to endometrial polyps, which could be benign or malignant, and hysteroscopic tis-sue sampling is often required to establish the diagnosis (Fig. 2b).

Morphological features of the endometrium associated with malignancy have been described. They include heterogeneous echotexture, hyperechoic echotexture with irregular borders, and a heterogeneous intraluminal mass. Using these criteria, Weigel et al. concluded that a combined assessment of endometrial thickness and morphology improves detection of endometrial pathology on TVUS (16).

As TVUS is used as a first step to triage patients with postmenopausal bleeding for tissue sampling, criteria for an abnormal endometrium should be optimized to maximize sensitivity for cancer detection. Thus, all patients with postmenopausal bleeding with abnormal endometrial thickness or morphology on TVUS should undergo histologic sampling.

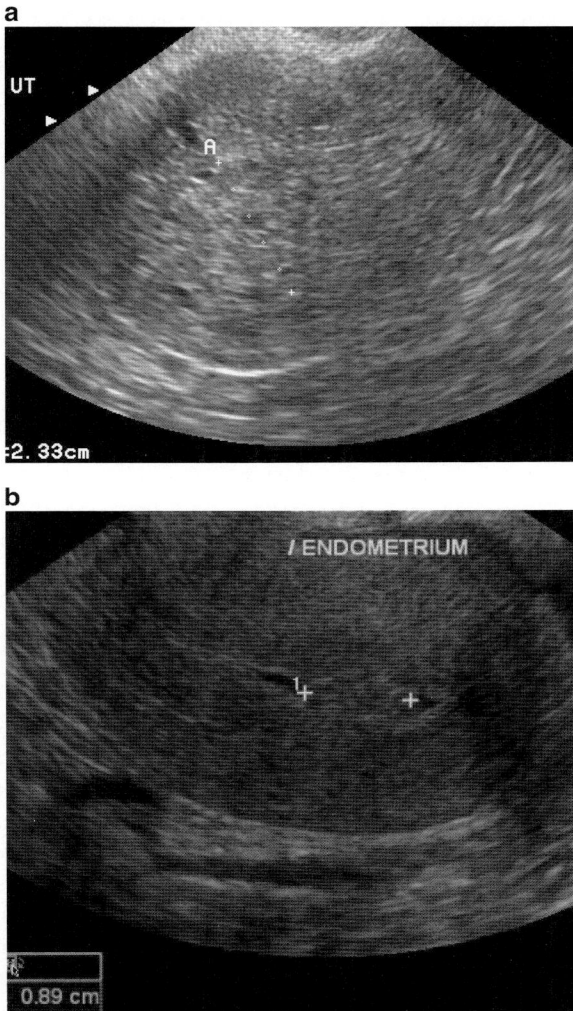

Fig. 2 Transvaginal ultrasound of abnormally thickened endometrium. Sagittal images of the uterus demonstrate diffuse (**a**) and focal (**b**) endometrial thickening (calipers) pathologically confirmed to be endometrial cancer and a benign endometrial polyp, respectively.

Cancer Staging

Although the International Federation of Gynecology and Obstetrics (FIGO) staging for endometrial cancer is based on surgery (Table 3), imaging is frequently used for preoperative treatment planning and to predict prognosis. The high resolution afforded by TVUS readily allows for assessment of extent of tumor spread within

Table 3. International Federation of Gynecology and Obstetrics (FIGO) staging of endometrial cancer: Preoperative evaluation with MRI[a]

I.	Confined to corpus
	a. Limited to endometrium
	b. < one half myometrial invasion
	c. **≥ one half myometrial invasion**
II.	Cervical involvement
	a. **Endocervical glands**
	b. **Stromal invasion**
III.	Extrauterine extension but confined to true pelvis
	a. **Serosal or adnexal extension** or positive peritoneal cytology
	b. Vaginal metastasis
	c. **Pelvic or para-aortic nodal involvement**
IV.	Extension beyond true pelvis into adjacent organs
	a. **Bladder or bowel involvement**
	b. Distant metastasis

[a]Bold lettering indicates tumor involvement best assessed preoperatively with MRI

the uterus. However, because of the limitations in tissue penetration, neither transabdominal nor TVUS can accurately assess extrauterine spread or nodal involvement by tumor.

To assess the utility of TVUS for tumor staging, accuracies of TVUS in detecting deep myometrial invasion (≥50% myometrial thickness) and cervical extension have been studied (17–20). In a series of 69 patients, Artner et al. reported high levels of accuracy in detecting deep myometrial invasion (99%) and cervical extension (96%) using TVUS (18), although in the latter, TVUS was noted to have missed three of nine cases of cervical extension. In a study of 90 patients, Sawicki et al. reported slightly lower accuracies of 84% for myometrial invasion and 86% for cervical extension (21). Studies comparing TVUS and MRI have not found comparable TVUS performance in tumor staging with reported accuracies of 68% (20) and 69% (19). This wide range in reported accuracies, likely explained in part by variations in patient body habitus and operator expertise, results in TVUS being a modality whose reliability in tumor staging is difficult to assess.

The technical factors limiting TVUS performance as a staging tool are well known. TVUS can both under- and overestimate the extent of myometrial tumor invasion. Overestimation can occur when coexisting myometrial processes, for example, adenomyosis, leiomyomas, or endometrial cavity distension from tumor or hematometra are present. Underestimation is usually seen in cases of microscopic or lymphovascular invasion.

Intrauterine sonography involving transcervical insertion of a high-frequency microtip probe has also been used as a staging tool. Probe placement does not require cervical dilatation or anesthesia. Improved accuracies for depth of tumor invasion when compared to TVUS have been reported (22) in a single series of 48 patients.

Sonohysterography

This is a minimally invasive procedure in which saline is instilled in the uterine cavity prior to TVUS through a catheter positioned in the cervical canal. The saline separates the two walls of the uterus facilitating sonographic evaluation of the endometrium. Endometrium suspicious for malignancy demonstrates irregularities in thickness or echotexture or a broad-based poorly marginated endoluminal mass (Fig. 3a). Benign endometrium is characterized as either normal, that is homogeneous echotexture or uniform thickness, or demonstrating a polyp, that is a smoothly marginated pedunculated endoluminal mass (Fig. 3b).

This technique is recommended when TVUS cannot adequately assess the endometrium. In patients with non- or poor visualization of the endometrium with TVUS, usually due to fibroids or adenomyosis, SHG can delineate the endometrial cavity. It is also extremely useful in assessing patients with postmenopausal bleeding on tamoxifen, many of whom demonstrate apparent endometrial thickening on TVUS due to cystic subendometrial atrophy (23). Because SHG can discriminate between endometrial and subendometrial processes, an endometrial lesion, for example polyp or cancer, can be visualized separate from the subendometrial tamoxifen-related changes after the instillation of saline (Fig. 3c).

Sonohysterography accurately identifies endometrial pathology with reported sensitivities of 89–98% and specificities of 46–88% (Table 1) (10, 24). As with TVUS, SHG demonstrates higher sensitivity than specificity, thereby a highly reliable negative predictive value. While SHG is more sensitive than TVUS in detecting focal endometrial pathology, there is no data to suggest that SHG is more sensitive in cancer detection when the endometrium has been adequately visualized with TVUS. Thus, based on the current evidence, the primary role of SHG in evaluating patients with postmenopausal bleeding should be to identify etiologies other than cancer (Table 2).

Sonohysterography is recommended in patients with abnormal endometrial thickness on TVUS or with persistent postmenopausal bleeding only after a non-focal endometrial biopsy has proven negative for cancer (25). Because SHG demonstrates sensitivity for endometrial pathology comparable to that reported for hysteroscopy (Table 1), it represents a less invasive alternative for evaluating patients with a negative biopsy.

Doppler Ultrasound

Cancer Detection

Color Doppler is used in conjunction with TVUS in the evaluation of women with postmenopausal bleeding. Presence of Doppler signal within an endometrial lesion eliminates blood clot as a possible etiology. Color Doppler can also assess the

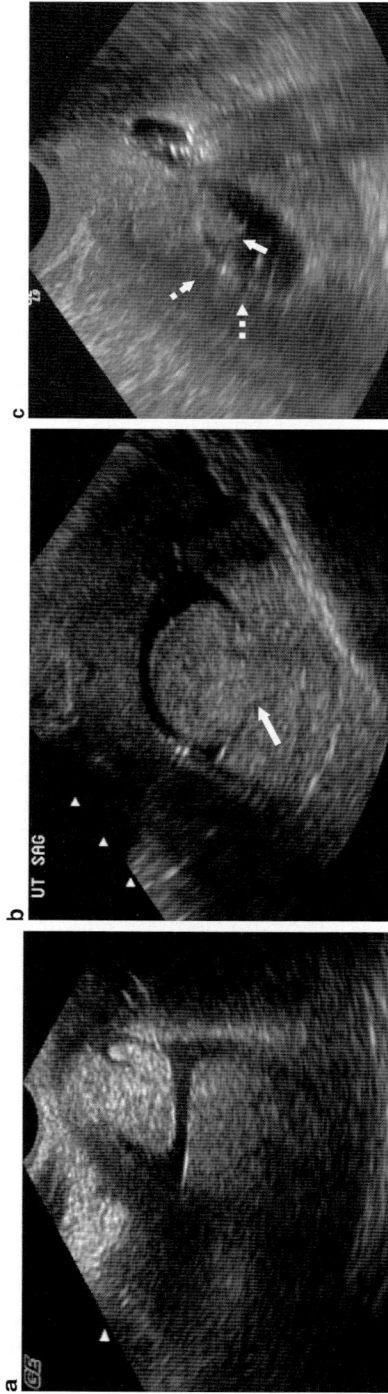

Fig. 3 Sonohysterography of abnormally thickened endometrium. Sagittal images of the uterus after intracavitary saline infusion delineate the morphology and location of the underlying endometrial lesion. Endometrial cancer (**a**) typically demonstrates a broad base of attachment to the uterine wall and involves the majority of the endometrial cavity; a polyp (**b**) demonstrates a narrow base of attachment (arrow), in this case, originating from the posterior fundal wall. Evaluation of the tamoxifen endometrium (**c**) demonstrates a polyp (solid arrow) originating from the anterior uterine body and the subendometrial location of the cysts (dashed arrows) both accounting for the apparent thickening seen on transvaginal ultrasound.

pattern of vascularity of an endometrial mass. Malignant lesions are usually broad-based and with diffuse high level of vascularity (Fig. 4a, b), whereas a single feeding vessel in a lesion of relatively low overall vascularity is associated with benign polyps on a stalk (Fig. 4c, d).

Various spectral Doppler indices have been proposed for the detection of an endometrial malignancy. A resistive index < 0.7 has been reported to represent abnormal vascularity associated with malignancy (26). Pulsatility index values ranging from <1.00 to <2.00 have also been associated with malignancy (26–28). However, none of these indices are accurate in determining the histologic diagnosis, with significant overlap observed between benign and malignant lesions. Comparison of Doppler analysis to conventional gray-scale TVUS demonstrated that abnormal endometrial thickness alone is a better predictor of endometrial pathology than Doppler velocity of the uterine arteries (29–31).

Cancer Staging

The association of tumor angiogenesis with the aggressive endometrial tumors has led to the hypothesis that Doppler TVUS could be used to detect abnormal intratumoral vessels and thereby predict prognostic factors such as nodal spread or depth of myometrial invasion. Color Doppler assesses the distribution of blood vessels (peripheral, central, or mixed) and vascular density. Tumor angiogenesis is associated with high vascular density with a peripheral or mixed distribution (30). Spectral Doppler characterizes the features of the blood flow such as peak systolic velocity and the resistive index, a measure of impedance. Abnormal intratumoral arteries are characterized by high-velocity low-impedance blood flow.

Current available data on the effectiveness of Doppler to preoperatively stage endometrial cancer patients is inconclusive. Testa et al. showed that while overall intratumoral blood flow is higher in patients with > 50% myometrial invasion, spectral Doppler analysis is not predictive of surgical stage, tumor grade, or nodal metastases (31). In contrast, Sawicki et al. found a statistically significant association between pelvic lymph node metastases and vascular density (30). These differences likely reflect the variability inherent to ultrasound, a modality whose performance is often subject to nontechnical factors such as patient habitus and operator expertise.

Magnetic Resonance Imaging

Magnetic resonance imaging is primarily used in staging endometrial cancer after the initial diagnosis has been made. The inherent soft tissue resolution and multi-planar imaging capability of MRI make it an effective modality to assess disease extent both within and outside the pelvis and to evaluate for nodal metastases. Because of its limited availability, MRI does not play a significant role in cancer

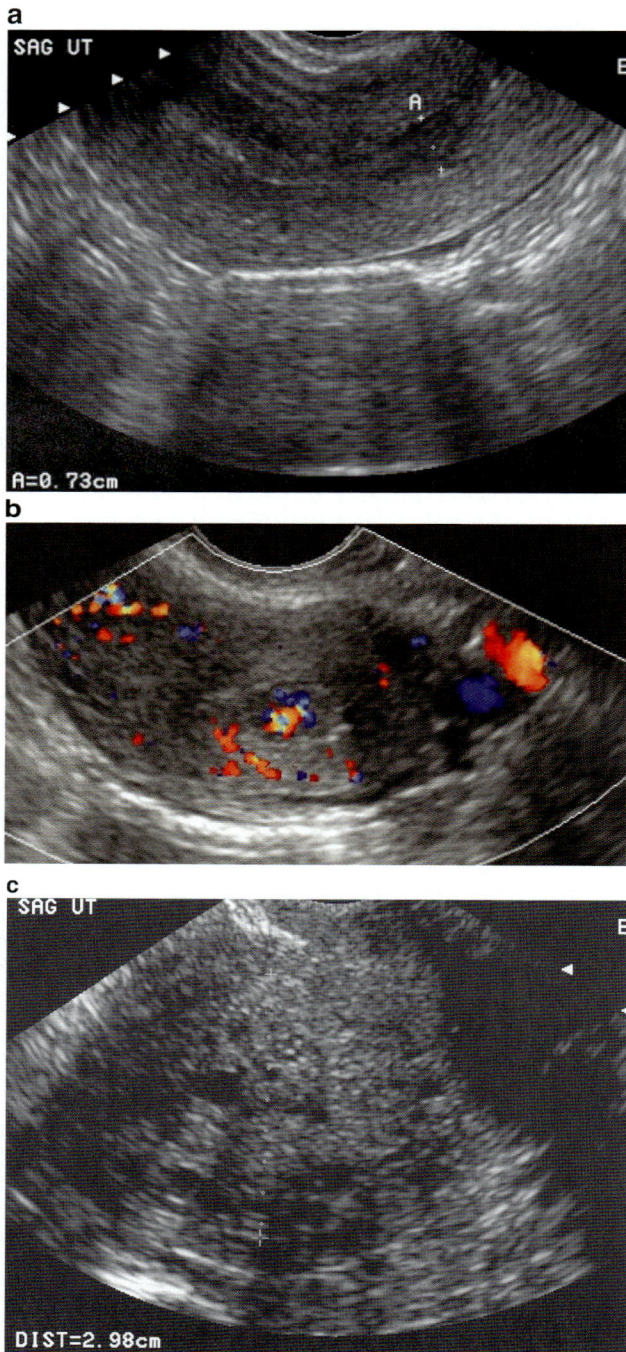

Fig. 4 Doppler ultrasound of abnormally thickened endometrium. Gray scale (**a** and **c**) and color Doppler (**b** and **d**) transvaginal ultrasound evaluation demonstrates a diffusely increased vascularity of the thickened endometrium typical for cancer (**a** and **b**) and a single feeding vessel in an endometrium of overall low vascularity characteristic of a polyp (**c** and **d**).

d

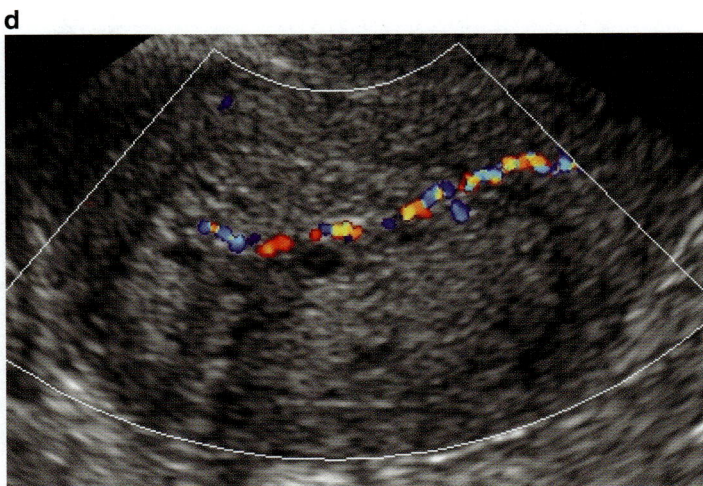

Fig. 4   (continued).

detection. It can be used as a problem-solving tool in evaluating patients with cervical or vaginal stenosis where adequate assessment of the endometrium with TVUS or biopsy is precluded.

Technique

Protocols for imaging patients with endometrial cancer include triplane T2-weighted fast spin echo images to be performed along the uterine axis, axial T1-weighted images up to the renal hilum to evaluate regional lymph nodes, sagittal dynamic gadolinium-enhanced fat-saturated T1-weighted images, and triplane postcontrast fat-saturated T1-weighted images (Fig. 5). For purposes of tumor staging, gadolinium should be routinely administered. High-resolution images usually are required to evaluate an atrophic endometrium. The study is performed with a phased array body coil. To decrease artifact from bowel motion, patients may be asked to fast for 4–6 h prior to imaging and glucagon may be administered.

Cancer Detection

The normal endometrium is isointense on T1-weighted images, very hyperintense on T2-weighted images, and enhances more slowly than the myometrium after dynamic gadolinium administration. Endometrial pathology, including cancer,

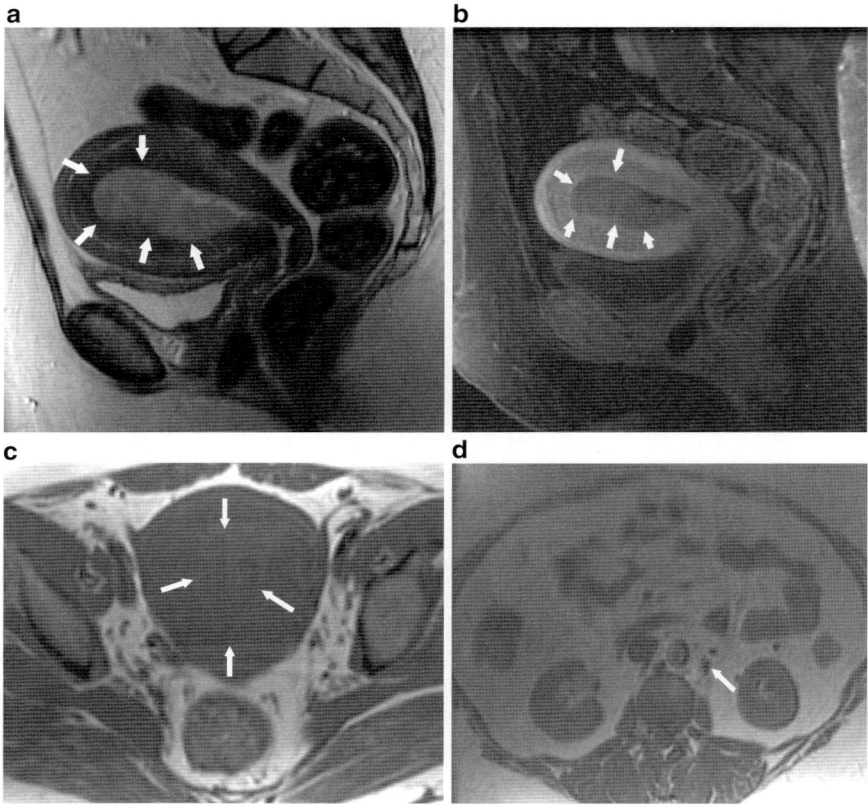

Fig. 5 Magnetic resonance imaging (MRI) of endometrial cancer. Sagittal T2-weighted (**a**) and postgadolinium T1-weighted fat-saturated (**b**) images of the uterus demonstrate a mass (arrows) extending throughout the uterine cavity which is T2-hypointense and enhances with gadolinium more avidly when compared to normal endometrium. Note that the cancer does not enhance as avidly as normal myometrium. Axial pregadolinium T1-weighted images through the pelvis (**c**) and the renal hila (**d**) show tumor isointense to myometrium (arrows) and a normal 5-mm node with a fatty hilum (arrow), respectively.

appears hypointense on T2-weighted images and enhances faster after dynamic gadolinium administration relative to normal endometrium (Fig. 5). Blood clots can be distinguished from endometrial pathology as they typically demonstrate portions that are T1 hyperintense and no enhancement with gadolinium. However, in the absence of tumor extension outside the endometrial cavity, MRI cannot discriminate cancer from other endometrial pathologies such as hyperplasia or polyps (32). Thus, endometrial lesions identified on MRI require histology for definitive diagnosis.

Cancer Staging

Magnetic resonance imaging is the most effective imaging modality for preoperative staging of patients with endometrial cancer (Table 3). A recent meta-analysis demonstrated that contrast-enhanced MRI performs better than noncontrast MRI, CT, or US in detecting myometrial invasion (33). In comparison with gross visual inspection of a surgical specimen, MRI compares favorably with accuracy of 93%, sensitivity of 80%, and specificity of 100% in detecting deep myometrial invasion (Stage IC) and accuracy of 80%, sensitivity of 33%, and specificity of 100% for cervical invasion (Stage II). Thus, MRI can be used as a "one-stop imaging examination" with the highest accuracy to triage a patient diagnosed with endometrial cancer to lymphadenectomy, medical hormonal therapy for fertility preservation, radical hysterectomy, or preoperative radiotherapy. MRI is also routinely used to stage patients who are not candidates for surgery.

Staging with MRI has been shown to have important therapeutic and prognostic implications. It is well known that tumor grade and depth of myometrial invasion are associated with prevalence of lymph node metastases and patient survival (34). Frei et al. have reported that findings on contrast-enhanced MRI examination significantly affect the posttest probability of deep myometrial invasion in patients with all grades of endometrial cancer. This, in turn, affects the probability of lymph node metastases (35). Thus, MRI is an effective tool to preoperatively assess whether a patient with endometrial cancer will require lymphadenectomy.

Myometrial Invasion

Assessment of myometrial invasion with MRI requires evaluation of both T2-weighted and postgadolinium administration images. Any disruption or irregularity of the myometrial junctional zone by an isointense mass on T2-weighted images is diagnostic of myometrial invasion. An intact junctional zone with a sharp tumor–myometrium interface suggests a noninvasive malignancy. MRI detects deep myometrial invasion with reported accuracies of 74–91% (Fig. 6) (36, 37). When compared side-by-side to TVUS, MRI demonstrates similar accuracies with noncontrast imaging (37), but higher accuracies when gadolinium is administered (38).

Typically, errors are in over- rather than underestimating the extent of myometrial invasion (39). Coexisting myometrial conditions, such as leiomyomas or thinned myometrium due to atrophy or endometrial canal distention, can decrease the accuracy of MRI in assessing tumor invasion. In patients with adenomyosis who demonstrate a thickened junctional zone, an indistinct junctional zone on T2-weighted images corresponds to myometrial invasion only in 22% of cases. With gadolinium administration, accuracy is reported to increase considerably to 92% (40).

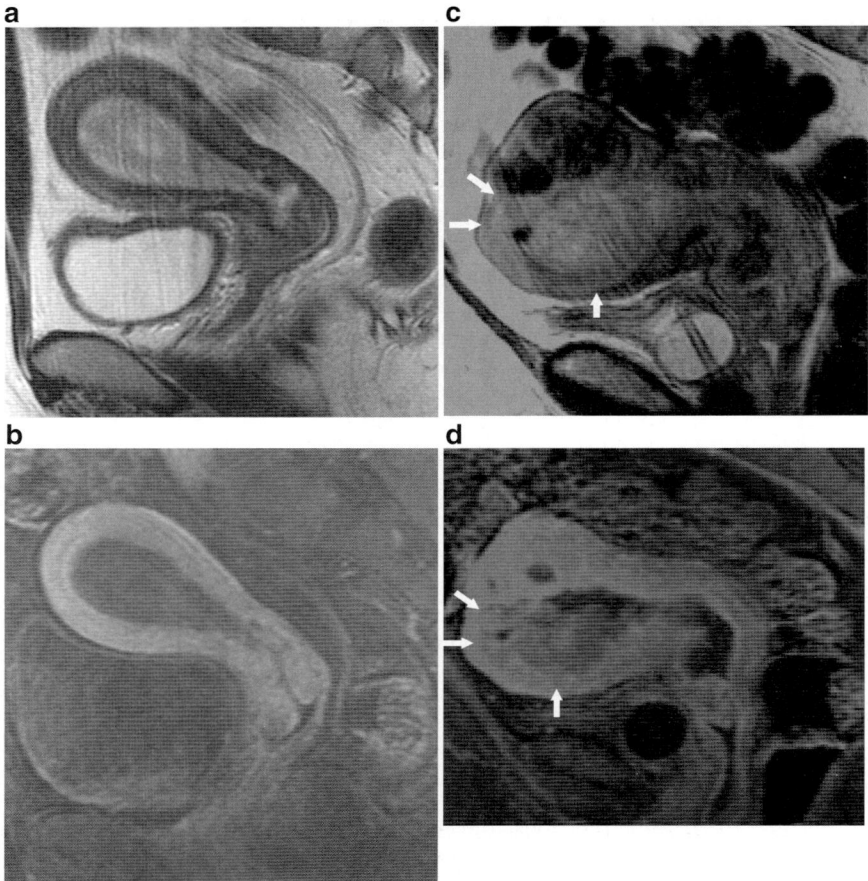

Fig. 6 MRI evaluation of the depth of myometrial invasion. Sagittal T2-weighted (**a** and **c**) and postgadolinium T1-weighted fat-saturated images of the uterus demonstrate a cancer with no myometrial invasion (**a** and **b**) and one with invasion of >50% myometrial depth (**c** and **d**, arrows). Imaging findings were confirmed with surgical pathology.

Cervical Invasion

Tumor extending into the cervix appears as widening of the internal os and the endocervical canal. Disruption of the cervical stroma is seen as loss of the fibrous black line around the cervix on T2-weighted images (Fig. 7). If the tumor extends into the cervix but the stroma is intact then the tumor is considered Stage IIA; stromal disruption is considered Stage II B (Table 1). While accuracies of up to 92% have been reported (41), sensitivity maybe lower because microscopic cervical invasion extension can be missed.

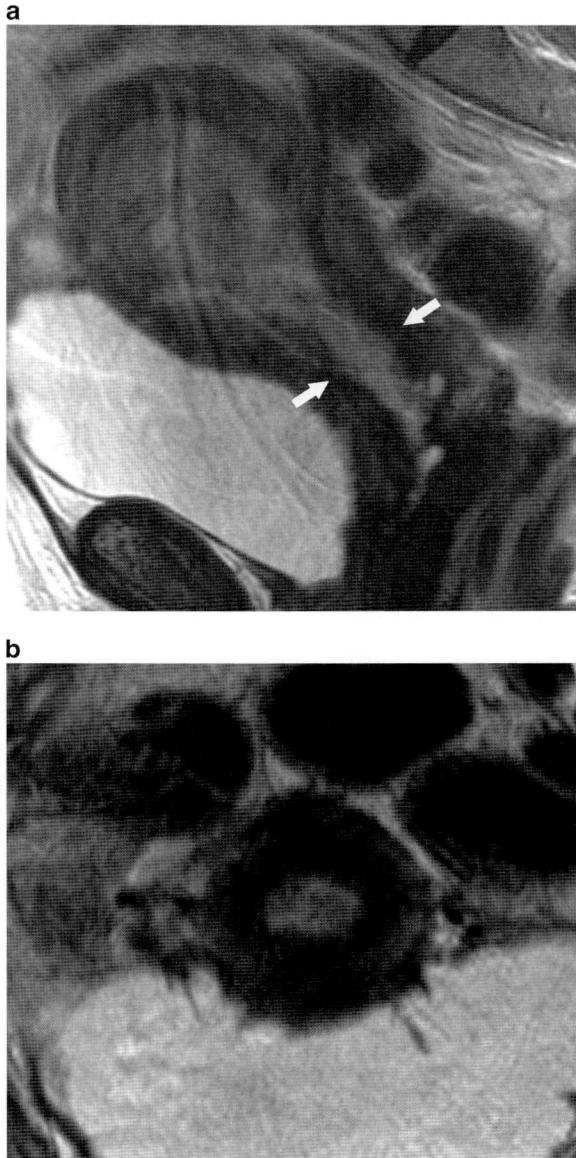

Fig. 7 MRI evaluation of cervical invasion. Sagittal T2-weighted image of the uterus (**a**) demonstrates a mass involving the endometrial cavity and the endocervical canal (arrows). A long-axis oblique T2-weighted image of the cervix reveals no evidence of gross stromal or parametrial invasion by tumor. Imaging findings were confirmed with surgical pathology.

Extrauterine Spread

Disruption or irregularities of the outer layer of the myometrium indicate extrauterine spread. There maybe direct extension of the tumor into parametrial fat or adnexa (Stage IIIA) (Fig. 8a). Ovaries can also be involved by discrete metastases. While gross tumor extension into the vaginal tissue (Stage IIIB) can be seen on gadolinium-enhanced images, mucosal vaginal involvement is more readily established by direct visualization and biopsy.

Extension into the bladder or rectum is best determined on gadolinium-enhanced sagittal images and can be corroborated on axial imaging. Loss of the normal fat plane between the tumor and the bladder or rectum indicates invasion (Stage IVA) (Fig. 8b). While this finding signifies tumor invasion of the bladder or rectal serosa, it does not necessary imply mucosal involvement, which is more accurately assessed by endoscopic visualization and biopsy.

Lymph Nodes

As a cross-sectional imaging modality, MRI enables detection of pelvic and retroperitoneal lymphadenopathy (Stage IIIC). Typically, endometrial cancer spreads to regional pelvic nodes, but it can metastasize to abdominal nodes with normal pelvic nodes. Consequently, a pelvic MRI examination for endometrial cancer staging includes a large field of view T1-weighted images from the pelvic floor to the renal hilum to assess for retroperitoneal as well as pelvic sidewall lymphadenopathy. Size and morphology have traditionally been used as criteria for lymphadenopathy with an oval node > 1 cm in the short axis and a rounded node > 8 mm labeled as concerning for malignancy (Fig. 9) (42).

While relatively specific, size as used on current cross-sectional imaging is an insensitive criterion for assessing nodal involvement by tumor (41, 43–46) (Table 4). Normal size nodes can harbor micrometastatic disease, whereas enlarged nodes may be reactive in nature. This has led to the development of a lymph node-specific contrast agent, Ferumoxtran-10, which evaluates nodal function rather than size (47, 48). Molecular imaging using these agents, called lymphotropic nanoparticle-enhanced MRI (LNMRI), has demonstrated greater accuracy than conventional gadolinium-enhanced MRI in predicting nodal involvement by tumor (Fig. 10). A recent evaluation of 15 patients with endometrial cancer found LNMRI to be 93% sensitive and 100% specific, while conventional MRI was only 29% sensitive and 99% specific (46).

Computed Tomography

Computed tomography (CT) plays no role in primary tumor detection or in staging early disease. It is predominantly used for preoperative staging of advanced disease and evaluation of nodal (Stage IIIC) and distant metastases (Stage IVB). Compared

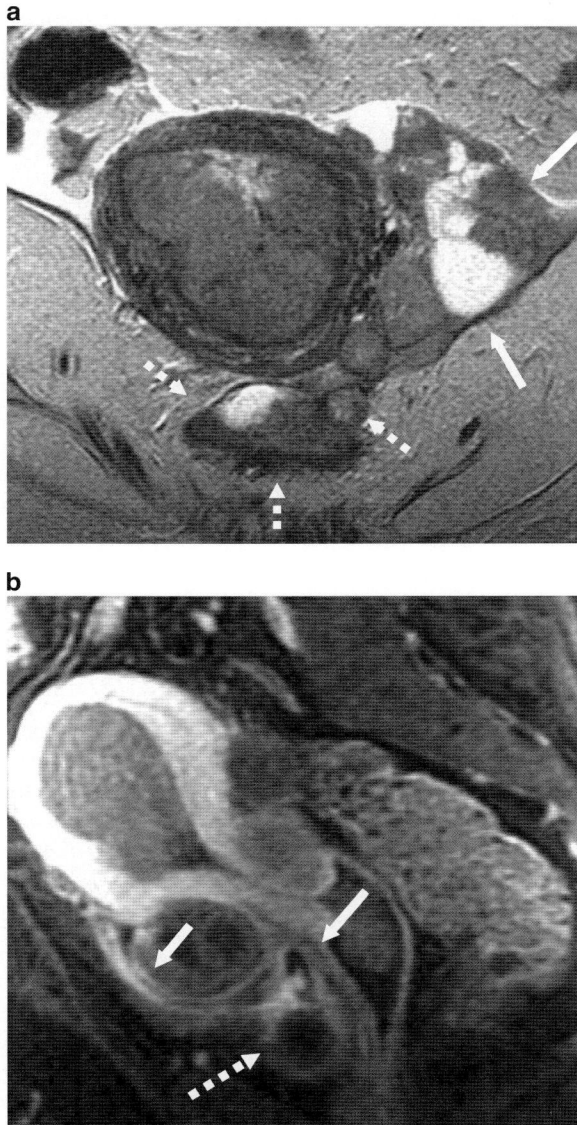

Fig. 8 MRI evaluation of extrauterine spread. Axial T2-weighted image of the uterus (**a**) shows cancer involving the endometrial cavity with metastasis to the left ovary (solid arrows). Tumor implants in the cul-de-sac (dashed arrows) are also noted. Sagittal postgadolinium T1-weighted image with fat saturation (**b**) illustrates a foley catheter balloon in a collapsed bladder (dashed arrow) and tumor involving the bladder dome and trigone (solid arrows). Imaging findings were confirmed with surgical evaluation and biopsies.

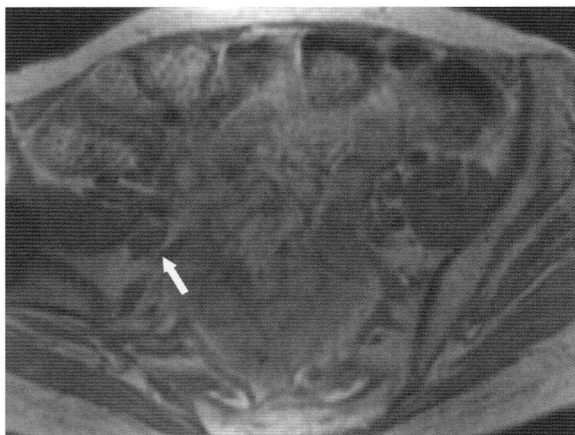

Fig. 9 MRI evaluation of nodal involvement. Axial T1-weighted image of the pelvis reveals an abnormally enlarged 1.8 cm right obturator node (arrow) shown to be involved by tumor on pathologic evaluation.

to MRI, whose resolution is sometimes compromised by bowel or patient motion, contrast-enhanced CT more reliably detects distant parenchymal metastases, peritoneal implants, and malignant ascites (Stage IVB) (49) (Fig. 11).

Because of its multiplanar and greater tissue-specific imaging capabilities, MRI performs better than CT in staging early disease (Stages I and II) and in evaluating tumor invasion into adjacent organs (Stage IVA) (33, 50–52). A side-by-side comparison of the two modalities found that, to detect myometrial invasion, CT demonstrates 83% sensitivity and 42% specificity, while MR demonstrates 92% sensitivity and 90% specificity. To detect cervical invasion, CT demonstrates 25% sensitivity and 70% specificity, while MR demonstrates 86% sensitivity and 97% specificity (53).

Positron Emission Tomography

Positron emission tomography (PET) with the radioactive glucose analogue 18-2-fluorodeoxy-2-deoxy-D-glucose (18-FDG) has proven to be a powerful tool to detect nodal involvement by various malignancies. Cells with elevated glycolysis avidly take up this glucose analogue. 18-FDG is phosphorylated to 18-FDG-6P, which is trapped in tumor cells that are relatively deficient in glucose-6-phosphatase during the time interval in which images are acquired. Following a ≥ 6 h fast, patients are injected with the 18-FDG (average dose, 555 MBq [15 mCi]). Images are obtained 45–60 min after intravenous injection of the tracer. This increased 18-FDG uptake can be detected on PET and corresponds to tissue with increased metabolic activity, such as malignancy or inflammation.

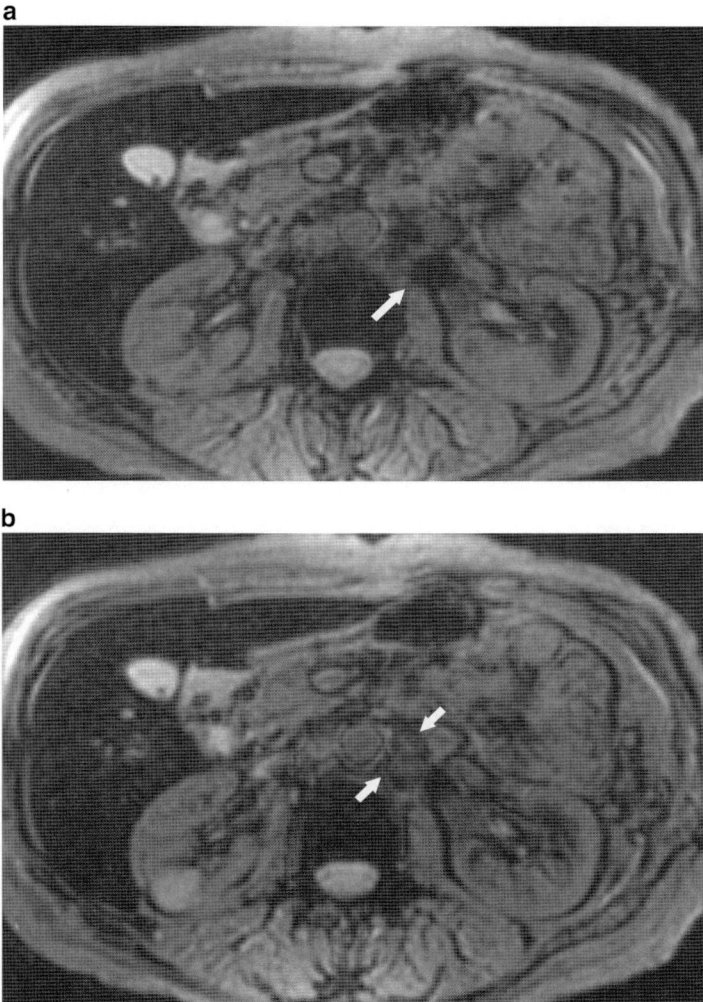

Fig. 10 Lymphotrophic nanoparticle-enhanced MRI evaluation of nodal involvement. Axial T2* images at level of renal hila (**a**) show a normal node (arrow) that takes up the lymphotrophic contrast agent, Ferumoxtran-10, and is consequently hypointense with susceptibility artifact. A cranial image (**b**) reveals similar-sized <1 cm nodes (arrows) that are hyperintense because they are involved by tumor and thereby do not take up the contrast agent. Imaging findings of nodal tumor involvement were confirmed with biopsies.

Preliminary studies in patients with endometrial cancer suggest that FDG-PET, in the absence of concurrent high-resolution cross-sectional imaging, is unlikely to be useful in staging. It lacks the spatial resolution to define extent of the primary tumor. Because a significant proportion of endometrial cancers are low grade, that

Table 4. Imaging for nodal metastases

Modality	Sensitivity (%)	Specificity (%)
CT (43, 44)	30–57	92–95.5
MRI (44)	50	95
PET (45)	63	98
LNMRI (46)	93	100

CT computed tomography; MRI magnetic resonance imaging; PET positron emission tomography; LNMRI lymphotropic nanoparticle-enhanced MRI

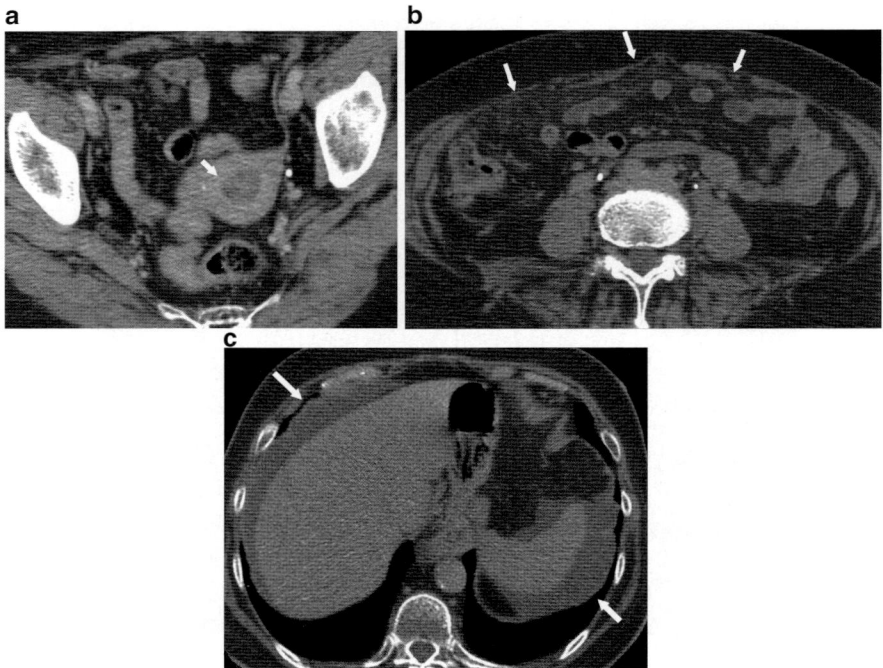

Fig. 11 Computed tomography (CT) of advanced endometrial cancer. Axial contrast-enhanced image through the pelvis (**a**) demonstrates an enhancing mass (arrow) enlarging the uterine endometrial cavity. Image through the mid-abdomen above the iliac crests (**b**) reveals omental carcinomatosis (arrows). Image of the upper abdomen at the level of the liver (**c**) shows ascites (arrows). Pathologic examination demonstrated a clear cell endometrial carcinoma.

is Grade I, and not markedly FDG-avid, PET is only moderately sensitive in detecting lymph node metastases. In a study of 19 patients, a high proportion of primary uterine corpus tumors demonstrated increased uptake. However, because of its limited ability in detecting micrometastases in normal-sized nodes, the sensitivity of FDG-PET for nodal metastases was 63% with a specificity of 98% (45).

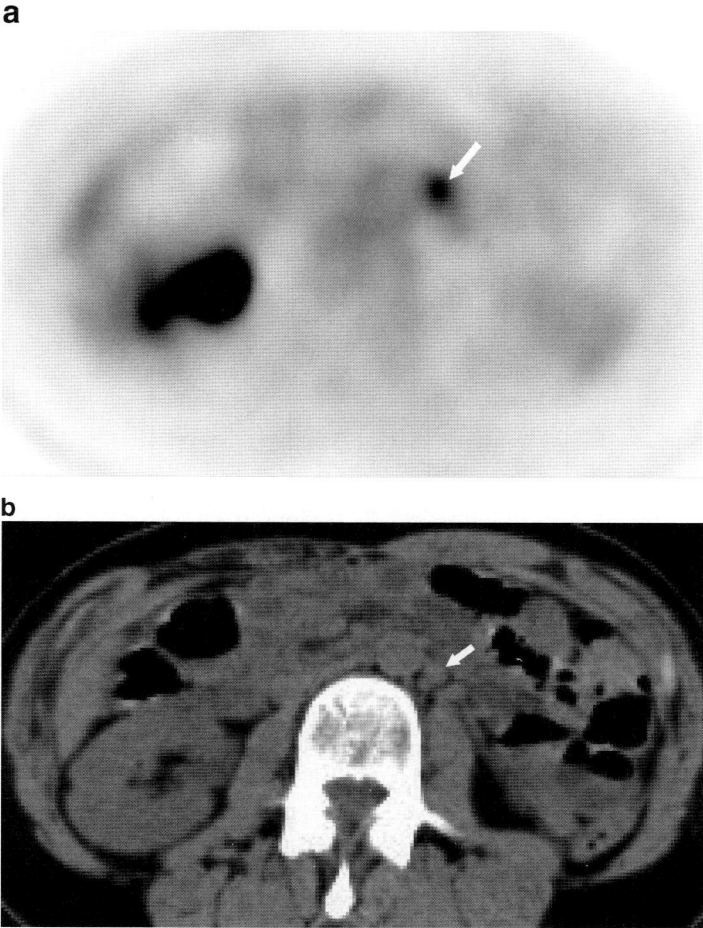

Fig. 12 Positron emission tomography (PET) of endometrial cancer. Axial FDG-PET image (**a**) of a patient with endometrial cancer demonstrates abnormal tracer uptake (arrow) medial to the left kidney. CT image at the same level (**b**) reveals a 9-mm-left para-aortic node (arrow) in that location. Tumor involvement of the node was pathologically confirmed.

A recent study in 49 patients evaluating the clinical impact of FDG-PET images interpreted in conjunction with CT or MRI suggested that FDG-PET performed concurrently with high-resolution cross-sectional imaging may prove more useful than FDG-PET alone. Only 30% of patients with an elevated CA-125 were found to derive any clinical benefit from FDG-PET alone. However, MRI or CT images interpreted concurrently with the FDG-PET images performed much better (accuracy 97% vs 94%, respectively) than MRI or CT alone in detecting extrapelvic and nodal metastases (Fig. 12) (54). With fusion PET-CT scanners becoming more widely available, future research will likely focus on the usefulness of fusion PET-CT in endometrial cancer staging.

Post-treatment Surveillance

Early detection of recurrent endometrial cancer poses unique challenges. Postoperative scarring and changes due to radiation therapy make early detection

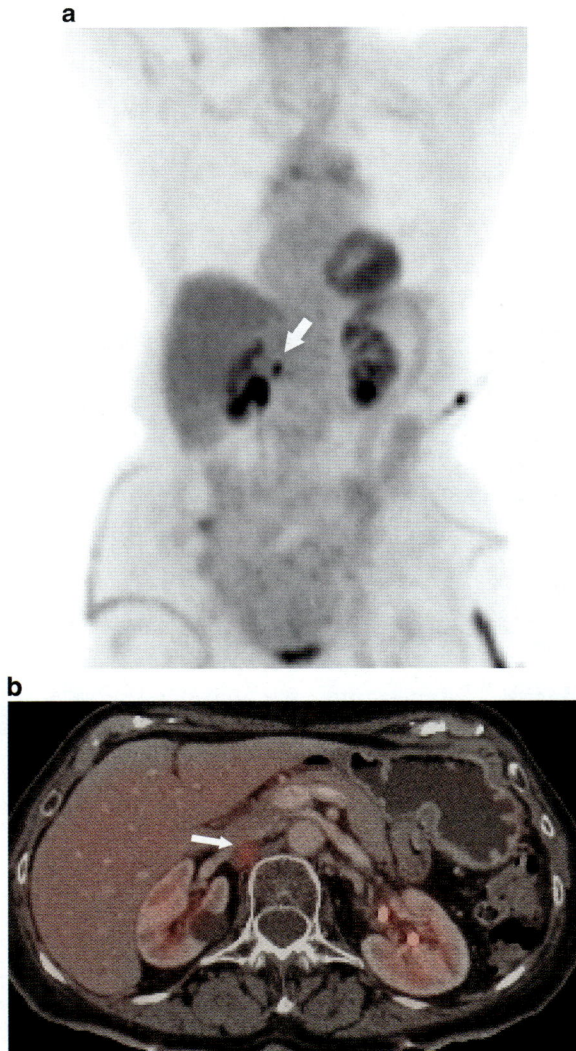

Fig. 13 Fusion positron emission tomography-computed tomography (PET-CT) detecting endometrial cancer recurrence. Coronal FDG-PET image (**a**) of a patient with a history of grade 2 endometrial cancer demonstrates a focus of abnormal tracer uptake (arrow) medial to the right kidney. Fusion PET-CT image (**b**) reveals a corresponding 1 cm retrocaval node which was not identified as abnormal on a standard CT examination 7 days before. Tumor involvement of the node was pathologically confirmed.

of small pelvic relapses difficult. Clinical methods used for postoperative surveillance include clinical history, pelvic examination, and vaginal cytology. Imaging is used as an adjunct to evaluate for recurrences not amenable to detection by physical examination. TVUS with color Doppler is an inexpensive but nonspecific tool for postoperative surveillance allowing for detection of recurrences at the vaginal apex. Color Doppler aids in differentiating hypoechoic pelvic masses from surrounding bowel (55). In discriminating postoperative fibrosis from tumor recurrence, contrast-enhanced MRI has been shown to be useful, with an accuracy of 83% in patients with gynecologic malignancies (56).

Despite its limited utility in preoperative imaging, FDG-PET is of great value in post-therapy surveillance (54, 57, 58) with reported sensitivity of 96%, specificity of 78%, and diagnostic accuracy of 90%. FDG-PET has demonstrated a high likelihood ratio for a positive test result and a low likelihood ratio for a negative result signifying a role in both detecting recurrence as well as ruling it out (58). A study measuring the added value of FDG-PET in addition to CT or MRI for post-therapy surveillance found that FDG-PET showed better diagnostic performance (accuracy 93.3%) compared to combined conventional imaging (accuracy 85%) and tumor markers (accuracy 83.3%) (57) (Fig. 13).

Conclusions

- Transvaginal ultrasound is the initial imaging modality of choice in the evaluation of patients presenting with postmenopausal bleeding and has a reliable negative predictive value.
- In evaluating patients with postmenopausal bleeding and a negative endometrial biopsy, sonohysterography is a less invasive alternative to hysteroscopy.
- Once the diagnosis of endometrial cancer is established, MRI is the most accurate and comprehensive modality for preoperative staging.
- In patients with advanced disease, CT is preferable for detection of distant metastases.
- Preliminary studies suggest that fusion PET-CT will likely be the most powerful imaging modality for post-treatment surveillance.

References

1. Fleischer AC, Kalemeris GC, Machin JE, Entman SS, James AE, Jr. Sonographic depiction of normal and abnormal endometrium with histopathologic correlation. J Ultrasound Med. 1986;5:445–452.
2. Fleischer AC, Mendelson EB, Bohm-Velez M, Entman SS. Transvaginal and transabdominal sonography of the endometrium. Semin Ultrasound CT MR. 1988;9:81–101.
3. Johnson MA, Graham MF, Cooperberg PL. Abnormal endometrial echoes: Sonographic spectrum of endometrial pathology. J Ultrasound Med. 1982;1:161–166.
4. Mendelson EB, Bohm-Velez M, Neiman HL, Russo J. Transvaginal sonography in gynecologic imaging. Semin Ultrasound CT MR. 1988;9:102–121.

5. Guy RL, King E, Ayers AB. The role of transvaginal ultrasound in the assessment of the female pelvis. Clin Radiol. 1988;39:669–672.
6. Coleman BG, Arger PH, Grumbach K, et al. Transvaginal and transabdominal sonography: Prospective comparison. Radiology. 1988;168:639–643.
7. Smith-Bindman R, Kerlikowske K, Feldstein VA, et al. Endovaginal ultrasound to exclude endometrial cancer and other endometrial abnormalities. JAMA. 1998;280:1510–1517.
8. Clark TJ, Mann CH, Shah N, Khan KS, Song F, Gupta JK. Accuracy of outpatient endometrial biopsy in the diagnosis of endometrial cancer: A systematic quantitative review. BJOG. 2002;109:313–321.
9. Clark TJ, Voit D, Gupta JK, Hyde C, Song F, Khan KS. Accuracy of hysteroscopy in the diagnosis of endometrial cancer and hyperplasia: A systematic quantitative review. JAMA. 2002;288:1610–1621.
10. Dubinsky TJ, Stroehlein K, Abu-Ghazzeh Y, Parvey HR, Maklad N. Prediction of benign and malignant endometrial disease: Hysterosonographic-pathologic correlation. Radiology. 1999;210:393–397.
11. Sheth S, Hamper UM, Kurman RJ. Thickened endometrium in the postmenopausal woman: Sonographic-pathologic correlation. Radiology. 1993;187:135–139.
12. Phillip H, Dacosta V, Fletcher H, Kulkarni S, Reid M. Correlation between transvaginal ultrasound measured endometrial thickness and histopathological findings in afro-caribbean jamaican women with postmenopausal bleeding. J Obstet Gynaecol. 2004;24:568–572.
13. Critchley HO, Warner P, Lee AJ, Brechin S, Guise J, Graham B. Evaluation of abnormal uterine bleeding: Comparison of three outpatient procedures within cohorts defined by age and menopausal status. Health Technol Assess. 2004;8:iii–iv, 1–139.
14. Affinito P, Palomba S, Pellicano M, et al. Ultrasonographic measurement of endometrial thickness during hormonal replacement therapy in postmenopausal women. Ultrasound Obstet Gynecol. 1998;11:343–346.
15. Weaver J, McHugo JM, Clark TJ. Accuracy of transvaginal ultrasound in diagnosing endometrial pathology in women with post-menopausal bleeding on tamoxifen. Br J Radiol. 2005;78:394–397.
16. Weigel M, Friese K, Strittmatter HJ, Melchert F. Measuring the thickness – is that all we have to do for sonographic assessment of endometrium in postmenopausal women? Ultrasound Obstet Gynecol. 1995;6:97–102.
17. Gordon AN, Fleischer AC, Reed GW. Depth of myometrial invasion in endometrial cancer: Preoperative assessment by transvaginal ultrasonography. Gynecol Oncol. 1990;39:321–327.
18. Artner A, Bosze P, Gonda G. The value of ultrasound in preoperative assessment of the myometrial and cervical invasion in endometrial carcinoma. Gynecol Oncol. 1994;54:147–151.
19. Del Maschio A, Vanzulli A, Sironi S, et al. Estimating the depth of myometrial involvement by endometrial carcinoma: Efficacy of transvaginal sonography vs MR imaging. AJR Am J Roentgenol. 1993;160:533–538.
20. Yamashita Y, Mizutani H, Torashima M, et al. Assessment of myometrial invasion by endometrial carcinoma: Transvaginal sonography vs contrast-enhanced MR imaging. AJR Am J Roentgenol. 1993;161:595–599.
21. Sawicki W, Spiewankiewicz B, Stelmachow J, Cendrowski K. The value of ultrasonography in preoperative assessment of selected prognostic factors in endometrial cancer. Eur J Gynaecol Oncol. 2003;24:293–298.
22. Gruessner SE. Intrauterine versus transvaginal sonography for benign and malignant disorders of the female reproductive tract. Ultrasound Obstet Gynecol. 2004;23:382–387.
23. Davis PC, O'Neill MJ, Yoder IC, Lee SI, Mueller PR. Sonohysterographic findings of endometrial and subendometrial conditions. Radiographics. 2002;22:803–816.
24. Bree RL, Bowerman RA, Bohm-Velez M, et al. US evaluation of the uterus in patients with postmenopausal bleeding: A positive effect on diagnostic decision making. Radiology. 2000;216:260–264.
25. Reinhold C, Khalili I. Postmenopausal bleeding: Value of imaging. Radiol Clin North Am. 2002;40:527–562.

26. Hata T, Hata K, Senoh D, et al. Doppler ultrasound assessment of tumor vascularity in gynecologic disorders. J Ultrasound Med. 1989;8:309–314.
27. Bourne TH, Campbell S, Whitehead MI, Royston P, Steer CV, Collins WP. Detection of endometrial cancer in postmenopausal women by transvaginal ultrasonography and colour flow imaging. BMJ. 1990;301:369.
28. Merce LT, Lopez Garcia G, de la Fuente F. Doppler ultrasound assessment of endometrial pathology. Acta Obstet Gynecol Scand. 1991;70:525–530.
29. Sladkevicius P, Valentin L, Marsal K. Endometrial thickness and doppler velocimetry of the uterine arteries as discriminators of endometrial status in women with postmenopausal bleeding: A comparative study. Am J Obstet Gynecol. 1994;171:722–728.
30. Sawicki V, Spiewankiewicz B, Stelmachow J, Cendrowski K. Color doppler assessment of blood flow in endometrial cancer. Eur J Gynaecol Oncol. 2005;26:279–284.
31. Testa AC, Ciampelli M, Mastromarino C, et al. Intratumoral color doppler analysis in endometrial carcinoma: Is it clinically useful? Gynecol Oncol. 2003;88:298–303.
32. Hricak H, Stern JL, Fisher MR, Shapeero LG, Winkler ML, Lacey CG. Endometrial carcinoma staging by MR imaging. Radiology. 1987;162:297–305.
33. Kinkel K, Kaji Y, Yu KK, et al. Radiologic staging in patients with endometrial cancer: A meta-analysis. Radiology. 1999;212:711–718.
34. Boronow RC, Morrow CP, Creasman WT, et al. Surgical staging in endometrial cancer: Clinical-pathologic findings of a prospective study. Obstet Gynecol. 1984;63:825–832.
35. Frei KA, Kinkel K, Bonel HM, Lu Y, Zaloudek C, Hricak H. Prediction of deep myometrial invasion in patients with endometrial cancer: Clinical utility of contrast-enhanced MR imaging: A meta-analysis and bayesian analysis. Radiology. 2000;216:444–449.
36. Sironi S, Taccagni G, Garancini P, Belloni C, DelMaschio A. Myometrial invasion by endometrial carcinoma: Assessment by MR imaging. AJR Am J Roentgenol. 1992;158:565–569.
37. Ascher SM, Reinhold C. Imaging of cancer of the endometrium. Radiol Clin North Am. 2002;40:563–576.
38. Nasi F, Fiocchi F, Pecchi A, Rivasi F, Torricelli P. MRI evaluation of myometrial invasion by endometrial carcinoma. Comparison between fast-spin-echo T2W and coronal-FMPSPGR gadolinium-dota-enhanced sequences. Radiol Med (Torino). 2005;110:199–210.
39. Ben-Shachar I, Vitellas KM, Cohn DE. The role of MRI in the conservative management of endometrial cancer. Gynecol Oncol. 2004;93:233–237.
40. Tanaka YO, Nishida M, Tsunoda H, Ichikawa Y, Saida Y, Itai Y. A thickened or indistinct junctional zone on T2-weighted MR images in patients with endometrial carcinoma: Pathologic consideration based on microcirculation. Eur Radiol. 2003;13:2038–2045.
41. Manfredi R, Mirk P, Maresca G, et al. Local-regional staging of endometrial carcinoma: Role of MR imaging in surgical planning. Radiology. 2004;231:372–378.
42. Jager GJ, Barentsz JO, Oosterhof GO, Witjes JA, Ruijs SJ. Pelvic adenopathy in prostatic and urinary bladder carcinoma: MR imaging with a three-dimensional TI-weighted magnetization-prepared-rapid gradient-echo sequence. AJR Am J Roentgenol. 1996;167:1503–1507.
43. Connor JP, Andrews JI, Anderson B, Buller RE. Computed tomography in endometrial carcinoma. Obstet Gynecol. 2000;95:692–696.
44. Pilka R, Kudela M, Dzvincuk P, Lubusky D. Preoperative detection of lymph nodes by means of computer tomography in patients with endometrial carcinoma. Ceska Gynekol. 2004;69:237–239.
45. Horowitz NS, Dehdashti F, Herzog TJ, et al. Prospective evaluation of FDG-PET for detecting pelvic and para-aortic lymph node metastasis in uterine corpus cancer. Gynecol Oncol. 2004;95:546–551.
46. Rockall AG, Sohaib SA, Harisinghani MG, et al. Diagnostic performance of nanoparticle-enhanced magnetic resonance imaging in the diagnosis of lymph node metastases in patients with endometrial and cervical cancer. J Clin Oncol. 2005;23:2813–2821.
47. Anzai Y, Piccoli CW, Outwater EK, et al. Evaluation of neck and body metastases to nodes with ferumoxtran 10-enhanced MR imaging: Phase III safety and efficacy study. Radiology. 2003;228:777–788.

48. Weissleder R, Elizondo G, Wittenberg J, Lee AS, Josephson L, Brady TJ. Ultrasmall super-paramagnetic iron oxide: An intravenous contrast agent for assessing lymph nodes with MR imaging. Radiology. 1990;175:494–498.
49. Russell AH, Anderson M, Walter J, Kinney W, Smith L, Scudder S. The integration of computed tomography and magnetic resonance imaging in treatment planning for gynecologic cancer. Clin Obstet Gynecol. 1992;35:55–72.
50. Pete I, Godeny M, Toth E, Rado J, Pete B, Pulay T. Prediction of cervical infiltration in stage II endometrial cancer by different preoperative evaluation techniques (D&C, US, CT, MRI). Eur J Gynaecol Oncol. 2003;24:517–522.
51. Kim SH, Kim HD, Song YS, Kang SB, Lee HP. Detection of deep myometrial invasion in endometrial carcinoma: Comparison of transvaginal ultrasound, CT, and MRI. J Comput Assist Tomogr. 1995;19:766–772.
52. Zerbe MJ, Bristow R, Grumbine FC, Montz FJ. Inability of preoperative computed tomography scans to accurately predict the extent of myometrial invasion and extracorporal spread in endometrial cancer. Gynecol Oncol. 2000;78:67–70.
53. Hardesty LA, Sumkin JH, Hakim C, Johns C, Nath M. The ability of helical CT to preoperatively stage endometrial carcinoma. AJR Am J Roentgenol. 2001;176:603–606.
54. Chao A, Chang TC, Ng KK, et al. (18)F-FDG PET in the management of endometrial cancer. Eur J Nucl Med Mol Imaging. 2006;33:36–44.
55. Savelli L, Testa AC, Ferrandina G, et al. Pelvic relapses of uterine neoplasms: Transvaginal sonographic and doppler features. Gynecol Oncol. 2004;93:441–445.
56. Kinkel K, Ariche M, Tardivon AA, et al. Differentiation between recurrent tumor and benign conditions after treatment of gynecologic pelvic carcinoma: Value of dynamic contrast-enhanced subtraction MR imaging. Radiology. 1997;204:55–63.
57. Saga T, Higashi T, Ishimori T, et al. Clinical value of FDG-PET in the follow up of post-operative patients with endometrial cancer. Ann Nucl Med. 2003;17:197–203.
58. Belhocine T, De Barsy C, Hustinx R, Willems-Foidart J. Usefulness of (18)F-FDG PET in the post-therapy surveillance of endometrial carcinoma. Eur J Nucl Med Mol Imaging. 2002;29:1132–1139.

Uterine Cancer: Pathology

Robert A. Soslow and Esther Oliva

Abstract Endometrioid adenocarcinoma is the most common type of endometrial carcinoma (approximately 85%). By definition, it should resemble, at least focally, proliferative-type endometrium with tubular glands lined by mitotically active columnar cells. Common problems in diagnosis involve its distinction from complex atypical hyperplasia, endocervical adenocarcinoma, serous carcinoma, clear cell carcinoma, and carcinosarcoma. Pure serous carcinomas comprise about 10% of endometrial cancers. The term "serous" refers to shared characteristics with cells lining the fallopian tube, particularly the tumor cells' columnar shape, eosinophilic cytoplasm and tendency to form papillae. However, some serous carcinomas are not papillary but glandular. Importantly, all serous carcinomas exhibit marked nuclear pleomorphism and most demonstrate discrepancies between architectural differentiation and cytologic features. Clear cell carcinoma is the third most common endometrial carcinoma subtype, even though it represents < 5% of cases. Epidemiologic features of patients with clear cell carcinoma are obscure because of this tumor's rarity, difficulties in diagnostic reproducibility and accumulating evidence that there are perhaps several subtypes of clear cell carcinoma. Most clear cell carcinomas are composed of cells with clear cytoplasm, but this feature is not restricted to clear cell carcinoma and some clear cell carcinomas may contain cells with eosinophilic cytoplasm. Other subtypes of endometrial carcinoma are rare and include squamous, transitional, small cell, and mixed cell types. Among pure mesenchymal tumors of the uterus, leiomyosarcoma is the most common. Microscopic criteria to establish the diagnosis of leiomyosarcoma include the combination of two of the following: cytologic atypia, mitotic activity and tumor cell necrosis. The threshold for mitotic activity varies for spindled, epithelioid and myxoid subtypes. A variety of uterine tumors enter in the differential diagnosis, including several variants of leiomyoma (mitotically active, apoplectic, with bizarre nuclei, highly cellular, and hydropic). Low-grade endometrial stromal sarcomas are composed

R.A. Soslow and E. Oliva (✉)
Department of Pathology, Massachusetts General Hospital, Boston, MA
e-mail: eoliva@partners.org

F. Muggia and E. Oliva (eds.), *Uterine Cancer*, Current Clinical Oncology,
DOI: 10.1007/978-1-60327-044-1_4,
© Humana Press, a Part of Springer Science+Business Media, LLC 2009

of a homogenous population of small cells with scant cytoplasm resembling proliferative-type endometrial stroma. They show a diffuse growth and infiltrate the uterine wall in a permeative (not destructive) fashion and may have prominent intravascular growth. Carcinosarcomas (malignant mixed mullerian tumors) are biphasic tumors typically composed of highly malignant epithelial and stromal/ mesenchymal elements. The histogenesis of these tumors has evolved in recent years and it is now accepted that they either arise from a common pluripotential cell with divergent differentiation or that the sarcomatous component develops from the carcinomatous component by a metaplastic process or dedifferentiation. Other less common mixed or mesenchymal tumors include 1) low-grade müllerian adenosarcoma (composed of benign-appearing glands and malignant stroma); 2) PEComa, which is composed of epithelioid cells that are typically positive for HMB-45 and may be associated with tuberous sclerosis; and 3) intravenous leiomyomatosis which shows a proliferation of smooth muscle cells within vascular spaces. Even though the smooth muscle proliferation is benign it can behave aggressively from the clinical point of view.

Keywords endometrioid • serous • clear cell • mixed carcinomas • leiomyosarcoma • endometrial stromal sarcoma • carcinosarcoma • low-grade müllerian adenosarcoma • PEComa • intravenous leiomyomatosis

Endometrial Carcinoma and Precursor Lesions

Endometrioid Carcinoma

Endometrioid adenocarcinoma is the most common type of endometrial carcinoma (approximately 85%). They are considered type I endometrial cancers according to the Bokhman classification (1) because of their epidemiologic association with estrogen excess. The current model of estrogen-dependent endometrial carcinogenesis involves progression from hyperplasia with increasingly degrees of architectural and cytologic atypia (complex atypical hyperplasia). The development of an invasive neoplasm heralds the emergence of "adenocarcinoma" in this context.

Gross Features

The typical endometrioid adenocarcinoma forms a grossly visible mass that protrudes into the endometrial cavity or causes a diffuse thickening of the endometrial stripe, making it difficult to appreciate a dominant mass. Most tumors arise in the fundus; less commonly, they are found in one of the cornua or in the lower uterine segment, and in some cases, the lesion is centered in an endometrial polyp. Endometrioid adenocarcinomas are usually tan in color and soft in consistency. A good gross description will include an estimate of the depth of invasion into the myometrium as well as involvement of the cervix, uterine serosa, fallopian tubes, or ovaries. These tissues may be involved by direct extension or metastasis.

Histologic Features

Endometrioid adenocarcinomas by definition should resemble, at least focally, proliferative-type endometrium showing tubular glands with smooth luminal surfaces, lined by mitotically active columnar cells (Fig. 1). Based on the degree of glandular differentiation, these tumors are divided into three Federation International Gynecologic Oncologists (FIGO) categories: grade 1 shows ≤ 5% of solid nonglandular growth (Figs. 1–4), grade 2 is defined by finding between 6% and 50% of

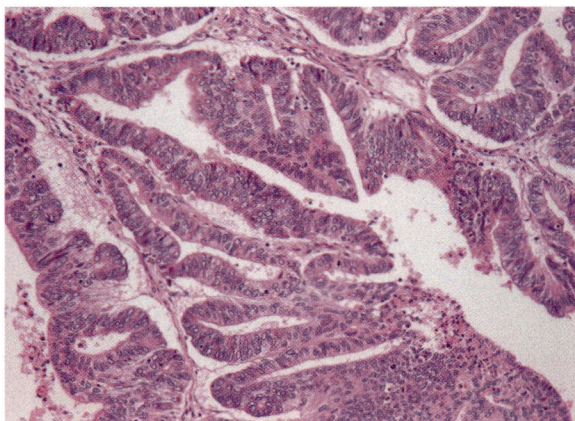

Fig. 1 Endometrioid adenocarcinoma. This typical well-differentiated adenocarcinoma (FIGO grade 1) is composed of well-formed endometrioid glands.

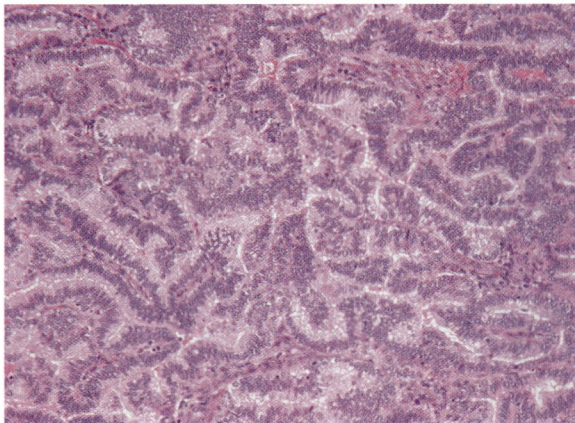

Fig. 2 Endometrioid adenocarcinoma. This well-differentiated adenocarcinoma (FIGO grade 1) features a highly complex proliferation of fused and branched glands that excludes endometrial stroma.

Fig. 3 Endometrioid
adenocarcinoma, well
differentiated (FIGO grade 1),
displaying papillary
architecture. Note the smooth
luminal contours and
low-grade cytologic
appearance of the tumor
cells.

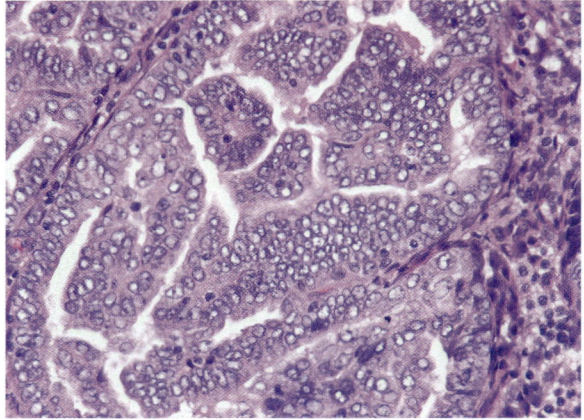

Fig. 4 Endometrioid
adenocarcinoma, well
differentiated (FIGO grade 1),
displaying secretory changes
(cytoplasmic clearing). Note
the absence of hobnail change
and the low-grade cytologic
appearance of the tumor cells.

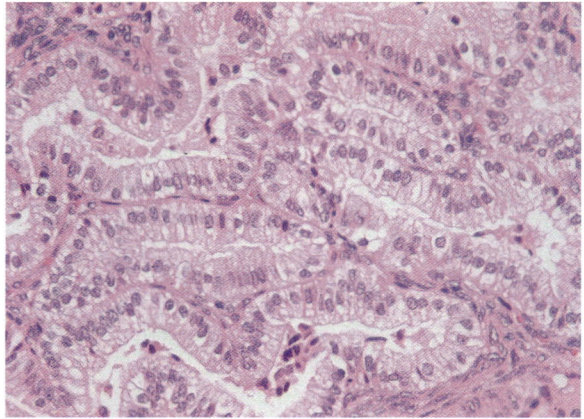

Fig. 5 Endometrioid
adenocarcinoma, poorly
differentiated (FIGO grade 3).
In contrast to FIGO grade 1
tumors, these neoplasms are
predominantly solid.

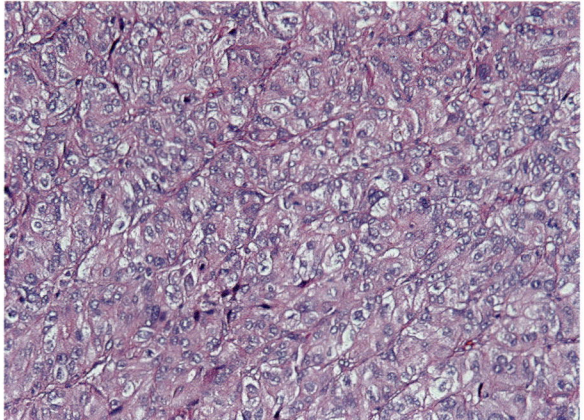

solid non-glandular growth, and grade 3 contains >50% of solid growth (Fig. 5). The presence of marked cytologic atypia increases the grade by one. Solid components showing overt squamous differentiation are not counted as "solid" for the purposes of tumor grading. Histologic features considered typical of endometrioid carcinoma include keratinizing squamous metaplasia or morular metaplasia (nonkeratinizing). Additional features commonly encountered in both nonneoplastic and neoplastic endometrium include tubal and/or mucinous metaplasia, and secretory/clear cell change (with subnuclear or supranuclear cytoplasmic vacuoles) (Fig. 4).

Differential Diagnosis

The differential diagnosis of uterine endometrioid adenocarcinoma includes other uterine carcinomas such as serous and clear cell carcinomas. Strategies for distinguishing between these entities are summarized in Table 1. Other common problems in diagnosis involve the distinction of complex atypical hyperplasia from endometrioid adenocarcinoma (Table 2), endocervical from endometrial adenocarcinoma (Table 3), and carcinosarcoma from endometrioid adenocarcinoma, which will be discussed subsequently in this chapter.

Table 1. Histologic and immunohistochemical summary useful in the differential diagnosis of endometrial carcinoma subtypes

Endometrioid adenocarcinoma:
  Endometrial hyperplasia
  Squamous, morular, mucinous metaplasia
  Smooth luminal contours
  ER, PR, vimentin positive; p53, p16, CEA negative (FIGO grades 1 and 2)

Serous carcinoma:
  No squamous, morular, mucinous metaplasia
  Jagged luminal contours
  Slit-like spaces
  Cytologic pleomorphism
  p53 overexpression, p16 and vimentin positive; ER, PR, CEA negative or weakly positive

Clear cell carcinoma:
  Hobnail cells
  Hyaline stroma
  Cytologic pleomorphism
  Vimentin positive; ER, PR, CEA negative or weakly positive; variable p16 and p53 positivity

Table 2. Features favoring adenocarcinoma over complex atypical hyperplasia

Extensive papillary architecture
Extensive gland fusion with exclusion of endometrial stroma
Extensive macroglands with internal complexity and exclusion of endometrial stroma
Marked cytologic atypia

Table 3. Endometrioid endometrial adenocarcinoma versus endocervical adenocarcinoma[a]

Endometrial adenocarcinoma:

Postmenopausal patient
Imaging and clinical examination favor corpus primary
More tissue in endometrial than in endocervical curettage
Endometrial hyperplasia
Stromal foam cells
Squamous metaplasia
Expression of ER, PR, and vimentin

Endocervical adenocarcinoma:

Pre- or perimenopausal patient
Imaging and clinical examination favor cervical primary
History of abnormal pap smears
More tissue in endocervical than in endometrial curettage
Endocervical adenocarcinoma in situ or squamous dysplasia
Large, elongated, pseudostratified darkly stained nuclei
Abundant mitotic activity, including forms toward the apical portion of the cells
Abundant apoptotic bodies
Diffuse expression of CEA and p16

[a]The phenotypes described pertain only to FIGO grades 1 and 2 endometrioid adenocarcinoma and endocervical adenocarcinoma of the usual type. These guidelines do *not* pertain to high-grade endometrial carcinomas (FIGO grade 3 endometrioid, serous, and clear cell) and unusual types of endocervical adenocarcinomas (adenoma malignum, intestinal mucinous, clear cell, mesonephric, and serous carcinoma).

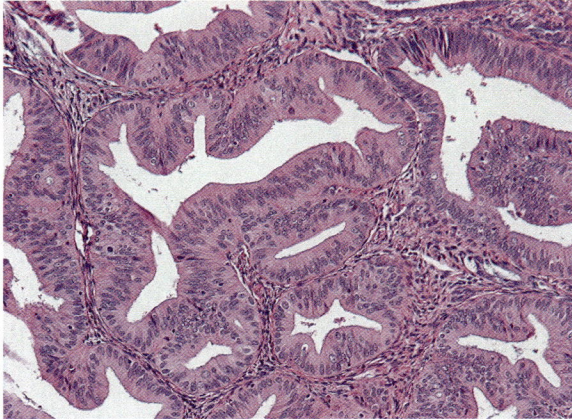

Fig. 6 Complex atypical hyperplasia. Note the preserved endometrial stroma between abnormal endometrioid glands.

Since complex atypical hyperplasia and well-differentiated (FIGO grade 1) endometrial endometrioid carcinoma are both differentiated neoplasms, endometrioid tubular glands generally predominate in both. Conceptually, hyperplasia is separated from adenocarcinoma by the absence of endometrial stromal invasion (Fig. 6) (2–4). Squamous metaplasia may be seen in both (Fig. 7). In practice, the

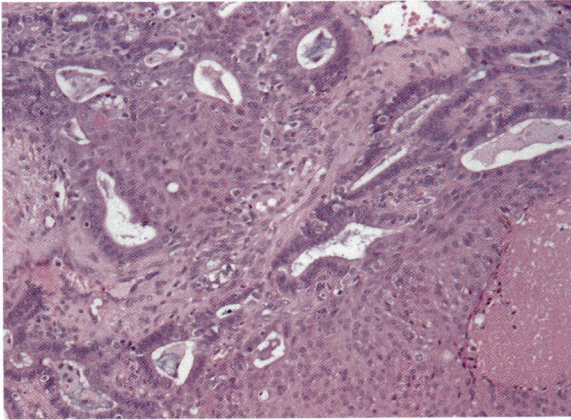

Fig. 7 Complex atypical hyperplasia exhibiting squamous metaplasia. Squamous metaplasia is typical of neoplastic endometrioid proliferations, either hyperplasia or carcinoma

presence of extensive confluent papillary growth, macroglands, and cribriform architecture is sufficient to categorize a lesion as adenocarcinoma (2–4). Marked cytologic atypia also disqualifies the diagnosis of hyperplasia (3). Another challenge concerns the differential diagnosis with endocervical adenocarcinoma. The latter may demonstrate features that resemble those of endometrial endometrioid adenocarcinoma, but there are usually subtle histologic differences. Clinical presentation, precursor lesions (endocervical adenocarcinoma in situ versus endometrial hyperplasia), and immunophenotype differ and can be used to establish the correct diagnosis (Table 3).

Related Carcinomas

As mentioned earlier, endometrioid adenocarcinomas can demonstrate mucinous differentiation and can contain ciliated cells and cells with secretory features. When mucinous differentiation predominates (intracytoplasmic but not luminal mucin; present in > 50% of cells), the tumor is referred to as "mucinous carcinoma" (5, 6). Likewise, "ciliated carcinoma" (7) and "secretory carcinoma" (8) have been described but are rare. Endometrioid adenocarcinomas may also feature papillary architecture. The tumor is referred to as "villoglandular carcinoma" (9) when the papillae are long, slender with delicate fibrovascular cores, and lined by pseudostratified columnar cells perpendicular to the basement membrane. Other findings that can be seen in endometrioid adenocarcinomas include psammomatous calcifications (10), cells with clear cytoplasm, spindled cells (10), trabeculae resembling sex cord ovarian tumors (10), hyalinized and myxoid stroma (10), and, exceptionally, heterologous elements (11) such as osteoid and lobules of cartilage.

Immunophenotype

The immunophenotype of endometrioid carcinoma tends to vary with degrees and types of differentiation. In general, endometrioid adenocarcinomas coexpress pan-cytokeratin and vimentin (12, 13) and they rarely show diffuse cytoplasmic staining with carcinoembryonic antigen (CEA) (14, 15, 16). Almost all endometrioid neoplasms express CK7 and are largely negative for CK20 (17, 18). Other commonly expressed antigens include CA125 (19), BerEP4 (20), and B72.3 (21). The expression of estrogen and progesterone receptors (ER, PR) is ubiquitous among FIGO grade 1 adenocarcinomas, but this feature is present in < 50% of FIGO grade 3 tumors (22, 23). Overexpression of p53 (expression in > 50–75% of nuclei) is seen in about one-third of FIGO grade 3 adenocarcinomas, but almost never in FIGO grade 1 tumors (24, 25). The expression of p16 also tends to accumulate with increasing histological grade (22). High molecular weight cytokeratins, p63, and nuclear β-catenin are preferentially expressed in areas demonstrating squamous differentiation (26, 27).

Serous Carcinoma

Pure serous carcinomas comprise about 10% of endometrial cancers. They are epidemiologically, biologically, histologically, and clinically distinct. The mean age of women with serous carcinoma is approximately one decade older than women with endometrioid adenocarcinoma. Instead of being related to hyperestrinism, serous carcinomas arise in the setting of atrophy and, as such, correspond to Bokhman's type II endometrial cancers (1). Other associations with serous carcinoma include a personal history of breast cancer (28, 29), treatment with tamoxifen (30, 31), and pelvic radiation therapy (32, 33). Serous carcinomas are aggressive neoplasms that have a tendency to present at high stage (34, 35).

Gross Features

Uteri harboring serous carcinomas tend to be small and lack the endometrial thickening that is more characteristic of endometrioid adenocarcinomas. Instead, many serous carcinoma uteri contain endometrial polyps. When carcinomas are confined to the polyp, the tumor itself may not be grossly apparent. More advanced tumors frequently demonstrate obvious myometrial permeation and either extension or metastasis to tissues included in the resection specimen. Uterine serous carcinomas have a predilection for peritoneal dissemination, just like ovarian serous carcinomas.

Histologic Features

The term "serous" refers to shared characteristics with cells lining the fallopian tube, particularly the tumor cells' columnar shape, eosinophilic cytoplasm and

Fig. 8 Serous carcinoma. Typical low-power appearance demonstrating papillary architecture and slit-like spaces.

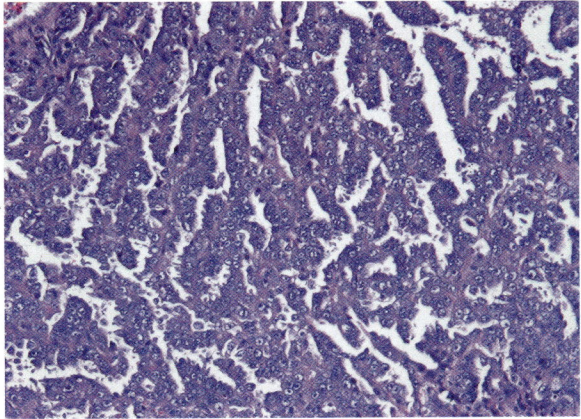

Fig. 9 Serous carcinoma. This high power shows the ragged luminal profiles and highly atypical nuclei.

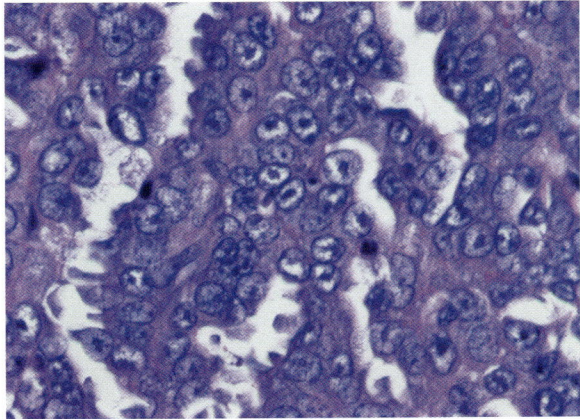

tendency to form papillae (Fig. 8). However, not all serous carcinomas are papillary and not all papillary carcinomas are serous. Essentially, all serous carcinomas exhibit marked nuclear pleomorphism and most demonstrate discrepancies between architectural differentiation and cytologic features. Serous carcinoma cells have high nuclear to cytoplasmic ratios with enlarged nuclei that tend to be irregularly shaped. They may be hyperchromatic or contain large, red macronucleoli (Fig. 9). Brisk mitotic activity and atypical mitoses are common. In contrast to endometrioid carcinoma, the luminal surfaces are irregular and jagged (Fig. 8), the cells are less cohesive with frequent cellular tufting, and detached small cell aggregates. Unlike endometrioid adenocarcinomas, serous carcinomas do not show squamous or mucinous metaplasia, or ciliated cells.

The earliest serous carcinomas may consist solely of neoplastic epithelium colonizing preexisting atrophic endometrium, particularly on the surface of endometrial polyps (36, 37). This has been referred to as intraepithelial serous carcinoma or endometrial intraepithelial carcinoma (36, 37). Importantly, intraepithelial serous carcinoma can metastasize despite the absence of myometual invasion. At low power, these minimal carcinomas appear hyperchromatic and display abrupt transition with the nonneoplastic epithelium. Serous carcinomas may be difficult to diagnose when they replace atrophic endometrial glands and papillary architecture is not apparent (38). Correct classification as serous carcinoma centers on appreciation of the cytologic features, jagged luminal profiles, absence of confirmatory endometrioid characteristics (including squamous and mucinous metaplasia), and background atrophy. Architectural patterns encountered in established serous carcinomas include papillae, tubular glands, slit-like glands, and solid nests and sheets. Since these patterns are not specific for serous carcinoma, attention directed to the cytologic characteristics is essential to make the correct diagnosis.

Immunophenotype

Like endometrioid adenocarcinomas, serous carcinomas coexpress pan-cytokeratins and vimentin and rarely express diffuse cytoplasmic CEA. They also express CK7, CA125, BerEP4, and B72.3 and are largely negative for CK20. The expression of ER and PR is less common than in endometrioid adenocarcinomas and is found in < 50% of cases (22, 23, 39). Overexpression of p53 (expression in > 50–75% of nuclei) is seen in nearly 90% of serous carcinomas and is related to the near universal presence of *p53* mutations (25, 40). p16 expression is also very common (22).

Clear Cell Carcinoma

Clear cell carcinoma is the third most common endometrial carcinoma subtype, even though it represents < 5% of cases. The epidemiologic features of patients with clear cell carcinoma are obscure because of this tumor's rarity, difficulties in diagnostic reproducibility, and accumulating evidence that there are perhaps several subtypes of clear cell carcinoma. The subtypes include 1) tumors admixed with endometrioid adenocarcinoma; 2) those mixed with or histologically resembling serous carcinoma, and 3) pure clear cell carcinoma (41, 42). There are emerging data that suggest that clear cell carcinomas might be overrepresented in patients with hereditary nonpolyposis colorectal cancer syndrome (43).

Gross Features

There are no gross features that are distinctive of clear cell carcinoma. Tumors combined with endometrioid adenocarcinomas may be associated with a thickened endometrium. Pure clear cell carcinomas as well as those mixed with serous carcinomas are often associated with endometrial polyps and deep myometrial invasion.

Histologic Features

Most clear cell carcinomas are composed of cells with clear cytoplasm, but this feature is not restricted to this subtype of endometrial cancer (*see* "Discussion" of endometrioid adenocarcinomas). Furthermore, some clear cell carcinomas may contain cells with eosinophilic cytoplasm. As with other endometrial carcinoma subtypes, the combination of the low-power architectural features and cytologic characteristics permits a diagnosis of clear cell carcinoma. These tumors classically demonstrate varied architectural patterns that include papillary, tubular, tubulocystic, solid, and mixtures thereof. The papillae of clear cell carcinoma are small and round in comparison to those of either serous carcinoma or villoglandular endometrioid adenocarcinomas. Characteristically, the stroma of the papillae is densely hyalinized (Fig. 10). The lining epithelium is only one or two cells thick, without prominent tufting. The cells are large, generally contain ample clear cytoplasm filled with glycogen, and show sharply defined cytoplasmic boundaries. Hobnail cells may be seen lining papillae or glands. The nuclei are large and pleomorphic with prominent macronucleoli (Fig. 10). Like serous carcinoma, clear cell carcinoma usually arises in the setting of atrophic endometrium and in endometrial polyps (36).

Immunophenotype

Most clear cell carcinomas coexpress pan-cytokeratins and vimentin and rarely show diffuse cytoplasmic CEA positivity. They also express CK7 and are largely negative for CK20. Data regarding expression of ER, PR, and p53 are contradictory, while results of p16 expression in clear cell carcinoma are now just emerging. ER and PR

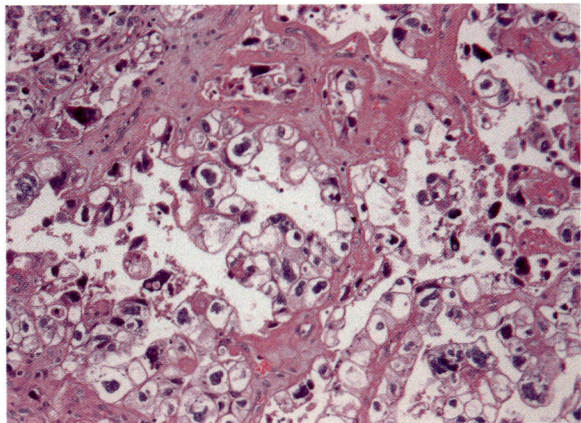

Fig. 10 Clear cell carcinoma. The tumor cells have cytoplasmic clearing, hobnail features, striking cytologic atypia, and hyalinized stroma is seen.

expression is uncommon and, when present, is weak and focal (22, 42, 44). p53
overexpression can be seen, but the rate (approximately at the 50% level) is significantly less than in serous carcinoma (41, 42, 44). The degree of ER, PR, and p53
expression might be related to an individual tumor's pathogenesis (41, 42, 44). For
example, clear cell carcinomas associated with endometrioid adenocarcinomas
might preferentially express ER and PR, while those resembling or associated with
serous carcinomas might overexpress p53. p16 expression is also commonly found
in clear cell carcinomas, being more common than in endometrioid adenocarcinomas but less frequent than in serous carcinomas (22).

Mixed (Mixed Epithelial) Carcinomas

With only one exception (mucinous carcinoma), mixed epithelial carcinomas are
diagnosed when at least two endometrial carcinoma subtypes are present and the
minor component (s) constitute at least 10% of the tumor. As mucinous differentiation is so commonly encountered in endometrioid adenocarcinomas, there is a
requirement for 50% mucinous differentiation before diagnosing a mixed mucinous and endometrioid adenocarcinoma. The term "mixed carcinoma" should not
be used for tumors that contain areas with subtle differences. For example, a
serous carcinoma with glandular architecture should not be considered a mixed
serous and endometrioid adenocarcinoma unless two distinctive morphologies
are present.

Squamous Cell Carcinoma

Primary squamous cell carcinoma of the endometrium is very rare and should only
be diagnosed in the absence of hyperplasia or any endometrioid glandular differentiation (45). They are histologically similar to squamous cell carcinomas of the
cervix and most are cytologically high grade. Extension from a cervical squamous
carcinoma or a history of a previous cervical squamous cell carcinoma excludes a
diagnosis of primary squamous carcinoma of the endometrium.

Transitional Cell Carcinoma

This extraordinarily rare tumor is by definition composed of cells resembling those
of urothelial transitional cell carcinoma (46, 47). The architecture is papillary, just
like the urothelial counterparts. Extension and metastasis from an urothelial primary carcinoma should always be excluded. These tumors can occur in pure form
or be mixed with other carcinoma subtypes.

Small Cell Carcinoma

The histologic appearance of this tumor is essentially identical to that of small cell neuroendocrine carcinomas of other organs (48). These tumors can occur in pure form or be mixed with other carcinoma subtypes.

Undifferentiated Carcinoma

Undifferentiated carcinomas by definition lack any evidence of differentiation. As such, their appearance may simulate high-grade sarcoma, lymphoma, melanoma, and metastases to the uterus. Universal, but frequently only focal expression of cytokeratins and epithelial membrane antigen (EMA) is seen (48, 49).

Uterine Sarcomas and Mixed Müllerian Tumors

Leiomyosarcoma

Uterine leiomyosarcoma constitutes 1% of all uterine malignancies, it is the most common uterine sarcoma, and represents approximately 40% of all uterine sarcomas, and 40% of leiomyosarcomas among women at all sites (50) (Table 4). The incidence of uterine leiomyosarcoma is approximately 0.67/100,000 women per year (51). Even though uterine leiomyomas are the most common tumor of the female genital tract, the incidence of leiomyosarcoma originating from leiomyoma is very low, ranging between 0.13 and 0.80 (52). As occurs with leiomyomas, uterine leiomyosarcomas are more frequent among black women (50). There is at least one familial cancer syndrome characterized by retinoblastoma, hereditary leiomyomatosis, and renal cell cancer which has an increased incidence of uterine leiomyosarcoma (53).

Table 4. Classification of malignant mesenchymal tumors of the uterus

Leiomyosarcoma
    Spindled
    Epithelioid
    Myxoid
Perivascular epithelioid tumor (PEComa) [a]
Low-grade endometrial stromal sarcoma
Undifferentiated endometrial sarcoma
Low-grade müllerian adenosarcoma
Malignant mixed müllerian tumor
Others

[a]Not all tumors in this category behave in a malignant fashion

Gross Features

Leiomyosarcoma occurs most commonly as a single nodule in almost 90% of cases and if multiple nodules are present in the uterus, it is usually the largest nodule (54, 55). Leiomyosarcoma typically forms an intramyometrial mass with either well-circumscribed or irregular infiltrative growth into the surrounding myometrium. On sectioning, the tumors appear fleshy, gray to pink, and are frequently associated with areas of hemorrhage and necrosis (54, 56). If the tumor has a prominent gelatinous appearance, it should raise suspicion for a myxoid leiomyosarcoma (56).

Histologic Features

The diagnosis of malignancy in a smooth muscle tumor is based on three histologic features: 1) tumor cell necrosis; 2) moderate to severe cytologic atypia; and 3) mitotic activity (57). Tumor cell necrosis is defined by the finding of an abrupt transition between the nonviable and viable tumor. The viable tumor frequently grows around vessels (perivascular distribution). Pleomorphic cells may still be identified in viable and devitalized areas. In most cases, tumor cell necrosis is accompanied by tumor cells showing increased mitotic activity and marked cellular atypia. Moderate to severe cytologic atypia is defined by cellular pleomorphism, nuclear enlargement and/or irregular outlines, hyperchromatism, as well as prominent nucleolus. Cytologic atypia should be identified at medium power (10×). Finally, counting mitotic activity in smooth muscle tumors may be difficult but it is important not to misinterpret apoptotic cells as mitotic figures. Apoptotic cells are typically characterized by refractile dense eosinophilic cytoplasm and coarse clumped chromatin, which contrasts with the delicate and thin appearance of the dividing chromatin. Even though mitotic activity had been considered the most important criterion to establish a diagnosis of malignancy in a smooth muscle tumor, it has been demonstrated that mitotic activity in the absence of one of the other two histologic features previously described is insufficient to establish the diagnosis of leiomyosarcoma. Furthermore, it is important to keep in mind that the threshold for mitotic activity is higher in smooth muscle tumors of the uterus than that used in soft tissue tumors (58). This is due to the mitogenic effect of estrogen and progesterone on gynecologic tumors and in particular on spindle cell smooth muscle tumors of the uterus.

Leiomyosarcomas can be classified into grade I, II, and III or low and high grade based on the degree of cellular differentiation, mitotic activity, and tumor cell necrosis, but this classification is subjective. A tumor showing marked cytologic atypia associated with brisk mitotic activity and tumor cell necrosis is classified as high grade while a tumor that at low-power displays mild cytologic atypia but has brisk mitotic activity and focal tumor necrosis can be classified as low-grade or grade I leiomyosarcoma. Most malignant smooth muscle tumors are high-grade.

Leiomyosarcomas are divided into three main categories depending on their morphologic appearance: (a) spindled, (b) epithelioid, and (c) myxoid; and not

Fig. 11 Spindle cell leiomyosarcoma. The neoplastic cells form intersecting fascicles and display pleomorphic and hyperchromatic nuclei.

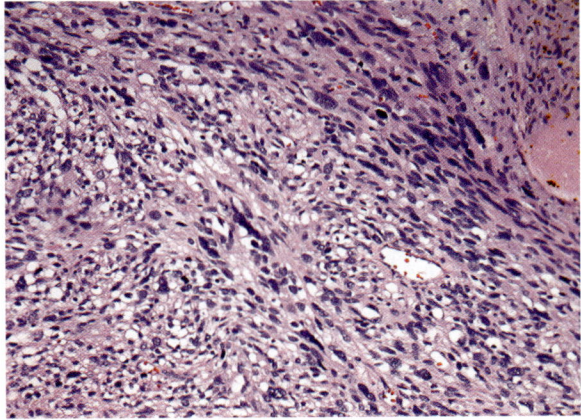

Fig. 12 Spindle cell leiomyosarcoma. The tumor cells grow around vessels and there is an abrupt transition from viable to nonviable tumor (tumor cell necrosis).

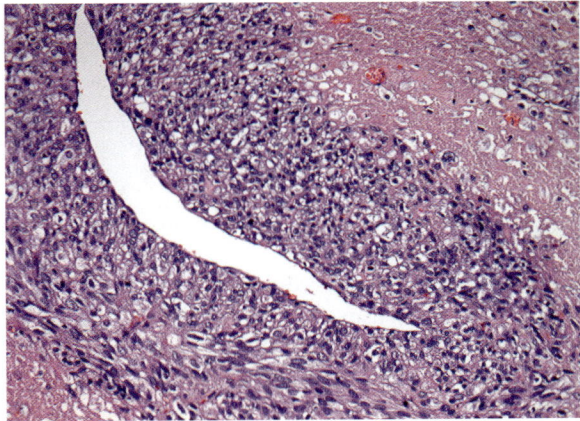

infrequently, they show more than one component. Rarely, leiomyosarcomas can contain xanthomatous or giant cells.

1. Spindle cell leiomyosarcoma is composed of fusiform cells showing central elongated nuclei with blunted ends occasionally indented by a clear vacuole (Fig. 11). The cytoplasm is deeply eosinophilic due to the presence of myofilaments that are disposed parallel to the cell axis (best seen in a Masson trichrome stain). The cells form long well-oriented intersecting fascicles (59). The combination of any two of the following three features establishes the diagnosis of spindled leiomyosarcoma: diffuse moderate to severe atypia, >10 mitoses/10 high-power fields (HPFs), and tumor cell necrosis (Fig. 12; Table 5) (58). Vascular invasion is detected in approximately 20% of leiomyosarcomas and some tumors may have a prominent intravascular growth (60, 61).

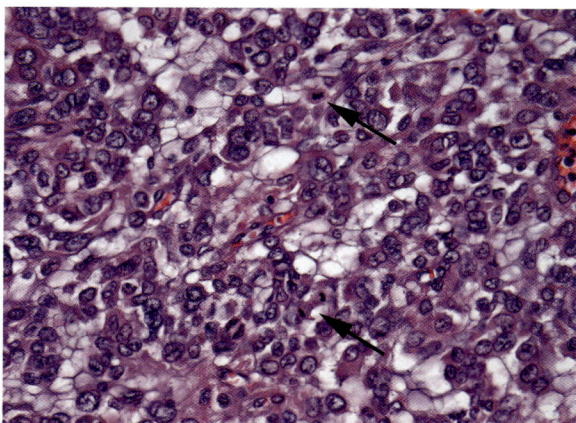

Fig. 13 Epithelioid leiomyosarcoma. The tumor cells grow in sheets. They have abundant eosinophilic cytoplasm, focal moderate nuclear atypia and mitoses are easy to identify (*arrows*).

Table 5. Diagnostic criteria for the different subtypes of leiomyosarcoma

	Cytologic atypia		Tumor cell necrosis		Mitoses
Spindled	+	and/or	+	and/or	>10/10HPFs[a]
Epithelioid	+	and/or	+	or	>4/10HPFs
Myxoid	+	or	+	or	≥2/10HPFs

[a]In spindled leiomyosarcomas, two of the three features need to be present

2. Epithelioid leiomyosarcoma is composed of sheets, nests, or cords of cells with abundant cytoplasm. To establish the diagnosis of epithelioid leiomyosarcoma, at least 50% of the cells should display epithelioid features. The cells show a centrally located round nucleus and eosinophilic cytoplasm (Fig. 13) but in up to 25% of the tumors, the cytoplasm is clear. Variable amounts of collagen deposition may be seen. The criteria to establish the diagnosis of malignancy in epithelioid smooth muscle tumors are not well established. However, as a general rule, the diagnosis of epithelioid leiomyosarcoma is warranted when there are ≥5 mitoses/10 HPFs and diffuse moderate to severe cytologic atypia or tumor cell necrosis (Table 5) (62, 63, 64, 65).

3. Myxoid leiomyosarcoma is a rare variant of uterine leiomyosarcoma. It is characterized by the presence of abundant myxoid matrix that is positive for Alcian Blue or colloidal iron histochemical stains. The tumors are typically hypocellular in contrast to most spindled and epithelioid leiomyosarcomas. Most tumors show infiltrative growth into the surrounding myometrium (Fig. 14a). At higher magnification, the degree of cytologic atypia and mitotic activity is quite variable (66–69). The diagnosis of myxoid leiomyosarcoma is made when either marked cytologic atypia or tumor cell necrosis is identified. In their absence, the finding of ≥ 2 mitoses/10 HPFs separates myxoid leiomyosarcoma from myxoid leiomyoma (Fig. 14b; Table 5) (70).

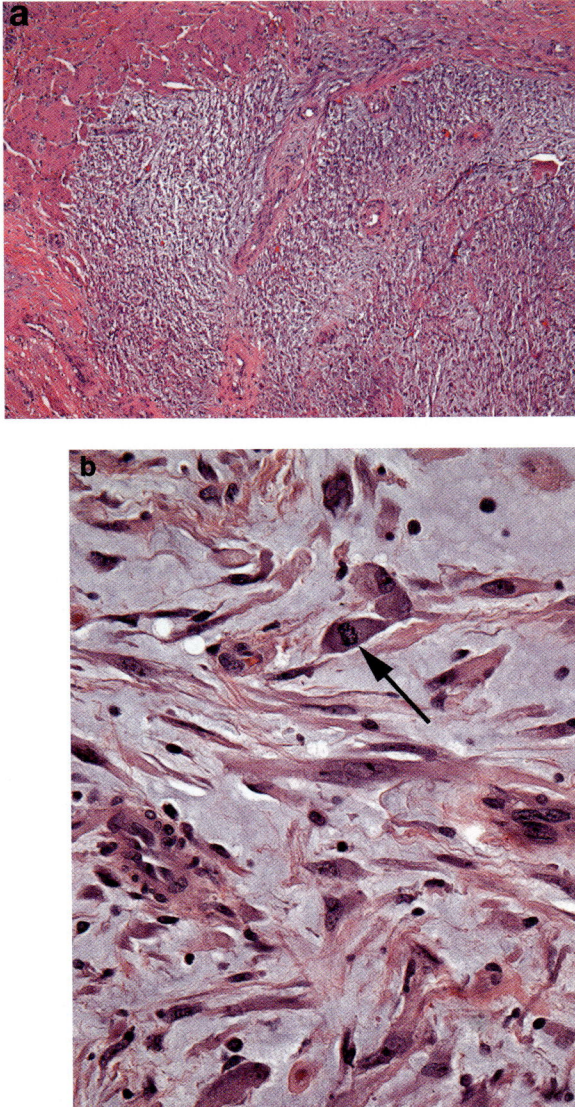

Fig. 14 Myxoid leiomyosarcoma. The tumor has an infiltrative margin and it is hypocellular with a prominent myxoid background (**a**). At higher magnification, the cells show nuclear pleomorphism and mitotic activity (*arrow*) (**b**).

Immunophenotype

Leiomyosarcomas are typically positive for actin, desmin, and h-caldesmon. They also frequently express CD10, oxytocin, ER, PR, and androgen receptor (71). Epithelioid leiomyosarcomas frequently express keratin and EMA, and both epithelioid and myxoid leiomyosarcomas are less frequently positive for smooth muscle markers. Leiomyosarcomas display p53 and c-kit positivity; however, no associated c-kit mutations have been reported (72, 73, 74).

Differential Diagnosis

Spindle cell leiomyosarcoma should be distinguished from leiomyoma variants including mitotically active leiomyoma, apoplectic leiomyoma, and leiomyoma with bizarre nuclei. Mitotically active leiomyoma displays brisk mitotic activity; however, it lacks cytologic atypia and tumor cell necrosis (75, 76, 77). Leiomyoma with apoplectic change may show areas of hypercellularity associated with slight cytologic atypia and brisk mitotic activity surrounding the areas of hemorrhage, thus causing concern for malignancy. However, away from these areas, the tumor has the appearance of a conventional leiomyoma (78, 79). Finally, worrisome features associated with leiomyoma with bizarre nuclei include the presence of mono- or multinucleated cells which may show prominent nuclei, nuclear pseudoinclusions, karyorrhectic nuclei (that may mimic atypical mitotic figures), and some degree of mitotic activity. It is important to notice that in most cases, the bizarre cells have a patchy distribution in the tumor, mitotic activity is low, and there is no tumor cell necrosis (80). Rare malignant tumors in the differential diagnosis include spindle cell rhabdomyosarcoma and undifferentiated endometrial sarcoma. The former may be very difficult to distinguish from a spindle cell leiomyosarcoma. The finding of cytoplasmic cross striations and positivity for skeletal muscle markers (myoglobin, myoD1 and myogenin) are helpful in this differential diagnosis. Undifferentiated endometrial sarcoma is a diagnosis of exclusion based on histologic and immunohistochemical findings (59).

Epithelioid leiomyosarcoma should be distinguished from a poorly differentiated carcinoma, trophoblastic tumors (placental site trophoblastic tumor and epithelioid trophoblastic tumor) (81), PEComa (discussed below) (82), uterine tumor resembling an ovarian sex-cord stromal tumor (83–85), the rare alveolar soft part sarcoma (86, 87), and metastatic melanoma (88). In order to establish the correct diagnosis, it is important to consider the patient's clinical history and to sample the tumor extensively. In difficult cases, the use of a battery of immunohistochemical markers including those for epithelial, smooth muscle, sex cord, and intermediate trophoblast differentiation may be helpful.

Myxoid leiomyosarcoma must be distinguished from its benign counterpart, the myxoid leiomyoma. This is an extremely rare tumor that typically shows well-circumscribed margins, no cytologic atypia, absent tumor cell necrosis, and mitotic counts < 2/10 HPFs (70). Leiomyoma with hydropic change may also be considered in the differential diagnosis of a myxoid leiomyosarcoma; however, the background matrix is composed of edema fluid which is Alcian Blue and colloidal iron negative (89).

Low-Grade Endometrial Stromal Sarcoma

Endometrial stromal neoplasms are divided into two main groups: (a) endometrial stromal nodule and (b) low-grade endometrial stromal sarcoma. Low-grade endometrial stromal sarcoma accounts for approximately 80% of all stromal neoplasms and it represents the second most common pure uterine sarcoma of the homologous type following leiomyosarcoma. The old term, high-grade endometrial stromal sarcoma, has been replaced in the most recent WHO classification with undifferentiated stromal sarcoma, as in contrast to low-grade endometrial endometrial stromal sarcoma, it is associated with a very poor prognosis and shows no resemblance to endometrial stroma (59).

Gross Features

Low-grade endometrial stromal sarcomas commonly appear as multiple coalescent tan to yellow soft nodules involving the endometrium and myometrium. The tumors typically show a permeative growth into the myometrial wall and myometrial veins and, not infrequently, may be identified grossly, outside the uterus in parametrial veins. They may show areas of necrosis and hemorrhage (90).

Histologic Features

These tumors infiltrate the myometrium as irregular islands without any associated stromal response (Fig. 15). The tumor cells are small, uniform with scant cytoplasm, and round to oval nuclei and indistinct nucleoli. The tumor cells may whorl around the vessels, which are small and reminiscent of endometrial-type arterioles (Fig. 16). Histiocytes, single or in groups, collagen plaques, and cholesterol clefts

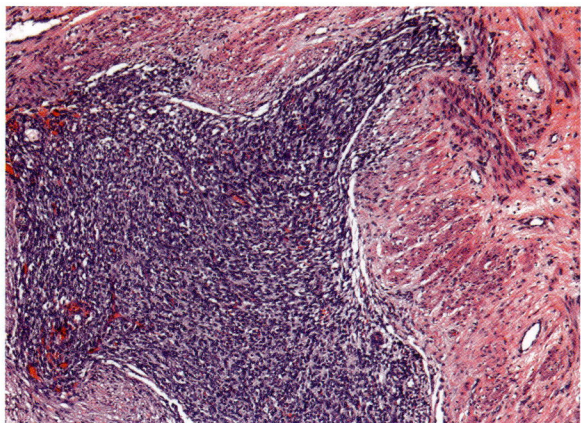

Fig. 15 Low-grade endometrial stromal sarcoma. The tumor is hypercellular and infiltrates the myometrium as irregular tongues.

Fig. 16 Low-grade endometrial stromal sarcoma. The tumor cells are small and uniform and focally whorl around arterioles.

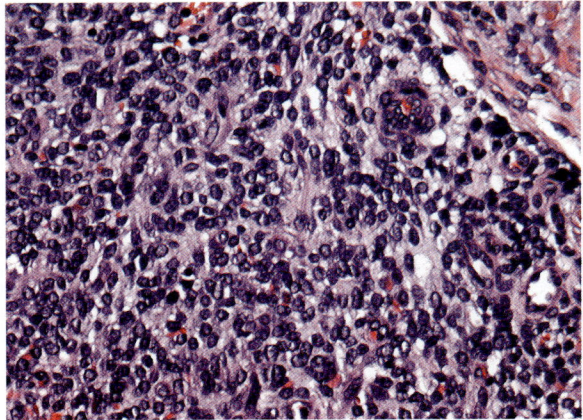

are common associated findings (91). Low-grade endometrial stromal sarcomas may show morphologic variations or unusual features including smooth muscle (92), skeletal muscle (93) or adipose differentiation (93), fibrous and/or myxoid background (94, 95), endometrioid glandular (96, 97) and sex cord-like differentiation (98), cells with granular eosinophilic or clear cytoplasm (99, 100), cells with a rhabdoid phenotype (101), and finally, cells with bizarre nuclei (93).

To establish the diagnosis of low-grade endometrial stromal sarcoma, the tumor must resemble proliferative-type endometrial stroma regardless of the mitotic index. The diagnosis of high-grade endometrial stromal sarcoma should only be made when a tumor with high-grade cytologic atypia or undifferentiated appearance arises in the context of a low-grade endometrial stromal sarcoma (59).

Immunophenotype

The neoplastic endometrial stromal cells are typically immunoreactive for vimentin, muscle-specific and smooth muscle actin, keratin, and CD10 (102–104). However, it is important to note that positive CD10 staining can be seen in other uterine tumors. Some degree of positivity for desmin and caldesmon may be seen particularly if the tumor shows smooth muscle differentiation (103–108). Areas of sex cord-like differentiation may be positive for inhibin, calretinin, CD99, WT1, and Melan A as well as demonstrate positivity for epithelial and smooth muscle markers (84, 109, 110). Areas of rhabdomyoblastic differentiation are positive for myoD1, myoglobin, and myogenin (93). C-kit has been reported to be positive in low-grade endometrial stromal sarcomas; however, no associated mutations have been noted (111). Some low-grade endometrial stromal sarcomas may show aromatase expression which may be used for therapeutic purposes (112).

Differential Diagnosis

The main entities in the differential diagnosis of low-grade endometrial stromal sarcomas include endometrial stromal nodule and highly cellular leiomyoma. An endometrial stromal nodule shares the same cytologic features described in low-grade endometrial stromal sarcoma. The main difference is the finding of a well-defined tumor–myometrium interface. Focal irregularities in the form of small finger-like projections or small islands not exceeding 3 mm are allowed; however, no vascular invasion should be seen (113). It is important to extensively sample the tumor–myometrium interface in order to identify subtle permeation into the myometrium that may escape the naked eye (113). Clinicians should be made aware that the pathologist cannot distinguish between an endometrial stromal nodule and a low-grade endometrial stromal sarcoma in a curettage specimen in most instances, as it is not possible to assess the entire margin, which is the most important feature in this differential diagnosis. The other important differential diagnosis is with a highly cellular leiomyoma. This benign smooth muscle tumor is characterized by dense uniform cellularity, prominent vascularity, and sometimes a pseudoinfiltrative growth into the surrounding myometrium, features that overlap with those described in endometrial stromal tumors. However, the tumor cells frequently form fascicles, the vessels are typically large with thick walls, and there is transition from the tumor to the myometrium, features that are lacking in a low-grade endometrial stromal sarcoma. The distinction is important, as it has prognostic implications, especially in a curettage specimen from a young woman. If the diagnosis is that of highly cellular leiomyoma, the patient may retain her uterus, whereas if the diagnosis is that of endometrial stromal neoplasm, the patient requires a hysterectomy in most cases (114). Other neoplastic and nonneoplastic processes that rarely enter into the differential diagnosis include gland poor adenomyosis (115) and cellular intravenous leiomyomatosis (116). When low-grade endometrial stromal sarcomas show unusual features, the differential diagnosis is broader including endometrioid adenomyoma (if there is prominent smooth muscle differentiation) (117), myxoid smooth muscle tumor (if there is prominent myxoid change) (91), uterine tumor resembling an ovarian sex cord tumor (if there is prominent sex cord-like differentiation) (83), and finally, adenomyosis and low-grade müllerian adenosarcoma (if there is glandular differentiation) (118).

Undifferentiated Endometrial Sarcoma

This is a high-grade sarcoma without specific histologic features. This diagnosis should only be made after poorly differentiated carcinoma, leiomyosarcoma, rhabdomyosarcoma, adenosarcoma with sarcomatous overgrowth, and malignant mixed müllerian tumor have been excluded by extensive sampling, careful histologic examination, and use of immunohistochemical stains if needed (59).

Table 6. Mixed müllerian tumors of the uterus

Müllerian adenofibroma
Low-grade Müllerian adenosarcoma
Homologous
Heterologous
Carcinosarcoma (malignant mixed müllerian tumor)
Homologous
Heterologous
Müllerian adenomyoma
Endometrioid-type
Endocervical-type
Atypical polypoid adenomyoma

As mentioned earlier, a diagnosis of high-grade endometrial stromal sarcoma can be applied only in cases in which a component of low-grade endometrial stromal sarcoma is identified. Otherwise, the diagnosis is that of undifferentiated endometrial sarcoma. This nomenclature conveys the highly aggressive nature of the tumor which contrasts with the much better prognosis associated with a low-grade endometrial stromal sarcoma (59).

Low-grade Müllerian Adenosarcoma

This tumor belongs to the biphasic müllerian category of tumors (Table 6). It is typically composed of benign appearing glands and a low-grade malignant mesenchymal component. It has been reported to represent approximately 7% of all uterine sarcomas in a large series (119). It most commonly affects perimenopausal women and has a similar incidence in white and black women. These tumors have been reported in women receiving tamoxifen therapy or after pelvic radiation therapy (120).

Gross Features

Most low-grade müllerian adenosarcomas appear as large polypoid masses filling the endometrial cavity, but rarely arise in the myometrium. On sectioning, they may be predominantly solid or have a spongy appearance with cysts of different sizes. The cysts are filled with clear fluid or hemorrhage and are separated by variable amounts of tan to brown tissue (118).

Histologic Features

On low-power examination, the key histologic features include the finding of marked condensation of the low-grade malignant stromal component around cystically dilated glands (Fig. 17a) or glands with a phyllodes-type morphology. Also characteristic is the finding of intraluminal protrusions of the neoplastic stroma. The malignant mesenchymal component is a low-grade homologous sarcoma reminiscent of a low-grade endometrial stromal sarcoma or fibrosarcoma in most cases. The greatest degree of cytologic atypia and mitotic activity is seen in the areas of stromal condensation. The glandular component is commonly of endometrioid-type although mucinous or tubal-type epithelium and squamous differentiation may be found. The epithelium is typically benign, but it may on occasion appear atypical. The diagnosis of adenosarcoma is generally established by the finding of >4 mitoses/10 HPFs in the stromal component surrounding the glands. Even though, tumors showing prominent periglandular condensation, stromal atypia, and <4 mitoses/10 HPFs are not uniformly diagnosed as adenosarcoma, tumors with these features frequently recur (118). The mesenchymal component may show bizarre nuclei, foamy histiocytes, smooth muscle, and sex cord-like differentiation (118, 120, 121). Rhabdomyoblastic, cartilaginous, or fatty differentiation is more commonly seen outside the uterine corpus and is present in 10–15% of cases (118, 122). Finally, 10% of these tumors show sarcomatous overgrowth, defined by the presence of pure sarcoma involving approximately 25% of the tumor (Fig. 17b) (123).

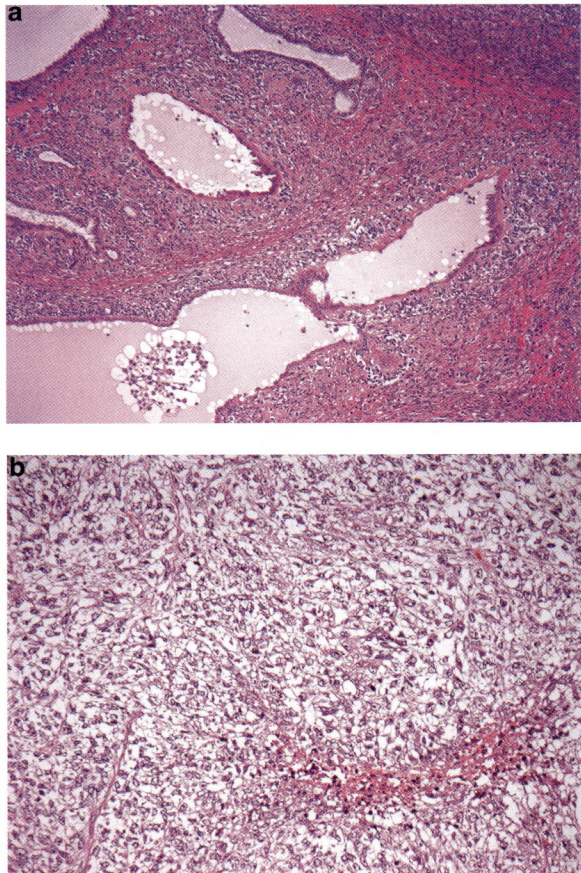

Fig. 17 Low-grade müllerian adenosarcoma. The neoplastic stromal cells condensate around the müllerian-type glands ("collaring") (**a**). Sarcomatous overgrowth. A high-grade sarcoma is associated with focal necrosis and has overgrown areas of conventional low-grade müllerian adenosarcoma (**b**).

In most cases, the sarcomatous overgrowth is composed of a high-grade sarcoma but it has also been reported as a low-grade sarcoma. Sarcomatous overgrowth is associated with destructive invasion of the myometrium not accompanied by glands. This is in contrast to typical low-grade müllerian adenosarcomas which show a low incidence of myometrial invasion with both epithelial and stromal components forming part of the invasive tumor (118).

Immunophenotype

The low-grade malignant stromal component is typically positive for vimentin, WT1, CD10, ER, and PR with variable expression of cytokeratin, muscle actin, and AR. This immunohistochemical profile overlaps with that reported in low-grade endometrial stromal sarcomas. Areas of sarcomatous overgrowth show decreased or absent CD10, ER, and PR expression (124).

Carcinosarcoma (Malignant mixed müllerian tumor)

Even though it represents < 5% of all malignant uterine tumors, this highly malignant mixed tumor was previously considered the most common uterine sarcoma (125). The histogenesis of these tumors has evolved in recent years. It is now widely accepted that carcinosarcomas either arise from a common pluripotential cell with divergent differentiation or that the sarcomatous component develops from the carcinomatous component by a metaplastic process or dedifferentiation (126, 127). These tumors occur typically in postmenopausal women and have a higher incidence in black women (125).

Gross Features

These are typically large, bulky polypoid tumors filling and distending the endometrial cavity. On sectioning, they show a fleshy heterogeneous cut-surface with extensive areas of hemorrhage and necrosis. Deep and destructive infiltration of the myometrium is easily identified in most cases. While most tumors originate in the uterine corpus, approximately 5% arise in the cervix (128–130).

Histologic Features

These tumors are characterized by an intimate admixture of high-grade malignant epithelial and mesenchymal elements. However, in some cases, the two elements do not appear admixed but they are juxtaposed. The high-grade carcinoma is more frequently either of serous or endometrioid type (with or without squamous differentiation) (Fig. 18), although any type of endometrial carcinoma can be seen. If the tumor

Fig. 18 Malignant mixed
müllerian tumor.
The epithelial and
sarcomatous components of
the tumor are intimately
admixed. The sarcomatous
component shows
rhabdomyoblastic
differentiation (*arrows*).

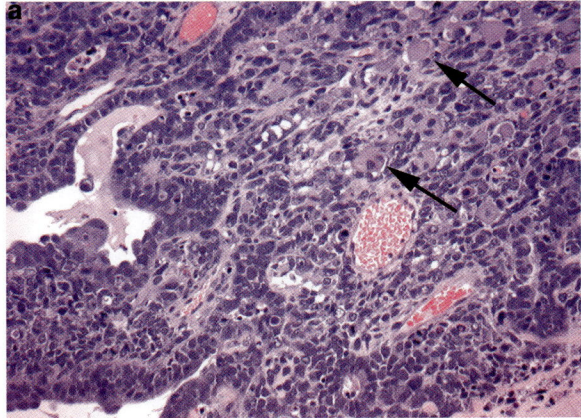

arises in the cervix, the epithelial component is typically squamous and can be found
adjacent to high-grade squamous dysplasia. The high-grade sarcoma is often of the
homologous type, resembling high-grade leiomyosarcoma, malignant fibrous histio-
cytoma, or undifferentiated endometrial sarcoma. Heterologous differentiation
[including in order of frequency rhabdomyosarcoma (Fig. 18), chondrosarcoma,
liposarcoma, and rarely osteosarcoma and neuroectodermal differentiation] is seen in
approximately 50% of cases (129, 131, 132).

Immunophenotype

The high-grade carcinoma typically coexpresses epithelial markers (keratin and
EMA) and vimentin. The high-grade sarcoma is positive for vimentin and frequently
for smooth muscle actin and epithelial markers. This overlapping profile of epithelial
and mesenchymal components supports a common histogenesis. Synaptophysin,
neuron specfic enolase, Leu-7, and CD10 may be expressed in the mesenchymal as
well as in the epithelial components. The rhabdomyosarcomatous component is
positive for myoglobin, myogenin, and MyoD1. p53 is frequently positive in both
components (129, 133, 134).

Perivascular Epithelioid Cell Tumor (PEComa)

These are rare uterine tumors that belong to the family of neoplasms thought to originate from the perivascular epithelioid cell. The latter cell type is defined by the presence of abundant clear to eosinophilic granular cytoplasm, positive staining for
HMB-45, as well as frequent expression of muscle markers (135). Other tumors that
belong to this family include clear cell "sugar" tumors of the lung and pancreas, some
forms of angiomyolipoma, and the clear cell myelomelanocytic tumor of ligamentum

teres/falciform ligament (136–139). These tumors show a particular association with lymphangiomyomatosis as well as tuberous sclerosis (82, 137).

Gross Features

Most tumors are solitary and can be well circumscribed with a white and whorled cut-surface or show poorly defined margins, often with a fleshy and soft, gray-white to tan or yellow cut-surface (82, 140, 141).

Histologic Features

On low-power examination, some tumors have a tongue-like infiltrative growth similar to that seen in a low-grade endometrial stromal sarcoma, while in others, the interface between the tumor and the surrounding tissue is smooth (140). The tumor cells grow in sheets or small nests with scant intervening stroma. The cells have abundant clear or eosinophilic cytoplasm and oval to round nuclei (Fig. 19a). The tumors not infrequently show, at least focally, a fascicular growth and in these areas, the cells have elongated nuclei with an appearance similar to that described in smooth muscle tumors. The degree of nuclear atypia is variable and the mitotic rates are low in most cases (82, 140–142).

Immunophenotype

The tumors are characteristically positive for HMB-45 (Fig. 19b), Melan-A, micro-phthalmia transcription factor (MiTF), and are negative for S-100. They frequently express muscle markers, including smooth muscle actin and desmin, and may be positive for CD10, but they are negative for inhibin and keratin. The coexpression of HMB-45 and muscle markers is highly specific for this tumor (82, 140, 141).

Intravenous Leiomyomatosis

Although this is a rare, histologically benign condition, characterized by a predominant intravascular proliferation of smooth muscle cells, it is included in this chapter because it may pursue an aggressive behavior, growing along the inferior vena cava into the right heart (143–146). As intravenous leiomyomatosis is frequently associated with uterine leiomyomas, a diagnosis of intravenous leiomyomatosis should only be made when the intravascular growth is present beyond the confines or in the absence of a leiomyoma (116). Extrauterine extension is most common within the broad ligament veins (up to 80% of cases) and into the right heart (up to 40% of cases) (116, 146). This condition may occur at any age, but it is more common in middle-aged women.

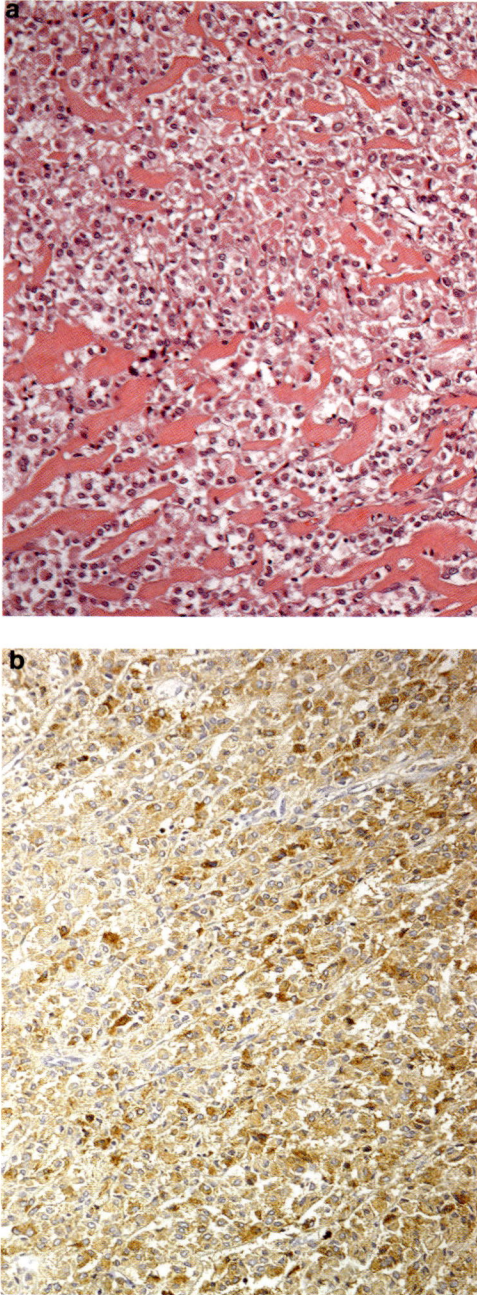

Fig. 19 PEComa. The tumor cells have abundant pale cytoplasm and grow in sheets and cords (**a**) and are diffusely positive for HMB-45 (**b**).

Gross Features

In some occasions, the gross appearance is similar to that seen in a leiomyoma being more often multinodular (147). White to yellow and firm to soft worm-like plugs of tumor may be seen filling and distending the myometrial veins, sometimes with extrauterine extension; however, not infrequently, it is not appreciated on initial gross examination of the uterus (116, 147, 148).

Histologic Features

On low-power examination, intravenous leiomyomatosis shows a prominent growth into vascular spaces. On high power, its appearance closely overlaps with that seen in typical leiomyomas (116). The bland tumor cells form intersecting fascicles and display elongated nuclei with "blunt ends," eosinophilic cytoplasm, and rare to absent mitotic activity (116, 147–149). Leiomyoma variants have also been described including hydropic change, myxoid, epithelioid, highly cellular, lipoleiomyoma, and with bizarre nuclei (150–152).

Conclusions

- Endometrioid adenocarcinomas resemble, at least focally, proliferative-type endometrium showing tubular glands with smooth luminal surfaces, lined by mitotically active columnar cells.
- Based on the degree of glandular differentiation, endometrioid carcinomas are divided into three FIGO categories: grade 1: ≤ 5% of solid non-glandular growth; grade 2: 6–50% of solid non-glandular growth; and grade 3: >50% of solid growth. The presence of marked cytologic atypia increases the grade by one.
- The presence of extensive confluent papillary growth, macroglands or cribriform architecture as well as marked cytologic atypia is diagnostic of adenocarcinoma and excludes endometrial hyperplasia.
- The distinction between endometrial carcinoma and endocervical carcinoma or between high-grade endometrial carcinoma and serous carcinoma may be very difficult on a curettage specimen.
- Mucinous, ciliated, secretory, and villoglandular carcinomas are related to endometrioid carcinomas.
- Serous carcinomas may be very small or even confined to a polyp or the endometrium but they are always high grade and frequently have extrauterine spread. They typically show p53 overexpresion and they are ER and PR positive in <50% of cases.
- Clear cell carcinoma is uncommonly ER and PR positive and p53 overexpression is significantly less frequent than in serous carcinoma.
- The specific diagnostic criteria for the different subtypes of leiomyosarcomas differ as it appears that epithelioid and myxoid tumors are in general more aggressive.

- A combination of any two of the following three features establishes the diagnosis of spindled leiomyosarcoma: diffuse moderate to severe atypia, >10 mitoses/10 HPFs, and tumor cell necrosis.
- The criteria to establish the diagnosis of malignancy are not well established in epithelioid smooth muscle tumors. As a general rule, this diagnosis is warranted when there are ≥5 mitoses/10 HPFs and diffuse moderate to severe cytologic atypia or tumor cell necrosis.
- The diagnosis of myxoid leiomyosarcoma is made when either marked cytologic atypia or tumor cell necrosis is identified. In their absence, the finding of ≥ 2 mitoses/10 HPFs separates myxoid leiomyosarcoma from myxoid leiomyoma.
- Clinicians should be made aware that pathologists cannot distinguish between endometrial stromal nodule and low-grade endometrial stromal sarcoma in a curettage specimen in most instances; the most important feature in this differential diagnosis, the status of the tumor myometrial interface, cannot be assessed in this setting.
- A diagnosis of high-grade endometrial stromal sarcoma can only be applied when the tumor has arisen in the context of a low-grade endometrial stromal sarcoma.
- The diagnosis of undifferentiated endometrial sarcoma is a diagnosis of exclusion as this is a high-grade sarcoma without specific histologic features.
- The most important histologic parameters in the prognosis of low-grade müllerian adenosarcoma are myometrial invasion and sarcomatous overgrowth.
- Malignant mixed müllerian tumors arise either from a common pluripotential cell with divergent differentiation or by progression from the carcinomatous component by a metaplastic process or dedifferentiation, coexpressing epithelial and mesenchymal markers.
- PEComas are rare uterine tumors that belong to the family of neoplasms thought to originate from the perivascular epithelioid cell, which is defined by the presence of abundant clear to eosinophilic granular cytoplasm, positive staining for HMB-45, as well as frequent expression of muscle markers.
- Intravenous leiomyomatosis is a proliferation of histologically benign smooth muscle growing in vascular spaces. It may be seen in the absence of leiomyomas or outside the confines of leiomyomas. It has commonly extrauterine extension which may be responsible of an aggressive behavior.

References

1. Bokhman JV. Two pathogenetic types of endometrial carcinoma. Gynecol Oncol 1983;15(1):10–7.
2. Kurman RJ, Norris HJ. Evaluation of criteria for distinguishing atypical endometrial hyperplasia from well-differentiated carcinoma. Cancer 1982;49(12):2547–59.
3. Longacre TA, Chung MH, Jensen DN, et al. Proposed criteria for the diagnosis of well-differentiated endometrial carcinoma. A diagnostic test for myoinvasion. Am J Surg Pathol 1995;19(4):371–406.

4. Norris HJ, Tavassoli FA, Kurman RJ. Endometrial hyperplasia and carcinoma. Diagnostic considerations. Am J Surg Pathol 1983;7(8):839–47.
5. Melhem MF, Tobon H. Mucinous adenocarcinoma of the endometrium: a clinico-pathological review of 18 cases. Int J Gynecol Pathol 1987;6(4):347–55.
6. Ross JC, Eifel PJ, Cox RS, et al. Primary mucinous adenocarcinoma of the endometrium. A clinicopathologic and histochemical study. Am J Surg Pathol 1983;7(8):715–29.
7. Hendrickson MR, Kempson RL. Ciliated carcinoma–a variant of endometrial adenocarcinoma: a report of 10 cases. Int J Gynecol Pathol 1983;2(1):1–12.
8. Tobon H, Watkins GJ. Secretory adenocarcinoma of the endometrium. Int J Gynecol Pathol 1985;4(4):328–35.
9. Chen JL, Trost DC, Wilkinson EJ. Endometrial papillary adenocarcinomas: two clinicopathological types. Int J Gynecol Pathol 1985;4(4):279–88.
10. Parkash V, Carcangiu ML. Endometrioid endometrial adenocarcinoma with psammoma bodies. Am J Surg Pathol 1997;21(4):399–406.
11. Murray SK, Clement PB, Young RH. Endometrioid carcinomas of the uterine corpus with sex cord-like formations, hyalinization, and other unusual morphologic features: a report of 31 cases of a neoplasm that may be confused with carcinosarcoma and other uterine neoplasms. Am J Surg Pathol 2005;29(2):157–66.
12. Ronnet BM ZR, Ellenson LG, Kurman RJ. Endometrial carcinoma. In: Kurman RJ, ed. Blaustein's Pathology of the Female Genital Tract. New York: Verlag; 2002:508.
13. Dabbs DJ, Geisinger KR, Norris HT. Intermediate filaments in endometrial and endocervical carcinomas. The diagnostic utility of vimentin patterns. Am J Surg Pathol 1986;10(8):568–76.
14. Dabbs DJ, Sturtz K, Zaino RJ. The immunohistochemical discrimination of endometrioid adenocarcinomas. Hum Pathol 1996;27(2):172–7.
15. Dallenbach-Hellweg G, Lang-Averous G, Hahn U. The value of immunohistochemistry in the differential diagnosis of endometrial carcinomas. Apmis 1991;23:91–9.
16. McCluggage WG, Sumathi VP, McBride HA, et al. A panel of immunohistochemical stains, including carcinoembryonic antigen, vimentin, and estrogen receptor, aids the distinction between primary endometrial and endocervical adenocarcinomas. Int J Gynecol Pathol 2002;21(1):11–5.
17. Castrillon DH, Lee KR, Nucci MR. Distinction between endometrial and endocervical adenocarcinoma: an immunohistochemical study. Int J Gynecol Pathol 2002;21(1):4–10.
18. Wang N ZS, Zarbo R, et al. Coordinate expression of cytokeratins 7 and 20 subset analysis defines unique subsets of carcinomas. Appl Immunohistochem 1995;3:99–107.
19. Ginath S, Menczer J, Fintsi Y, et al. Tissue and serum CA125 expression in endometrial cancer. Int J Gynecol Cancer 2002;12(4):372–5.
20. Cherchi PL, Bosincu L, Dessole S, et al. Immunohistochemical expression of BerEP4, a new epithelial antigen, in endometrial carcinoma: correlation with clinical parameters. Eur J Gynaecolo Oncol 1999;20(5–6):393–5.
21. Katari RS, Fernsten PD, Schlom J. Characterization of the shed form of the human tumor-associated glycoprotein (TAG-72) from serous effusions of patients with different types of carcinomas. Cancer Res 1990;50(16):4885–90.
22. Reid-Nicholson M, Iyengar P, Hummer AJ, et al. Immunophenotypic diversity of endometrial adenocarcinomas: implications for differential diagnosis. Mod Pathol 2006;19(8):1091–100.
23. Soslow RA, Shen PU, Chung MH, et al. Cyclin D1 expression in high-grade endometrial carcinomas–association with histologic subtype. Int J Gynecol Pathol 2000;19(4):329–34.
24. Lax SF, Kendall B, Tashiro H, et al. The frequency of p53, K-ras mutations, and microsatellite instability differs in uterine endometrioid and serous carcinoma: evidence of distinct molecular genetic pathways. Cancer 2000;88(4):814–24.
25. Sherman ME, Bur ME, Kurman RJ. p53 in endometrial cancer and its putative precursors: evidence for diverse pathways of tumorigenesis. Hum Pathol 1995;26(11):1268–74.
26. Brachtel EF, Sanchez-Estevez C, Moreno-Bueno G, et al. Distinct molecular alterations in complex endometrial hyperplasia (CEH) with and without immature squamous metaplasia (squamous morules). Am J Surg Pathol 2005;29(10):1322–9.

27. Schlosshauer PW, Ellenson LH, Soslow RA. Beta-catenin and E-cadherin expression patterns in high-grade endometrial carcinoma are associated with histological subtype. Mod Pathol 2002;15(10):1032–7.
28. Gehrig PA, Bae-Jump VL, Boggess JF, et al. Association between uterine serous carcinoma and breast cancer. Gynecol Oncol 2004;94(1):208–11.
29. Geisler JP, Sorosky JI, Duong HL, et al. Papillary serous carcinoma of the uterus: increased risk of subsequent or concurrent development of breast carcinoma. Gynecol Oncol 2001;83(3):501–3.
30. Magriples U, Naftolin F, Schwartz PE, Carcangiu ML. High-grade endometrial carcinoma in tamoxifen-treated breast cancer patients. J Clin Oncol 1993;11(3):485–90.
31. Olson SH, Finstad CL, Harlap S, et al. A case-case analysis of factors related to overexpression of p53 in endometrial cancer following breast cancer. Cancer Epidemiol Biomarkers Prev 1997;6(10):815–7.
32. Parkash V, Carcangiu ML. Uterine papillary serous carcinoma after radiation therapy for carcinoma of the cervix. Cancer 1992;69(2):496–501.
33. Pothuri B, Ramondetta L, Martino M, et al. Development of endometrial cancer after radiation treatment for cervical carcinoma. Obstet Gynecol 2003;101:941–5.
34. Carcangiu ML, Chambers JT. Uterine papillary serous carcinoma: a study on 108 cases with emphasis on the prognostic significance of associated endometrioid carcinoma, absence of invasion, and concomitant ovarian carcinoma. Gynecol Oncol 1992;47(3):298–305.
35. Hendrickson M, Ross J, Eifel P, et al. Uterine papillary serous carcinoma: a highly malignant form of endometrial adenocarcinoma. Am J Surg Pathol 1982;6(2):93–108.
36. Ambros RA, Sherman ME, Zahn CM, et al. Endometrial intraepithelial carcinoma: a distinctive lesion specifically associated with tumors displaying serous differentiation. Hum Pathol 1995;26(11):1260–7.
37. Spiegel GW. Endometrial carcinoma in situ in postmenopausal women. Am J Surg Pathol 1995;19(4):417–32.
38. Darvishian F, Hummer AJ, Thaler HT, et al. Serous endometrial cancers that mimic endometrioid adenocarcinomas: a clinicopathologic and immunohistochemical study of a group of problematic cases. Am J Surg Pathol 2004;28(12):1568–78.
39. Demopoulos RI, Mesia AF, Mittal K, Vamvakas E. Immunohistochemical comparison of uterine papillary serous and papillary endometrioid carcinoma: clues to pathogenesis. Int J Gynecol Pathol 1999;18(3):233–7.
40. Tashiro H, Isacson C, Levine R, et al. p53 gene mutations are common in uterine serous carcinoma and occur early in their pathogenesis. Am J Pathol 1997;150(1):177–85.
41. An HJ, Logani S, Isacson C, Ellenson LH. Molecular characterization of uterine clear cell carcinoma. Mod Pathol 2004;17(5):530–7.
42. Lax SF, Pizer ES, Ronnett BM, Kurman RJ. Clear cell carcinoma of the endometrium is characterized by a distinctive profile of p53, Ki-67, estrogen, and progesterone receptor expression. Hum Pathol 1998;29(6):551–8.
43. Carcangiu ML DT, Radice P, Bertario L, Sala P. HNPCC-related endometrial carcinomas show a high frequency of non-endometrial types and of high FIGO grade endometrioid carcinomas. Mod Pathol; 2006:173A
44. Vang R, Whitaker BP, Farhood AI, et al. Immunohistochemical analysis of clear cell carcinoma of the gynecologic tract. Int J Gynecol Pathol 2001;20(3):252–9.
45. Goodman A, Zukerberg LR, Rice LW, et al. Squamous cell carcinoma of the endometrium: a report of eight cases and a review of the literature. Gynecol Oncol 1996;61(1):54–60.
46. Lininger RA, Ashfaq R, Albores-Saavedra J, Tavassoli FA. Transitional cell carcinoma of the endometrium and endometrial carcinoma with transitional cell differentiation. Cancer 1997;79(10):1933–43.
47. Spiegel GW, Austin RM, Gelven PL. Transitional cell carcinoma of the endometrium. Gynecol Oncol 1996;60(2):325–30.
48. Abeler VM, Kjorstad KE, Nesland JM. Undifferentiated carcinoma of the endometrium. A histopathologic and clinical study of 31 cases. Cancer 1991;68(1):98–105.

49. Altrabulsi B, Malpica A, Deavers MT, et al. Undifferentiated carcinoma of the endometrium. Am J Surg Pathol 2005;29(10):1316–21.
50. Toro JR, Travis LB, Wu HJ, et al. Incidence patterns of soft tissue sarcomas, regardless of primary site, in the surveillance, epidemiology and end results program, 1978–2001: An analysis of 26,758 cases. Int J Cancer 2006;119(12):2922–30.
51. Harlow BL, Weiss NS, Lofton S. The epidemiology of sarcomas of the uterus. J Natl Cancer Inst 1986;76(3):399–402.
52. Schwartz PE, Kelly MG. Malignant transformation of myomas: myth or reality? Obstet Gynecol Clin North Am 2006;33(1):183–98, xii.
53. Launonen V, Vierimaa O, Kiuru M, et al. Inherited susceptibility to uterine leiomyomas and renal cell cancer. Proc Natl Acad Sci U S A 2001;98(6):3387–92.
54. Rammeh-Rommani S, Mokni M, Stita W, et al. Uterine smooth muscle tumors: retrospective epidemiological and pathological study of 2760 cases. J Gynecol Obstet Biol Reprod (Paris) 2005;34(6):568–71.
55. Schwartz LB, Diamond MP, Schwartz PE. Leiomyosarcomas: clinical presentation. Am J Obstet Gynecol 1993;168 (1 Pt 1):180–3.
56. Oliva E, Clement PB, Young RH. Mesenchymal tumours of the uterus: selected topics emphasizing diagnostic pitfalls. Curr Diagn Pathol 2002;8:268–82.
57. Bell SW, Kempson RL, Hendrickson MR. Problematic uterine smooth muscle neoplasms. A clinicopathologic study of 213 cases. Am J Surg Pathol 1994;18(6):535–58.
58. Hornick JL, Fletcher CD. Criteria for malignancy in nonvisceral smooth muscle tumors. Ann Diagn Pathol 2003;7(1):60–6.
59. Tavassoli F, Devilee P, eds. Pathology and Genetics of Tumours of the Breast and Female Genital Organs. Lyon: IARC Press; 2003.
60. Burns B, Curry RH, Bell ME. Morphologic features of prognostic significance in uterine smooth muscle tumors: a review of eighty-four cases. Am J Obstet Gynecol 1979;135(1):109–14.
61. Coard KC, Fletcher HM. Leiomyosarcoma of the uterus with a florid intravascular component ("intravenous leiomyosarcomatosis"). Int J Gynecol Pathol 2002;21(2):182–5.
62. Atkins K, Bell S, Kempson R, Hendrickson M. Epithelioid smooth muscle tumors of the uterus. Mod Pathol 2001;14:132A.
63. Kurman RJ, Norris HJ. Mesenchymal tumors of the uterus. VI. Epithelioid smooth muscle tumors including leiomyoblastoma and clear-cell leiomyoma: a clinical and pathologic analysis of 26 cases. Cancer 1976;37(4):1853–65.
64. Oliva E, Nielsen PG, Clement PB, et al. Epithelioid smooth muscle tumors of the uterus. A clinicopathologic study of 80 cases. Mod Pathol 1997;10:107A.
65. Prayson RA, Goldblum JR, Hart WR. Epithelioid smooth-muscle tumors of the uterus: a clinicopathologic study of 18 patients. Am J Surg Pathol 1997;21(4):383–91.
66. Chen KT. Myxoid leiomyosarcoma of the uterus. Int J Gynecol Pathol 1984;3(4):389–92.
67. King ME, Dickersin GR, Scully RE. Myxoid leiomyosarcoma of the uterus. A report of six cases. Am J Surg Pathol 1982;6(7):589–98.
68. Pounder DJ, Iyer PV. Uterine leiomyosarcoma with myxoid stroma. Arch Pathol Lab Med 1985;109(8):762–4.
69. Salm R, Evans DJ. Myxoid leiomyosarcoma. Histopathol 1985;9(2):159–69.
70. Atkins K, Bell S, Kempson R, Hendrickson M. Myxoid smooth muscle tumors of the uterus. Mod Pathol 2001;14:132A.
71. Leitao MM, Soslow RA, Nonaka D, et al. Tissue microarray immunohistochemical expression of estrogen, progesterone, and androgen receptors in uterine leiomyomata and leiomyosarcoma. Cancer 2004;101(6):1455–62.
72. Anderson SE, Nonaka D, Chuai S, et al. p53, epidermal growth factor, and platelet-derived growth factor in uterine leiomyosarcoma and leiomyomas. Int J Gynecol Cancer 2006;16(2):849–53.
73. Raspollini MR, Pinzani P, Simi L, et al. Uterine leiomyosarcomas express KIT protein but lack mutation(s) in exon 9 of c-KIT. Gynecol Oncol 2005;98(2):334–5.

74. Leath CA, 3rd, Straughn JM, Jr., Conner MG, et al. Immunohistochemical evaluation of the c-kit proto-oncogene in sarcomas of the uterus: a case series. J Reprod Med 2004;49(2):71–5.
75. O'Connor DM, Norris HJ. Mitotically active leiomyomas of the uterus. Hum Pathol 1990;21(2):223–7.
76. Perrone T, Dehner LP. Prognostically favorable "mitotically active" smooth-muscle tumors of the uterus. A clinicopathologic study of ten cases. Am J Surg Pathol 1988;12(1):1–8.
77. Prayson RA, Hart WR. Mitotically active leiomyomas of the uterus. Am J Clin Pathol 1992;97(1):14–20.
78. Myles JL, Hart WR. Apoplectic leiomyomas of the uterus. A clinicopathologic study of five distinctive hemorrhagic leiomyomas associated with oral contraceptive usage. Am J Surg Pathol 1985;9(11):798–805.
79. Norris HJ, Hilliard GD, Irey NS. Hemorrhagic cellular leiomyomas ("apoplectic leiomyoma") of the uterus associated with pregnancy and oral contraceptives. Int J Gynecol Pathol 1988;7(3):212–24.
80. Downes KA, Hart WR. Bizarre leiomyomas of the uterus: a comprehensive pathologic study of 24 cases with long-term follow-up. Am J Surg Pathol 1997;21(11):1261–70.
81. Shih IM, Kurman RJ. Epithelioid trophoblastic tumor: a neoplasm distinct from choriocarcinoma and placental site trophoblastic tumor simulating carcinoma. Am J Surg Pathol 1998;22(11):1393–403.
82. Vang R, Kempson RL. Perivascular epithelioid cell tumor ('PEComa') of the uterus: a subset of HMB-45-positive epithelioid mesenchymal neoplasms with an uncertain relationship to pure smooth muscle tumors. Am J Surg Pathol 2002;26(1):1–13.
83. Clement PB, Scully RE. Uterine tumors resembling ovarian sex-cord tumors. A clinicopathologic analysis of fourteen cases. Am J Clin Pathol 1976;66(3):512–25.
84. Irving JA, Carinelli S, Prat J. Uterine tumors resembling ovarian sex cord tumors are polyphenotypic neoplasms with true sex cord differentiation. Mod Pathol 2006;19(1):17–24.
85. Krishnamurthy S, Jungbluth AA, Busam KJ, Rosai J. Uterine tumors resembling ovarian sex-cord tumors have an immunophenotype consistent with true sex-cord differentiation. Am J Surg Pathol 1998;22(9):1078–82.
86. Nielsen GP, Oliva E, Young RH, et al. Alveolar soft-part sarcoma of the female genital tract: a report of nine cases and review of the literature. Int J Gynecol Pathol 1995;14(4):283–92.
87. Roma AA, Yang B, Senior ME, Goldblum JR. TFE3 immunoreactivity in alveolar soft part sarcoma of the uterine cervix: case report. Int J Gynecol Pathol 2005;24(2):131–5.
88. Giordano G, Gnetti L, Ricci R, et al. Metastatic extragenital neoplasms to the uterus: a clinicopathologic study of four cases. Int J Gynecol Cancer 2006;16 Suppl 1:433–8.
89. Clement PB, Young RH, Scully RE. Diffuse, perinodular, and other patterns of hydropic degeneration within and adjacent to uterine leiomyomas. Problems in differential diagnosis. Am J Surg Pathol 1992;16(1):26–32.
90. Chang KL, Crabtree GS, Lim-Tan SK, et al. Primary uterine endometrial stromal neoplasms. A clinicopathologic study of 117 cases. Am J Surg Pathol 1990;14(5):415–38.
91. Oliva E, Clement PB, Young RH. Endometrial stromal tumors: an update on a group of tumors with a protean phenotype. Adv Anat Pathol 2000;7(5):257–81.
92. Oliva E, Clement PB, Young RH, Scully RE. Mixed endometrial stromal and smooth muscle tumors of the uterus: a clinicopathologic study of 15 cases. Am J Surg Pathol 1998;22(8):997–1005.
93. Baker PM, Moch H, Oliva E. Unusual morphologic features of endometrial stromal tumors: a report of 2 cases. Am J Surg Pathol 2005;29(10):1394–8.
94. Oliva E, Young RH, Clement PB, Scully RE. Myxoid and fibrous endometrial stromal tumors of the uterus: a report of 10 cases. Int J Gynecol Pathol 1999;18(4):310–9.
95. Yilmaz A, Rush DS, Soslow RA. Endometrial stromal sarcomas with unusual histologic features: a report of 24 primary and metastatic tumors emphasizing fibroblastic and smooth muscle differentiation. Am J Surg Pathol 2002;26(9):1142–50.
96. Clement PB, Scully RE. Endometrial stromal sarcomas of the uterus with extensive endometrioid glandular differentiation: a report of three cases that caused problems in differential diagnosis. Int J Gynecol Pathol 1992;11(3):163–73.

97. Levine PH, Abou-Nassar S, Mittal K. Extrauterine low-grade endometrial stromal sarcoma with florid endometrioid glandular differentiation. Int J Gynecol Pathol 2001;20(4):395–8.
98. McCluggage WG, Date A, Bharucha H, Toner PG. Endometrial stromal sarcoma with sex cord-like areas and focal rhabdoid differentiation. Histopathol 1996;29(4):369–74.
99. Oliva E, Clement PB, Young RH. Epithelioid endometrial and endometrioid stromal tumors: a report of four cases emphasizing their distinction from epithelioid smooth muscle tumors and other oxyphilic uterine and extrauterine tumors. Int J Gynecol Pathol 2002;21(1): 48–55.
100. Lifschitz-Mercer B, Czernobilsky B, Dgani R, et al. Immunocytochemical study of an endometrial diffuse clear cell stromal sarcoma and other endometrial stromal sarcomas. Cancer 1987;59(8):1494–9.
101. Kim YH, Cho H, Kyeom-Kim H, Kim I. Uterine endometrial stromal sarcoma with rhabdoid and smooth muscle differentiation. J Korean Med Sci 1996;11(1):88–93.
102. Chu P, Arber DA. Paraffin-section detection of CD10 in 505 nonhematopoietic neoplasms. Frequent expression in renal cell carcinoma and endometrial stromal sarcoma. Am J Clin Pathol 2000;113(3):374–82.
103. Farhood AI, Abrams J. Immunohistochemistry of endometrial stromal sarcoma. Hum Pathol 1991;22(3):224–30.
104. Lillemoe TJ, Perrone T, Norris HJ, Dehner LP. Myogenous phenotype of epithelial-like areas in endometrial stromal sarcomas. Arch Pathol Lab Med 1991;115(3):215–9.
105. de Leval L, Waltregny D, Boniver J, et al Use of histone deacetylase 8 (HDAC8), a new marker of smooth muscle differentiation, in the classification of mesenchymal tumors of the uterus. Am J Surg Pathol 2006;30(3):319–27.
106. Franquemont DW, Frierson HF, Jr., Mills SE. An immunohistochemical study of normal endometrial stroma and endometrial stromal neoplasms. Evidence for smooth muscle differentiation. Am J Surg Pathol 1991;15(9):861–70.
107. Oliva E, Young RH, Amin MB, Clement PB. An immunohistochemical analysis of endometrial stromal and smooth muscle tumors of the uterus: a study of 54 cases emphasizing the importance of using a panel because of overlap in immunoreactivity for individual antibodies. Am J Surg Pathol 2002;26(4):403–12.
108. Rush DS, Tan J, Baergen RN, Soslow RA. h-Caldesmon, a novel smooth muscle-specific antibody, distinguishes between cellular leiomyoma and endometrial stromal sarcoma. Am J Surg Pathol 2001;25(2):253–8.
109. Baker RJ, Hildebrandt RH, Rouse RV, et al. Inhibin and CD99 (MIC2) expression in uterine stromal neoplasms with sex-cord-like elements. Hum Pathol 1999;30(6):671–9.
110. Sumathi VP, Al-Hussaini M, Connolly LE, et al. Endometrial stromal neoplasms are immunoreactive with WT-1 antibody. Int J Gynecol Pathol 2004;23(3):241–7.
111. Geller MA, Argenta P, Bradley W, et al. Treatment and recurrence patterns in endometrial stromal sarcomas and the relation to c-kit expression. Gynecol Oncol 2004;95(3):632–6.
112. Reich O, Regauer S. Aromatase expression in low-grade endometrial stromal sarcomas: an immunohistochemical study. Mod Pathol 2004;17(1):104–8.
113. Dionigi A, Oliva E, Clement PB, Young RH. Endometrial stromal nodules and endometrial stromal tumors with limited infiltration: a clinicopathologic study of 50 cases. Am J Surg Pathol 2002;26(5):567–81.
114. Oliva E, Young RH, Clement PB, et al. Cellular benign mesenchymal tumors of the uterus. A comparative morphologic and immunohistochemical analysis of 33 highly cellular leiomyomas and six endometrial stromal nodules, two frequently confused tumors. Am J Surg Pathol 1995;19(7):757–68.
115. Goldblum JR, Clement PB, Hart WR. Adenomyosis with sparse glands. A potential mimic of low-grade endometrial stromal sarcoma. Am J Clin Pathol 1995;103(2):218–23.
116. Clement PB. Intravenous leiomyomatosis of the uterus. Pathol Annu 1988;23:153–83.
117. Gilks CB, Clement PB, Hart WR, Young RH. Uterine adenomyomas excluding atypical polypoid adenomyomas and adenomyomas of endocervical type: a clinicopathologic study of 30 cases of an underemphasized lesion that may cause diagnostic problems with brief

consideration of adenomyomas of other female genital tract sites. Int J Gynecol Pathol 2000;19(3):195–205.

118. Clement PB, Scully RE. Mullerian adenosarcoma of the uterus: a clinicopathologic analysis of 100 cases with a review of the literature. Hum Pathol 1990;21(4):363–81.

119. Major FJ, Blessing JA, Silverberg SG, et al. Prognostic factors in early-stage uterine sarcoma. A Gynecologic Oncology Group study. Cancer 1993;71(4 Suppl):1702–9.

120. Clement PB, Oliva E, Young RH. Mullerian adenosarcoma of the uterine corpus associated with tamoxifen therapy: a report of six cases and a review of tamoxifen-associated endometrial lesions. Int J Gynecol Pathol 1996;15(3):222–9.

121. Clement PB, Scully RE. Mullerian adenosarcomas of the uterus with sex cord-like elements. A clinicopathologic analysis of eight cases. Am J Clin Pathol 1989;91(6):664–72.

122. Ramos P, Ruiz A, Carabias E, et al. Mullerian adenosarcoma of the cervix with heterologous elements: report of a case and review of the literature. Gynecol Oncol 2002;84(1):161–6.

123. Clement PB. Mullerian adenosarcomas of the uterus with sarcomatous overgrowth. A clinicopathological analysis of 10 cases. Am J Surg Pathol 1989;13(1):28–38.

124. Soslow RA, Ali A, Oliva E. Mullerian adenosarcomas: an immunophenotypic analysis of 35 cases. Am J Surg Pathol 2008;32(7):1013–21.

125. Brooks SE, Zhan M, Cote T, Baquet CR. Surveillance, epidemiology, and end results analysis of 2677 cases of uterine sarcoma 1989–1999. Gynecol Oncol 2004;93(1):204–8.

126. McCluggage WG. Malignant biphasic uterine tumours: carcinosarcomas or metaplastic carcinomas? J Clin Pathol 2002;55(5):321–5.

127. Zelmanowicz A, Hildesheim A, Sherman ME, et al. Evidence for a common etiology for endometrial carcinomas and malignant mixed mullerian tumors. Gynecol Oncol 1998;69(3):253–7.

128. Clement PB, Zubovits JT, Young RH, Scully RE. Malignant mullerian mixed tumors of the uterine cervix: a report of nine cases of a neoplasm with morphology often different from its counterpart in the corpus. Int J Gynecol Pathol 1998;17(3):211–22.

129. Costa MJ, Khan R, Judd R. Carcinoma (malignant mixed mullerian [mesodermal] tumor) of the uterus and ovary. Correlation of clinical, pathologic, and immunohistochemical features in 29 cases. Arch Pathol Lab Med 1991;115(6):583–90.

130. Grayson W, Taylor LF, Cooper K. Carcinosarcoma of the uterine cervix: a report of eight cases with immunohistochemical analysis and evaluation of human papillomavirus status. Am J Surg Pathol 2001;25(3):338–47.

131. Fukunaga M, Nomura K, Endo Y, et al. Carcinosarcoma of the uterus with extensive neuroectodermal differentiation. Histopathol 1996;29(6):565–70.

132. Kempson RL, Hendrickson MR. Smooth muscle, endometrial stromal, and mixed Mullerian tumors of the uterus. Mod Pathol 2000;13(3):328–42.

133. George E, Manivel JC, Dehner LP, et al. Malignant mixed mullerian tumors: an immunohistochemical study of 47 cases, with histogenetic considerations and clinical correlation. Hum Pathol 1991;22(3):215–23.

134. Meis JM, Lawrence WD. The immunohistochemical profile of malignant mixed mullerian tumor. Overlap with endometrial adenocarcinoma. Am J Clin Pathol 1990;94(1):1–7.

135. Pea M, Martignoni G, Zamboni G, Bonetti F. Perivascular epithelioid cell. Am J Surg Pathol 1996;20(9):1149–53.

136. Bonetti F, Pea M, Martignoni G, et al. Clear cell ("sugar") tumor of the lung is a lesion strictly related to angiomyolipoma–the concept of a family of lesions characterized by the presence of the perivascular epithelioid cells (PEC). Pathol 1994;26(3):230–6.

137. Folpe AL, Goodman ZD, Ishak KG, et al. Clear cell myomelanocytic tumor of the falciform ligament/ligamentum teres: a novel member of the perivascular epithelioid clear cell family of tumors with a predilection for children and young adults. Am J Surg Pathol 2000;24(9):1239–46.

138. Pea M, Bonetti F, Zamboni G, et al. Melanocyte-marker-HMB-45 is regularly expressed in angiomyolipoma of the kidney. Pathol 1991;23(3):185–8.

139. Zamboni G, Pea M, Martignoni G, et al. Clear cell "sugar" tumor of the pancreas. A novel member of the family of lesions characterized by the presence of perivascular epithelioid cells. Am J Surg Pathol 1996;20(6):722–30.
140. Folpe AL, Mentzel T, Lehr HA, et al. Perivascular epithelioid cell neoplasms of soft tissue and gynecologic origin: a clinicopathologic study of 26 cases and review of the literature. Am J Surg Pathol 2005;29(12):1558–75.
141. Fukunaga M. Perivascular epithelioid cell tumor of the uterus: report of four cases. Int J Gynecol Pathol 2005;24(4):341–6.
142. Bosincu L, Rocca PC, Martignoni G, et al. Perivascular epithelioid cell (PEC) tumors of the uterus: a clinicopathologic study of two cases with aggressive features. Mod Pathol 2005;18(10):1336–42.
143. Burke M, Opeskin K. Death due to intravenous leiomyomatosis extending to the right pulmonary artery. Pathol 2004;36(2):202–3.
144. Topcuoglu MS, Yaliniz H, Poyrazoglu H, et al. Intravenous leiomyomatosis extending into the right ventricle after subtotal hysterectomy. Ann Thorac Surg 2004;78(1):330–2.
145. Virzi G, Ragazzi S, Bussichella F, et al. Intravenous leiomyomatosis extending from the inferior caval vein to the pulmonary artery. J Thorac Cardiovasc Surg 2007;133(3):831–2.
146. To WW, Ngan HY, Collins RJ. Intravenous leiomyomatosis with intracardiac involvement. Int J Gynaecol Obstet 1993;42(1):37–40.
147. Mulvany NJ, Slavin JL, Ostor AG, Fortune DW. Intravenous leiomyomatosis of the uterus: a clinicopathologic study of 22 cases. Int J Gynecol Pathol 1994;13(1):1–9.
148. Nogales FF, Navarro N, Martinez de Victoria JM, et al. Uterine intravascular leiomyomatosis: an update and report of seven cases. Int J Gynecol Pathol 1987;6(4):331–9.
149. Norris HJ, Parmley T. Mesenchymal tumors of the uterus. V. Intravenous leiomyomatosis. A clinical and pathologic study of 14 cases. Cancer 1975;36(6):2164–78.
150. Clement PB, Young RH, Scully RE. Intravenous leiomyomatosis of the uterus. A clinicopathological analysis of 16 cases with unusual histologic features. Am J Surg Pathol 1988;12(12):932–45.
151. Han HS, Park IA, Kim SH, Lee HP. The clear cell variant of epithelioid intravenous leiomyomatosis of the uterus: report of a case. Pathol Int 1998;48(11):892–6.
152. Jordan LB, Al-Nafussi A, Beattie G. Cotyledonoid hydropic intravenous leiomyomatosis: a new variant leiomyoma. Histopathol 2002;40(3):245–52.

Molecular Pathology and Cytogenetics of Endometrial Carcinoma, Carcinosarcoma, and Uterine Sarcomas

Jose Palacios and Paola Dal Cin

Abstract Molecular pathology and genetics are the subject of increasing focus since they are providing a link between etiologic factors and the heterogeneity of clinicopathologic manifestations that have been covered in the preceding chapters. In endometrial cancer, two divergent pathways have been delineated that may be thought as analogous to the hormone-dependent and -independent subtypes in breast and prostate cancers. The subtypes of endometrial adenocarcinoma reflect differences in the dysregulation of hormone-dependent and -independent pathways and may be subject to increasing manipulation described in Chapters 6 and 15. Knowledge on alterations in sarcomas will hopefully lead to advances in diagnosis and therapy that are urgently needed in women where spread beyond the uterus has occurred.

Keywords Molecular pathways • Microsatellite instability • PTEN inactivation β-catenin • Cytogenetics

Endometrial Carcinoma

Molecular Alterations

During the last years, it has been demonstrated that endometrioid (EEC) (type I) and nonendometrioid (type II) endometrial carcinomas (NEEC) not only differed from epidemiologic, clinical, and morphologic point of views but also regarding molecular alterations implicated in their initiation and progression. Four main genetic changes have been described in EEC including mutations in *PTEN* (phosphatase and tensin homologue

J. Palacios and P. Dal Cin (✉)
Pathology Department, Brigham and Women's Hospital, Boston, MA
e-mail: pdalcin@partners.org

F. Muggia and E. Oliva (eds.), *Uterine Cancer*, Current Clinical Oncology,
DOI: 10.1007/978-1-60327-044-1_5,
© Humana Press, a Part of Springer Science+Business Media, LLC 2009

deleted on chromosome 10), *KRAS*, *β-catenin*, and microsatellite instability (MSI) (Figs. 1–3). All these alterations have also been found in atypical endometrial hyperplasia, indicating their role in tumor initiation, but they are infrequent in NECC. In contrast, p53 mutations occur in a high percentage of NEEC, mainly in serous carcinomas and in its precursor lesion, endometrial intraepithelial carcinoma (Fig. 4), but are detected only in a subset of grade 3 EECs. In addition, it has been suggested that p53 inactivation may be

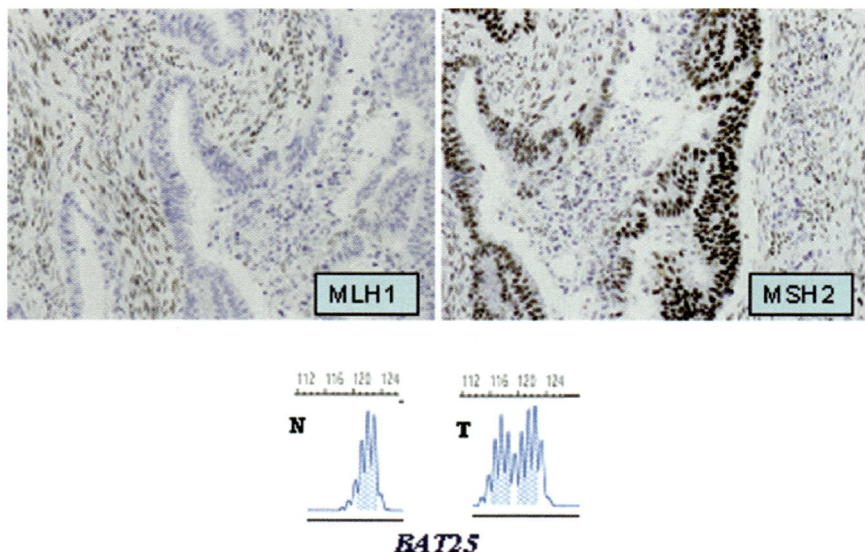

Fig. 1 Absence of MLH1 expression and preserved MSH2 expression in an EEC with microsatellite instability. Note abnormal size of BAT25 microsatellite in tumor tissue (T) with respect to normal tissue (N).

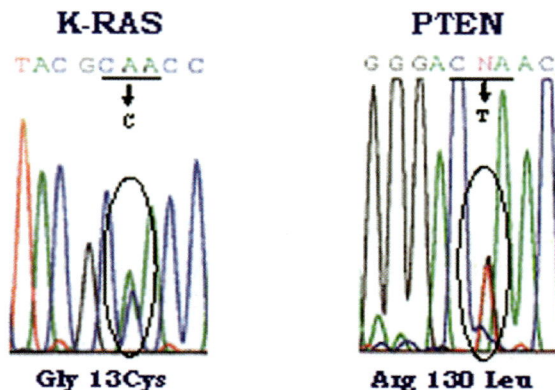

Fig. 2 Common single point mutations in *PTEN* and *K-RAS* genes.

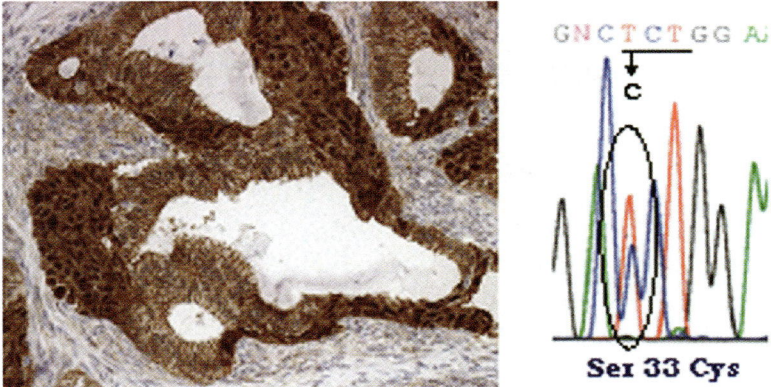

Fig. 3 β-Catenin nuclear accumulation in areas of squamous metaplasia in an EEC, which carry a single point mutation in codon 33.

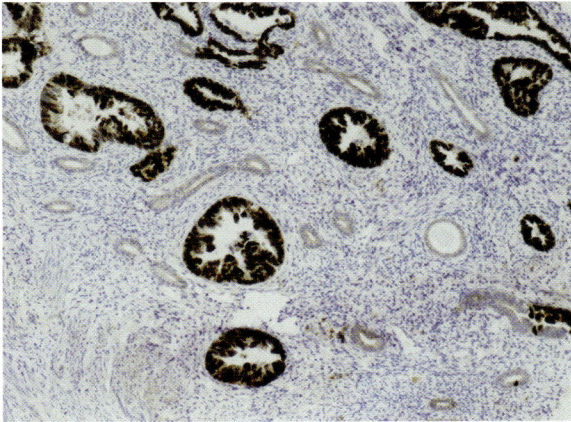

Fig. 4 p53-positive immunostaining in endometrial intraepithelial carcinoma. Note the admixture of atrophic (p53-negative) and neoplastic (p53-positive) glands.

implicated in the phenotypic change from EEC to NEEC as observed in some mixed carcinomas (1). Although *PTEN* mutation is the most frequent genetic alteration of EC, it will be discussed after MSI since some mutations in this gene are probably secondary to mismatch repair (MMR) deficiency status (Table 1).

Microsatellite Instability

Microsatellite instability represents a pattern of mutations in cells with a replication error phenotype due to deficient DNA MMR. This results in the addition or deletion

Table 1. Frequency of molecular alterations in different types of endometrial carcinoma as well as in atypical endometrial hyperplasia

Molecular alteration	Atypical endometrial hyperplasia (%)	Endometrioid endometrial carcinomas (%)	Nonendometrioid endometrial carcinomas (%)
PTEN mutation	20–55	24–83	<5
Microsatellite instability	10	15–45	<5
KRAS mutation	5–20	10–30	<5
β-Catenin mutation	0–14	15–20	<5
p53 mutation	–	10–20	50–80
HER2 amplification	–	10	40

of bases within nucleotide repeats known as microsatellite regions. Microsatellite loci contain repetitive elements of 1–6 nucleotides in length and are most commonly $(CA)_n$ or poly A/T sequences. MSI status can be detected by using a standard panel of five microsatellite markers. When at least two of the five markers show MSI, tumors are classified as MSI-high (MSI-H). In contrast, tumors without size alteration in microsatellites or those with only one altered marker are classified as microsatellite stable (MSS) and MSI-low (MSI-L), respectively (2). From a clinicopathologic point of view, MSI-L tumors should be included with MSS tumors (3).

Microsatellite instability was first reported in colorectal adenocarcinomas of patients with Lynch syndrome (hereditary nonpolyposis colorectal cancer, HNPCC). This status of high-frequency mutagenesis is caused by mutations in the main DNA MMR genes, such as *hMLH1* and *hMSH2* and less frequently *hMSH6*, *hPMS1*, and *hPMS2*. MSI is also seen in approximately 15% of sporadic colorectal carcinomas, usually reflecting loss of expression of hMLH1 associated with gene silencing by *hMLH1* promoter methylation (3).

Available data indicate that endometrial carcinoma (EC) is the most common extracolonic tumor in Lynch syndrome, with lifetime risk estimates ranging from 40% to 60% in female mutation carriers (4). As a result, the original Amsterdam criteria for Lynch syndrome was revised in 1999 to include EC among the diagnostic criteria (5). It has been suggested that EC is the most common malignancy among women carrying hMSH6 germ line mutations (6).

Microsatellite instability is seen in approximately 15–45% of sporadic EEC (7–12), usually reflecting loss of expression of hMLH1 associated with gene silencing by *hMLH1* promoter methylation. This change has been reported in 69–92% of EC with MSI (13, 14). In addition, it has been shown that the *hMLH1* promoter is frequently methylated in the histologically normal endometrium (15) and atypical endometrial hyperplasia (13) of patients with ECs and that the methylation status is similar to that in the carcinoma. These findings support the notion that, in a subset of tumors, epigenetic changes in DNA MMR genes might be the initial events that trigger the genetic alterations involved in endometrial carcinogenesis.

Immunohistochemistry can be used to explore MMR gene inactivation in EC. Currently, there are antibodies available to study the expression of the most important MMR proteins, such as hMLH1, hMSH2, hMSH6, and hPMS2. In colon cancer, large studies comparing immunohistochemistry and MSI genotyping have demonstrated a

93–100% sensitivity to detect MSI by immunohistochemistry analysis. Although there are not such larger series in EC, different studies have reported a 70–100% sensitivity when using immunohistochemistry when hMLH1 and hMSH2 are utilized together (Fig. 1) (14, 16, 17).

MMR deficiency in cancer produces instability not only in microsatellites that are located in noncoding sequences, such as those used for MSI genotyping, but also in mononucleotide tract repeats located in coding sequences of different genes. The proteins encoded by these genes participate in a variety of essential cellular processes like signal transduction (TGFβRII, IGFIIR, PTEN), apoptosis (BAX, caspase 5), DNA repair (hMSH3, hMSH6, MBD4), transcriptional regulation (TCF-4), protein translocation and modification (SEC63, OGT), or immune surveillance (β2M). It is generally believed that this subset of critical targets specifically promotes MSI carcinogenesis in a large proportion of tumors. Moreover, several studies have demonstrated that selection of target gene mutations in MSI cancers is a tissue-specific process. Whereas some of the genes were proposed to be real target genes for mutation in the most common types of cancers with MSI (colon, gastric, and endometrial cancer) (TGFβRII, BAX, IGFIIR, MSH3, MSH6, and GRB14), selection of other genes for mutation appeared to be dependent on the primary site of the tumor. MSI ECs accumulate significantly fewer mutations at coding repeats compared with gastrointestinal MSI tumors. For example, the almost systematic TGFβRII gene mutation in MSI gastrointestinal tumors was observed in only 0–10% of the MSI EC cases in different series (18–20).

Although MSI occurs in a substantial fraction of sporadic EC, data on whether these endometrial tumors differ from their MSI-negative counterparts in clinical characteristics, pathologic features, and survival is controversial; although some studies have reported favorable survival associated with MSI EEC (21), most large series did not find differences in grade, recurrence rate, and survival between MSI-positive and -negative EC (10, 11).

PTEN Inactivation

PTEN gene is located in 10q23, a region undergoing frequent somatic deletion in tumors. It encodes a 403-amino acid dual-specificity phosphatase containing a region of homology to tensin and auxilin, which are two cytoskeletal proteins. Among other activities, PTEN antagonizes the PI3K/AKT pathway, which results in downregulation of AKT phosphorylation activation. Thus, decreased expression of PTEN leads to increased levels of phospho-AKT, which results in both suppression of apoptosis and induction of cell cycle.

PTEN is mutated in the germ line of patients with Cowden's disease, a rare autosomal dominant cancer syndrome, which occasionally may be associated with EC. However, PTEN is also frequently somatically mutated in tumors from various tissues. PTEN may be also inactivated by deletion, as shown by the elevated frequency of loss of heterozygosity in different tumor types. Finally, a third proposed mechanism for PTEN inactivation is promoter hypermethylation. However, the true significance of PTEN promoter methylation is still under discussion.

PTEN is frequently abnormal in ECs. Loss of heterozygosity at chromosome 10q23 occurs in 40% of cases (22). Moreover, *PTEN* is the most frequently mutated gene in EEC (Fig. 2). The frequency of PTEN mutations in EEC varies between 24% and 50% (5, 23–25) in different series, although one study has reported an incidence as high as 83% (26). In addition, *PTEN* silencing may occur not only in EEC and endometrial hyperplasia (25–28) but also in isolated glands in up to 40% of premenopausal women (29), indicating a major role of this alteration in the initiation of some EEC.

PTEN mutations may occur throughout the entire coding region, but are more frequent in exons 5, 7, and 8. A high percentage of mutations in exon 5 (around 60%) are single base substitution, being more common in codon 130. In contrast, frameshift mutations are more frequent in exons 7 and 8, where two hot spots for deletion or insertion have been identified: two $(A)_6$ sequences in codons 265–267 and codons 321–323. Mutations in those sites are characteristic features of MSI tumors and suggest that some mutations in the *PTEN* gene are consequence of loss of DNA repair mechanism. Opinions differ, however, on the relationship between occurrence of *PTEN* gene mutations and the presence of MSI in EC. Thus, most series (24, 30, 31, 57) have demonstrated that *PTEN* gene mutations occur more frequently in EC with MSI (65–86%) than in carcinomas without this instability (20–36%). However, other authors failed to find any relationship between the high frequency of *PTEN* gene mutations and MSI in EC (26).

PTEN mutations have been detected more frequently in Caucasians relative to African-Americans, and have been correlated with young age, low FIGO-stage, low grade, and favorable prognosis (32–34).

It has been suggested that *PTEN* immunostaining may be an effective method to screen for abnormal *PTEN* expression in tumors and premalignant lesions. However, some variability has been observed with different antibodies and techniques, particularly when correlating the immunohistochemical results with the presence of molecular alterations. Recent studies have suggested that the monoclonal antibody 6.H2.1 is the only antibody that recognizes a pattern of PTEN expression that correlates with the presence of molecular alterations in *PTEN* (mutations, deletions, or promoter hypermethylation) (35).

Very recently, it has been demonstrated that the PI3K pathway can be activated in EC not only by PTEN mutations but also by mutations in the catalytic subunit alpha of PI3K (PIK3CA), which occurs in 36% of EC. Interestingly, these mutations are most common among EC with PTEN mutations (46%), and approximately one quarter of the tumors carry mutations in both genes. These results indicate that combinations of PTEN/PI3CA alterations might play an important role in the development of EC (36).

β-Catenin Mutations

The Wnt signaling pathway plays an important role in normal and tumoral cells. In the absence of an extracellular Wnt signal in normal cells, the free (cytoplasmic) β-catenin level is low since the protein is targeted for destruction in the ubiquitin–proteasome system after phosphorylation by glycogen synthase kinase-3β (GSK-3β). The latter forms a complex with the adenomatous polyposis coli (APC) protein and other proteins, such as *AXIN1*, *AXIN2*, and protein phosphatase 2A. The most common molecular alterations in tumor cells leading to disruption of β-catenin degradation are mutations that inactivate APC or activate β-catenin itself. These alterations produce an accumulation of cytoplasmic β-catenin that translocates into the nucleus and, interacting with members of the lymphoid enhancer factor-1/T-cell factor (Lef-1/Tcf), activates transcription of various genes, such as *cyclin D1* and *MYC*.

Regarding EC, the Wnt signaling pathway is altered only in EEC. In these tumors, mutations of APC have not been detected (37, 38), but β-catenin mutations occurred in approximately 15–20% of EEC (Fig. 3) (37–41), and in 14% of endometrial atypical hyperplasias (24). Most studies on β-catenin mutations have only analyzed the consensus sequence for GSK-3β phosphorylation in exon 3. Mutations affect the amino acids implicated in the downregulation of β-catenin through phosphorylation by this serine/threonine kinase (serine 33, serine 37, threonine 41, and serine 45) and two adjacent residues. Mutations in these residues render a fraction of cellular β-catenin insensitive to APC-mediated downregulation and are responsible for the upregulation of cytoplasmic β-catenin and its accumulation in the nuclei of tumor cells, which can be detected by immunohistochemistry.

Approximately 15% of tumors feature β-catenin nuclear accumulation without evidence of β-catenin mutations, suggesting alterations in molecules of the Wnt pathway other than β-catenin mutations. However no *APC*, *AXIN1*, or *AXIN2* mutations have been detected in EEC. In addition, alterations of genes involved in GSK-3-β regulation, such as *PTEN* and *KRAS*, have also been excluded as causes of β-catenin upregulation (38).

From a morphologic point of view, several studies have stressed the association between nuclear β-catenin accumulation and squamous metaplasia in EEC. Although nuclear β-catenin may be associated with usual squamous metaplasia, it is more characteristically associated with morular metaplasia and β-catenin mutations are found in 50% of atypical endometrial hyperplasias with squamous morules (28).

Some series have not found significant relationship between *β-catenin* gene mutations and clinicopathologic features, such as age, tumor grade, and stage. However, other series have shown an association with low-grade tumors and absence of lymph node metastases (41), suggesting that *β-catenin* mutations might occur in a subset of less-aggressive ECs.

KRAS Mutations

KRAS mutations in codons 12 and 13 have been identified in 10–30% of ECs (Fig. 2) (9, 38, 42–44). Although some authors have failed to demonstrate a correlation between *KRAS* mutations and stage, grade, depth of invasion, age, or clinical outcome in EC (45), others have reported associations between *KRAS* mutations and the presence of coexistent endometrial atypical hyperplasia (43), lymph node metastases, and clinical outcome in postmenopausal patients above 60 years (46).

An association between *KRAS* mutations and mucinous differentiation has also been reported (44). Several studies have tried to correlate *KRAS* mutations and MSI in EC, but results are contradictory.

BRAF, which encodes a *RAF* family member that functions downstream of RAS, has been reported to be somatically mutated in a number of human cancers. Recently, activating mutations of *BRAF* have been frequently observed in MSI colorectal carcinomas, in which mutations of *BRAF* and *KRAS* have been reported to be mutually exclusive (47). Several series have analyzed the frequency of *BRAF* mutations in EC. Although one of these studies reported a 21% incidence of *BRAF* mutations and suggested an association with MSI status (48), most studies have found a very low incidence of BRAF alterations (49–51), indicating a minor role of this gene in endometrial carcinogenesis.

p53 Inactivation

The *p53* tumor suppressor gene was initially identified as being essential for DNA damage checkpoint, but it was subsequently found to have a broader function after cellular stress, such as oncogene activation or hypoxia. The p53 protein is found at very low levels in normal unstressed cells. After stress, different pathways lead to post-translational modification of the protein and its stabilization. This accumulation activates the transcription of a wide range of genes involved in various activities, including cell cycle inhibition and apoptosis depending on the cellular context, the extent of damage, or other unknown parameters.

Inactivation of the *p53* gene is essentially due to small mutations (missense and nonsense mutations or insertions/deletions of several nucleotides), which lead to either expression of a mutant protein (90% of cases) or absence of protein (10% of cases). Thus, there is no a complete concordance between genotyping and immunohistochemistry in tumors with *p53* mutations. No inactivation of *p53* gene expression by hypermethylation of transcription promoters has been demonstrated. In many cases, these mutations are associated with loss of the wild-type allele of the *p53* gene located on the short arm of chromosome 17.

p53 mutations have been detected in approximately 20% of EECs, being more frequent among grade 3 or advanced stage EECs (52–56). In contrast, 50–80% of serous carcinomas (NEEC) and its precursor lesion, endometrial intraepithelial carcinoma, carry *p53* mutations, more frequently associated with protein overexpression (Fig. 4) (57, 58). For this reason, p53 immunohistochemistry may help in the differential diagnosis of uterine serous carcinoma when it exhibits glands without papillary architecture that make it difficult to distinguish from EEC (59).

p53 expression and mutations have been reported to be an adverse prognostic factor in EC in some studies, but not in others. It has been proposed that the functional activity of mutant p53 protein is a strong predictor of survival in patients with EC (56). Thus, the presence of dominant-negative *p53* mutations, those that produce mutated proteins that complex with and inactivate wild-type protein, are associated with poor prognosis in advanced EEC.

HER-2/neu Amplification and Overexpression

The human HER-2/neu gene located on 17q.12 encodes a protein (p185), which is a member of the epidermal growth factor receptor (EGFR) transmembrane receptor tyrosine kinase family. Overexpression of HER-2/neu plays a role in cellular transformation, tumorigenesis, and metastases. *HER-2/neu* gene has been extensively studied in breast cancer, where up to 20% of tumors show protein overexpression as a result of gene amplification. In these tumors, the use of the humanized anti-HER-2/neu antibody trastuzumab has proven to be of clinical benefit.

In EC, immunohistochemical or molecular studies addressing the HER/2-neu protein or gene status and the prognostic utility of these alterations are limited, in part due to methodology-related issues. Recent studies using standardized systems of immunohistochemical evaluation for protein expression have reported that approximately 15% of EEC and 20–60% of NEEC overexpressed HER-2/neu (60–62). Overexpression was defined as >10% of cells with complete membrane staining of weak to moderate (2+) or intense (3+) intensity. Gene amplification evaluated by fluorescent in situ hybridization (FISH) or chromogenic in situ hybridization (CISH) has been observed in 9% EEC and in 3–42% NEEC (60–62). Amplified cases more frequently showed 3+ expression. Differences in frequency of HER2–2/neu overexpression and amplification between different NEEC series are related to the number of mixed carcinomas included, as it is suggested that HER-2/neu overexpression is more characteristic of pure serous papillary carcinomas (62).

Although some studies have reported poor prognosis in patients with EC that overexpressed HER-2-neu, further studies are needed to better establish the prognostic significance of this alteration and its potential use as a pharmacodiagnostic and therapeutic marker.

Cytogenetic Abnormalities

Cytogenetic studies of EC have shown that most tumors have hyperdiploid karyotypes with relatively simple abnormalities, both numerical and structural, although cases also exist with complex chromosomal rearrangements (63). Although aberrations of chromosome 1 leading to trisomy/tetrasomy 1q are the most frequent abnormalities reported, no specific karyotypic changes have been detected. A recent comparative genomic hybridization (CGH) study revealed more complex chromosomal imbalances in hormone-independent, type II ECs than in hormone-related, type I carcinomas. Moreover, the same study showed increased karyotypic complexity in relation to tumor grade in type I ECs, supporting the idea that tumor-phenotype is altered with accumulation of genomic imbalances (64).

Uterine Carcinosarcomas (Malignant Mixed Müllerian Tumors)

Molecular Abnormalities

The histogenesis of carcinosarcomas (CSs) has long been a matter of speculation and dispute. Two main hypotheses have been proposed to explain carcinomatous and sarcomatous components. In the "collision theory," synchronous biclonal tumors are thought to blend together. The second, and most favored theory, is the "combination theory" which postulates that both elements originate from a single stem cell clone. According to this theory, the sarcomatous component arises in a carcinoma through evolution of subclones.

A number of recent immunohistochemical and molecular-genetic studies support the monoclonal nature of these neoplasms. For example, immunohistochemical studies have documented the expression of epithelial markers in the sarcomatous components of a large proportion of cases. More recently, X-chromosomal inactivation assays, p53 and KRAS mutational analyses, and LOH studies have all shown the carcinomatous and sarcomatous elements to share common genetic alterations (65, 66). LOH, mutations, or protein overexpression of p53 have been found in 32–80% of these tumors. In addition, 24% of CSs carry KRAS mutations. The same mutations were detected in the carcinomatous and sarcomatous components of the tumors, supporting the clonal origin of both components (65, 67, 68).

LOH at the *PTEN* locus is infrequent in CS but may occur late in the progression of these neoplasms (66). The frequency of PTEN mutations in CS is also low. Thus, Lancaster et al. (69) studied PTEN mutations in 24 CSs and were unable to detect any, while Amant et al. (70) analyzed 18 CSs and found PTEN mutations in 3 (17%) cases, all with an endometrioid-type carcinoma component.

HER-2/neu overexpression and gene amplification have been reported in 22–49% and 15–20% of endometrial CS, respectively (71, 72). Interestingly, protein expression was most commonly found in the epithelial than in the sarcomatous component. In contrast, the expression of EGFR, which is found in about 50% of CSs, predominates in the sarcomatous component (72). These findings may have treatment implications for patients with endometrial CS.

Cytogenetic Abnormalities

It has been reported that karyotypes and CGH profiles of CSs are very similar to uterine carcinomas and different from sarcomas. Genetic imbalance profiles of CSs frequently mirror those of the epithelial component present in the tumor (64).

Uterine Sarcomas

Leiomyosarcoma

Molecular Abnormalities

Several series, including a relatively low number of cases, have reported a 13–37% frequency of p53 mutations in these tumors (73–75). PTEN mutational status has been studied in uterine sarcomas since these tumors frequently show loss of heterozygosity of 10q23.3 (76); however, the incidence of PTEN mutations seems to be very low since only one mutation has been detected among 33 leiomyosarcomas (LMS) analyzed in two different series (69, 70).

Cytogenetic Abnormalities

Most reported karyotypes in LMSs are complex without consistent aberrations (Table 2). In addition, CGH studies have confirmed a high frequency of gains and losses of several chromosomal regions (77). This large number of nonrandom aberrations suggests that increased genetic instability plays a role in the origin of LMSs. The majority of molecular and cytogenetic data do not support an origin of LMS from its benign counterpart, leiomyoma. A recent study of a series of smooth muscle tumors showed a different gene expression profile for LMS and leiomyoma (78). However, an intriguing recent observation revealed that the transcriptional profile of a small group of cellular leiomyomas with a specific chromosome abnormality, e.g., del(1)(p11p36), is more similar to that seen in LMS than to profiles of normal myometrium and conventional leiomyoma (79).

Several uterine smooth muscle proliferations i.e., intravenous leiomyomatosis (IVL), disseminated peritoneal leiomyomatosis (DPL), and benign metastasizing leiomyoma (BML) are unusual because of their "aggressive" clinical behavior but they do not belong to the LMS category of smooth muscle tumors. However, several cytogenetic alterations have been detected that are worth discussing. A nonrandom pathogenetic event in IVL is the finding of a karyotype showing a der(14)t(12;14)(q15;q24) in addition to two normal copies of chromosome 12 (Table 2). The presence of t(12;14) in IVL, which is the most frequent abnormality in conventional leiomyomas, suggests a pathogenetic relationship between these two smooth muscle tumors (80).

Table 2. Most frequent/characteristic cytogenetic abnormalities in mesenchymal uterine tumors

Tumor type	Characteristic cytogenetic abnormality	Molecular event
Endometrial stromal tumor	t(7;17)(p15;q21)	*JAZF1–JJAZ1 fusion*
	t(6;7)(p21;p15)	*JAZF1–PHF1 fusion*
Intravenous leiomyomatosis	der(14)t(12;14)(q15;q24)	*HMGA2 rearrangement*
Leiomyosarcoma	complex karyotype	

Benign metastasizing leiomyoma is a controversial entity in which a benign appearing uterine smooth muscle tumor is associated with similarly appearing tumors at distant sites, most commonly involving lung and abdominal lymph nodes. No cytogenetic or molecular genetic studies have been reported except for a recent study using variable length of the polymorphic CAG repeat sequence within the human androgen receptor gene which supports the notion that BML is derived from uterine leiomyoma (81).

Finally, diffuse peritoneal leiomyomatosis, a rare condition presenting with multiple benign smooth muscle proliferations throughout omental and peritoneal surfaces, has been suggested to have a common pathogenesis with conventional leiomyoma because of similar chromosome aberrations involving chromosomes 7 and 12 (82).

Low-Grade Endometrial Stromal Sarcomas

Molecular Abnormalities

No mutations in p53, PTEN, KRAS, or β-catenin have been described in low-grade endometrial stromal sarcomas (LG-ESS); however, nuclear β-catenin expression is seen in up to 40% of these tumors (83). This immunohistochemical pattern might be related to the downregulation of SFRP4, a negative modulator of the Wnt pathway (84).

Cytogenetic Abnormalities

Cytogenetic abnormalities have been reported in at least 30 LG-ESSs showing wide karyotypic heterogeneity (85). The most common abnormality is a t(7;17)(p15;q21) (Fig. 5a), resulting in the fusion of *JAZF1* and *JJAZ1* genes at 7p15 and 17q21, respectively (86) (Table 2). So far, the reported frequency of *JAZF1–JJAZ1* fusion by RT-PCR analysis has ranged from 25% to 100%, mostly in endometrial nodules and LG-EESs (85–88). The variation in frequency of detection of this translocation by RT-PCR may reflect molecular heterogeneity of fusion transcripts and/or tumors carrying other chromosomal aberrations, as well as technical problems with RT-PCR. The second most frequent abnormality in these tumors is a t(6;7) (p21;p15) (Fig. 5b), a so-called variant translocation of the t(7;17), because of the involvement of 7p15 but not the 17q21.

Recently, Micci et al. have shown specific involvement of the PHD finger protein 1 (*PHF1*) gene, located in chromosome 6, band p21, in two tumors with a t(6;7). In these tumors, *PHF1* was rearranged with *JAZF1* from 7p15, resulting in a *JAZF1–PHF1* fusion gene. A third tumor in their series showed a t(6p;10q;10p) as the sole karyotypic abnormality, leading to fusion of *PHF1* with another partner, the enhancer of polycomb (*EPC1*) gene, which maps to 10p11 (89). These findings support the emerging concept that although endometrial stromal tumors are genetically

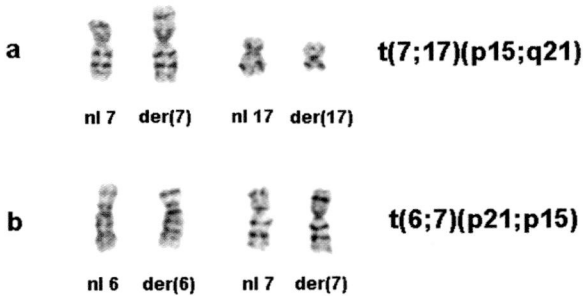

a   t(7;17)(p15;q21)

nl 7   der(7)   nl 17   der(17)

b   t(6;7)(p21;p15)

nl 6   der(6)   nl 7   der(7)

Fig. 5 Partial GTG-banding karyotype showing the two most frequent translocations seen in a low-grade endometrial stromal sarcoma: t(7;17)(p15;q21) (**a**) and t(6;7)(p21;p15) (**b**).

heterogeneous, the different genes involved in these tumors are probably functionally related. Finally, the most common cytogenetic alterations in these tumors have been recently observed using standardized FISH analysis which may be used for diagnostic purposes (90, 91).

Conclusions

- Four main genetic changes have been described in EECs including mutations in *PTEN*, *KRAS*, *β-catenin*, and MSI.
- p53 mutations occur in a high percentage of NEECs, mainly in serous carcinomas and in its precursor lesion, endometrial intraepithelial carcinoma, but are also detected in a subset of grade 3 EECs.
- MSI is seen in approximately 15–45% of sporadic ECs usually reflecting loss of expression of hMLH1 associated with gene silencing by *hMLH1* promoter methylation.
- EC is the most common extracolonic tumor in Lynch syndrome and it has been suggested that it is the most common malignancy among women carrying hMSH6 germ line mutations. As a result, the original Amsterdam criteria for Lynch syndrome include EC among the diagnostic criteria.
- Most large series have found no differences in grade, recurrence rate, and survival between MSI-positive and -negative EC.
- *PTEN* abnormalities are most common in EECs and some *PTEN* mutations are thought to be consequence of loss of DNA repair mechanism.
- *PTEN* mutations have been detected more frequently in Caucasians relative to African-Americans, and have been correlated with young age, low FIGO stage, low grade, and favorable prognosis.
- β-Catenin mutations occur in approximately 20% of EECs. However, immunohistochemical nuclear expression of β-catenin does not always correlate with β-catenin mutations.

- From a morphologic point of view, nuclear β-catenin accumulation is frequently seen in association with squamous metaplasia in EECs.
- Varied prognostic significance of KRAS in EC type I has been shown among different studies.
- HER-2/neu overexpression is more characteristic of pure serous papillary carcinomas. However, overexpression of HER-2-neu is not a well-established prognostic marker in EC.
- Molecular-genetic studies support the monoclonal nature of CSs, as they have shown that the carcinomatous and sarcomatous elements share common genetic alterations. Furthermore, CGH profiles of CSs are very similar to uterine carcinomas and different from sarcomas.
- Among sarcomas, the most common abnormality appears to occur in LG-ESS which show a t(7;17)(p15;q21) resulting in the fusion of *JAZF1* and *JJAZ1* genes at 7p15 and 17q21, respectively.

References

1. Matias-Guiu X, Catasus L, Bussaglia E, et al. Molecular pathology of endometrial hyperplasia and carcinoma. Hum Pathol. 2001;32(6):569–577.
2. Boland CR, Thibodeau SN, Hamilton SR, et al. A National Cancer Institute Workshop on Microsatellite Instability for cancer detection and familial predisposition: development of international criteria for the determination of microsatellite instability in colorectal cancer. Cancer Res. 1998;58(22):5248–5257.
2. Umar A, Boland CR, Terdiman JP, et al. Revised Bethesda Guidelines for hereditary nonpolyposis colorectal cancer (Lynch syndrome) and microsatellite instability. J Natl Cancer Inst. 2004;96(4):261–268.
4. Boyd J. Genetic basis of familial endometrial cancer: is there more to learn? J Clin Oncol. 2005;23(21):4570–4573.
5. Vasen HF, Watson P, Mecklin JP, Lynch HT. New clinical criteria for hereditary nonpolyposis colorectal cancer (HNPCC, Lynch syndrome) proposed by the International Collaborative group on HNPCC. Gastroenterology. 1999;116(6):1453–1456.
6. Wijnen J, de Leeuw W, Vasen H, et al. Familial endometrial cancer in female carriers of MSH6 germline mutations. Nat Genet. 1999;23(2):142–144.
7. Risinger JI, Berchuck A, Kohler MF, et al. Genetic instability of microsatellites in endometrial carcinoma. Cancer Res. 1993;53(21):5100–5103.
8. Burks RT, Kessis TD, Cho KR, Microsatellite instability in endometrial carcinoma. Oncogene. 1994;9(4):1163–1166.
9. Duggan BD, Felix JC, Muderspach LI, Tsao JL, Shibata DK. Early mutational activation of the c-Ki-ras oncogene in endometrial carcinoma. Cancer Res. 1994;54(6):1604–1607.
10. Basil JB, Goodfellow PJ, Rader JS, Mutch DG, Herzog TJ. Clinical significance of microsatellite instability in endometrial carcinoma. Cancer. 2000;89(8):1758–1764.
11. MacDonald ND, Salvesen HB, Ryan A, Iversen OE, Akslen LA, Jacobs IJ. Frequency and prognostic impact of microsatellite instability in a large population-based study of endometrial carcinomas. Cancer Res. 2000;60(6):1750–1752.
12. Goodfellow PJ, Buttin BM, Herzog TJ, et al. Prevalence of defective DNA mismatch repair and MSH6 mutation in an unselected series of endometrial cancers. Proc Natl Acad Sci U S A. 2003;100(10):5908–5913.

13. Esteller M, Catasus L, Matias-Guiu X, et al. hMLH1 promoter hypermethylation is an early event in human endometrial tumorigenesis. Am J Pathol. 1999;155(5):1767–1772.
14. Salvesen HB, MacDonald N, Ryan A, et al. Methylation of hMLH1 in a population-based series of endometrial carcinomas. Clin Cancer Res. 2000;6(9):3607–3613.
15. Kanaya T, Kyo S, Maida Y, et al. Frequent hypermethylation of MLH1 promoter in normal endometrium of patients with endometrial cancers. Oncogene. 2003;22(15):2352–2360.
16. Stefansson I, Akslen LA, MacDonald N, et al. Loss of hMSH2 and hMSH6 expression is frequent in sporadic endometrial carcinomas with microsatellite instability: a population-based study. Clin Cancer Res. 2002;8(1):138–143.
17. Hardisson D, Moreno-Bueno G, Sanchez L, et al. Tissue microarray immunohistochemical expression analysis of mismatch repair (hMLH1 and hMSH2 genes) in endometrial carcinoma and atypical endometrial hyperplasia: relationship with microsatellite instability. Mod Pathol. 2003;16(11):1148–1158.
18. Schwartz S, Yamamoto H, Navarro M, Maestro M, Reventos J, Perucho M. Frameshift mutations at mononucleotide repeats in caspase-5 and other target genes in endometrial and gastrointestinal cancer of the microsatellite mutator phenotype. Cancer Res. 1999;59(12):2995–3002.
19. Catasus L, Matias-Guiu X, Machin P, et al. Frameshift mutations at coding mononucleotide repeat microsatellites in endometrial carcinoma with microsatellite instability. Cancer. 2000;88(10):2290–2297.
20. Furlan D, Casati B, Cerutti R, et al. Genetic progression in sporadic endometrial and gastrointestinal cancers with high microsatellite instability. J Pathol. 2002;197(5):603–609.
21. Maxwell GL, Risinger JI, Alvarez AA, Barrett JC, Berchuck A. Favorable survival associated with microsatellite instability in endometrioid endometrial cancers. Obstet Gynecol. 2001;97(3):417–422.
22. Peiffer SL, Herzog TJ, Tribune DJ, Mutch DG, Gersell DJ, Goodfellow PJ. Allelic loss of sequences from the long arm of chromosome 10 and replication errors in endometrial cancers. Cancer Res. 1995;55(9):1922–1926.
23. Risinger JI, Hayes AK, Berchuck A, Barrett JC. PTEN/MMAC1 mutations in endometrial cancers. Cancer Res. 1997;57(21):4736–4738.
24. Moreno-Bueno G, Hardisson D, Sarrio D, et-al. Abnormalities of E- and P-cadherin and catenin (beta-, gamma-catenin, and p120ctn) expression in endometrial cancer and endometrial atypical hyperplasia. J Pathol. 2003;199(4):471–478.
25. Sun H, Enomoto T, Fujita M, et al. Mutational analysis of the PTEN gene in endometrial carcinoma and hyperplasia. Am J Clin Pathol. 2001;115(1):32–38.
26. Mutter GL, Lin MC, Fitzgerald JT, et al. Altered PTEN expression as a diagnostic marker for the earliest endometrial precancers. J Natl Cancer Inst. 2000;92(11):924–930.
27. Orbo A, Kaino T, Arnes M, Kopp M, Eklo K. Genetic derangements in the tumor suppressor gene PTEN in endometrial precancers as prognostic markers for cancer development: a population-based study from northern Norway with long-term follow-up. Gynecol Oncol. 2004;95(1):82–88.
28. Brachtel EF, Sanchez-Estevez C, Moreno-Bueno G, Prat J, Palacios J, Oliva E. Distinct molecular alterations in complex endometrial hyperplasia (CEH) with and without immature squamous metaplasia (squamous morules). Am J Surg Pathol. 2005;29(10):1322–1329.
29. Mutter GL, Ince TA, Baak JP, Kust GA, Zhou XP, Eng C. Molecular identification of latent precancers in histologically normal endometrium. Cancer Res. 2001;61(11):4311–4314.
30. Bussaglia E, del Rio E, Matias-Guiu X, Prat J. PTEN mutations in endometrial carcinomas: a molecular and clinicopathologic analysis of 38 cases. Hum Pathol. 2000;31(3):312–317.
31. Koul A, Willen R, Bendahl PO, Nilbert M, Borg A. Distinct sets of gene alterations in endometrial carcinoma implicate alternate modes of tumorigenesis. Cancer. 2002;94(9):2369–2379.
32. Risinger JI, Hayes K, Maxwell GL, et al. PTEN mutation in endometrial cancers is associated with favorable clinical and pathologic characteristics. Clin Cancer Res. 1998;4(12):3005–3010.
33. Maxwell GL, Risinger JI, Hayes KA, et al. Racial disparity in the frequency of PTEN mutations, but not microsatellite instability, in advanced endometrial cancers. Clin Cancer Res. 2000;6(8):2999–3005.

34. Salvesen HB, Stefansson I, Kretzschmar EI, et al. Significance of PTEN alterations in endometrial carcinoma: a population-based study of mutations, promoter methylation and PTEN protein expression. Int J Oncol. 2004;25(6):1615–1623.
35. Pallares J, Bussaglia E, Martinez-Guitarte JL, et al. Immunohistochemical analysis of PTEN in endometrial carcinoma: a tissue microarray study with a comparison of four commercial antibodies in correlation with molecular abnormalities. Mod Pathol. 2005;18(5):719–727.
36. Oda K, Stokoe D, Taketani Y, McCormick F. High frequency of coexistent mutations of PIK3CA and PTEN genes in endometrial carcinoma. Cancer Res. 2005;65(23):10669–10673.
37. Schlosshauer PW, Pirog EC, Levine RL, Ellenson LH. Mutational analysis of the CTNNB1 and APC genes in uterine endometrioid carcinoma. Mod Pathol. 2000;13(10):1066–1071.
38. Moreno-Bueno G, Hardisson D, Sanchez C, et al. Abnormalities of the APC/beta-catenin pathway in endometrial cancer. Oncogene. 2002;21(52):7981–7990.
39. Fukuchi T, Sakamoto M, Tsuda H, Maruyama K, Nozawa S, Hirohashi S. Beta-catenin mutation in carcinoma of the uterine endometrium. Cancer Res. 1998;58(16):3526–3528.
40. Mirabelli-Primdahl L, Gryfe R, Kim H, et al. Beta-catenin mutations are specific for colorectal carcinomas with microsatellite instability but occur in endometrial carcinomas irrespective of mutator pathway. Cancer Res. 1999;59(14):3346–3351.
41. Saegusa M, Hashimura M, Yoshida T, Okayasu I. Beta-catenin mutations and aberrant nuclear expression during endometrial tumorigenesis. Br J Cancer. 2001;84(2):209–217.
42. Sasaki H, Nishii H, Takahashi H, et al. Mutation of the Ki-ras protooncogene in human endometrial hyperplasia and carcinoma. Cancer Res. 1993;53(8):1906–1910.
43. Tsuda H, Jiko K, Yajima M, et al. Frequent occurrence of c-Ki-ras gene mutations in well differentiated endometrial adenocarcinoma showing infiltrative local growth with fibrosing stromal response. Int J Gynecol Pathol. 1995;14(3):255–259.
44. Lagarda H, Catasus L, Arguelles R, Matias-Guiu X, Prat J. K-ras mutations in endometrial carcinomas with microsatellite instability. J Pathol. 2001;193(2):193–199.
45. Caduff RF, Johnston CM, Frank TS. Mutations of the Ki-ras oncogene in carcinoma of the endometrium. Am J Pathol. 1995;146(1):182–188.
46. Ito K, Watanabe K, Nasim S, et al. K-ras point mutations in endometrial carcinoma: effect on outcome is dependent on age of patient. Gynecol Oncol. 1996;63(2):238–246.
47. Rajagopalan H, Bardelli A, Lengauer C, Kinzler KW, Vogelstein B, Velculescu VE. Tumorigenesis: RAF/RAS oncogenes and mismatch-repair status. Nature. 2002;418(6901):934.
48. Feng YZ, Shiozawa T, Miyamoto T, et al. BRAF mutation in endometrial carcinoma and hyperplasia: correlation with KRAS and p53 mutations and mismatch repair protein expression. Clin Cancer Res. 2005;11(17):6133–6138.
49. Mutch DG, Powell MA, Mallon MA, Goodfellow PJ. RAS/RAF mutation and defective DNA mismatch repair in endometrial cancers. Am J Obstet Gynecol. 2004;190(4):935–942.
50. Salvesen HB, Kumar R, Stefansson I, et al. Low frequency of BRAF and CDKN2A mutations in endometrial cancer. Int J Cancer. 2005;115(6):930–934.
51. Pappa KI, Choleza M, Markaki S, et al. Consistent absence of BRAF mutations in cervical and endometrial cancer despite KRAS mutation status. Gynecol Oncol. 2006;100(3):596–600.
52. Risinger JI, Dent GA, Ignar-Trowbridge D, et al. p53 gene mutations in human endometrial carcinoma. Mol Carcinog. 1992;5(4):250–253.
53. Enomoto T, Fujita M, Inoue M, et al. Alterations of the p53 tumor suppressor gene and its association with activation of the c-K-ras-2 protooncogene in premalignant and malignant lesions of the human uterine endometrium. Cancer Res. 1993;53(8):1883–1888.
54. Kihana T, Hamada K, Inoue Y, et al. Mutation and allelic loss of the p53 gene in endometrial carcinoma. Incidence and outcome in 92 surgical patients. Cancer. 1995;76(1):72–78.
55. Swisher EM, Peiffer-Schneider S, Mutch DG, et al. Differences in patterns of TP53 and KRAS2 mutations in a large series of endometrial carcinomas with or without microsatellite instability. Cancer. 1999;85(1):119–126.
56. Sakuragi N, Watari H, Ebina Y, et al. Functional analysis of p53 gene and the prognostic impact of dominant-negative p53 mutation in endometrial cancer. Int J Cancer. 2005;116(4):514–519.

57. Tashiro H, Blazes MS, Wu R, et al. Mutations in PTEN are frequent in endometrial carcinoma but rare in other common gynecological malignancies. Cancer Res. 1997;57(18):3935–3940.
58. Kovalev S, Marchenko ND, Gugliotta BG, Chalas E, Chumas J, Moll UM. Loss of p53 function in uterine papillary serous carcinoma. Hum Pathol. 1998;29(6):613–619.
59. Darvishian F, Hummer AJ, Thaler HT, et al. Serous endometrial cancers that mimic endometrioid adenocarcinomas: a clinicopathologic and immunohistochemical study of a group of problematic cases. Am J Surg Pathol. 2004;28(12):1568–1578.
60. Peiro G, Mayr D, Hillemanns P, Lohrs U, Diebold J. Analysis of HER-2/neu amplification in endometrial carcinoma by chromogenic in situ hybridization. Correlation with fluorescence in situ hybridization, HER-2/neu, p53 and Ki-67 protein expression, and outcome. Mod Pathol. 2004;17(3):227–287.
61. Slomovitz BM, Broaddus RR, Burke TW, et al. Her-2/neu overexpression and amplification in uterine papillary serous carcinoma. J Clin Oncol. 2004;22(15):3126–3132.
62. Santin AD, Bellone S, Van Stedum S, et al. Determination of HER2/neu status in uterine serous papillary carcinoma: comparative analysis of immunohistochemistry and fluorescence in situ hybridization. Gynecol Oncol. 2005;98(1):24–30.
63. Mitelman Database of Chromosome Aberrations in Cancer (2008). Mitelman F, Johansson B, and Mertens F (Eds.), http://cgap.nci.nih.gov/Chromosomes/Mitelman.
64. Micci F, Teixeira MR, Haugom L, Kristensen G, Abeler VM, Heim S. Genomic aberrations in carcinomas of the uterine corpus. Genes Chromosomes Cancer. 2004;40(3):229–246.
65. Wada H, Enomoto T, Fujita M, et al. Molecular evidence that most but not all carcinosarcomas of the uterus are combination tumors. Cancer Res. 1997;57(23):5379–5385.
66. Fujii H, Yoshida M, Gong ZX, et al. Frequent genetic heterogeneity in the clonal evolution of gynecological carcinosarcoma and its influence on phenotypic diversity. Cancer Res. 2000;60(1):114–120.
67. Abeln EC, Smit VT, Wessels JW, de Leeuw WJ, Cornelisse CJ, Fleuren GJ. Molecular genetic evidence for the conversion hypothesis of the origin of malignant mixed mullerian tumours. J Pathol. 1997;183(4):424–431.
68. Soong R, Knowles S, Hammond IG, Michael C, Iacopetta BJ. p53 protein overexpression and gene mutation in mixed Mullerian tumors of the uterus. Cancer Detect Prev. 1999;23(1):8–12.
69. Lancaster JM, Risinger JI, Carney ME, Barrett JC, Berchuck A. Mutational analysis of the PTEN gene in human uterine sarcomas. Am J Obstet Gynecol. 2001;184(6):1051–1053.
70. Amant F, de la Rey M, Dorfling CM, et al. PTEN mutations in uterine sarcomas. Gynecol Oncol. 2002;85(1):165–169.
71. Amant F, Vloeberghs V, Woestenborghs H, et al. ERBB-2 gene overexpression and amplification in uterine sarcomas. Gynecol Oncol. 2004;95(3):583–587.
72. Livasy CA, Reading FC, Moore DT, Boggess JF, Lininger RA. EGFR expression and HER2/neu overexpression/amplification in endometrial carcinosarcoma. Gynecol Oncol. 2006;100(1):101–106.
73. de Vos S, Wilczynski SP, Fleischhacker M, Koeffler P. p53 alterations in uterine leiomyosarcomas versus leiomyomas. Gynecol Oncol. 1994;54(2):205–208.
74. Jeffers MD, Farquharson MA, Richmond JA, McNicol AM. p53 immunoreactivity and mutation of the p53 gene in smooth muscle tumours of the uterine corpus. J Pathol. 1995;177(1):65–70.
75. Teneriello MG, Taylor RR, et al. Analysis of Ki-ras, p53, and MDM2 genes in uterine leiomyomas and leiomyosarcomas. Gynecol Oncol. 1997;65(2):330–335.
76. Quade BJ, Pinto AP, Howard DR, Peters WA, 3rd, Crum CP. Frequent loss of heterozygosity for chromosome 10 in uterine leiomyosarcoma in contrast to leiomyoma. Am J Pathol. 1999;154(3):945–950.
77. Levy B, Mukherjee T, Hirschhorn K. Molecular cytogenetic analysis of uterine leiomyoma and leiomyosarcoma by comparative genomic hybridization. Cancer Genet Cytogenet. 2000;121(1):1–8.
78. Quade BJ, Wang TY, Sornberger K, Dal Cin P, Mutter GL, Morton CC. Molecular pathogenesis of uterine smooth muscle tumors from transcriptional profiling. Genes Chromosomes Cancer. 2004;40(2):97–108.

79. Christacos NC, Quade BJ, Dal Cin P, Morton CC. Uterine leiomyomata with deletions of Ip represent a distinct cytogenetic subgroup associated with unusual histologic features. Genes Chromosomes Cancer. 2006;45(3):304–312.
80. Dal Cin P, Quade BJ, Neskey DM, Kleinman MS, Weremowicz S, Morton CC. Intravenous leiomyomatosis is characterized by a der(14)t(12;14)(q15;q24). Genes Chromosomes Cancer. 2003;36(2):205–206.
81. Patton KT, Cheng L, Papavero V, et al. Benign metastasizing leiomyoma: clonality, telomere length and clinicopathologic analysis. Mod Pathol. 2006;19(1):130–140.
82. Quade BJ, McLachlin CM, Soto-Wright V, Zuckerman J, Mutter GL, Morton CC. Disseminated peritoneal leiomyomatosis. Clonality analysis by X chromosome inactivation and cytogenetics of a clinically benign smooth muscle proliferation. Am J Pathol. 1997;150(6):2153–2166.
83. Ng TL, Gown AM, Barry TS, et al. Nuclear beta-catenin in mesenchymal tumors. Mod Pathol. 2005;18(1):68–74.
84. Hrzenjak A, Tippl M, Kremser ML, et al. Inverse correlation of secreted frizzled-related protein 4 and beta-catenin expression in endometrial stromal sarcomas. J Pathol. 2004;204(1):19–27.
85. Micci F, Walter CU, Teixeira MR, et al. Cytogenetic and molecular genetic analyses of endometrial stromal sarcoma: nonrandom involvement of chromosome arms 6p and 7p and confirmation of JAZF1/JJAZ1 gene fusion in t(7;17). Cancer Genet Cytogenet. 2003;144(2):119–124.
86. Koontz JI, Soreng AL, Nucci M, et al. Frequent fusion of the JAZF1 and JJAZ1 genes in endometrial stromal tumors. Proc Natl Acad Sci U S A. 2001;98(11):6348–6353.
87. Huang HY, Ladanyi M, Soslow RA. Molecular detection of JAZF1-JJAZ1 gene fusion in endometrial stromal neoplasms with classic and variant histology: evidence for genetic heterogeneity. Am J Surg Pathol. 2004;28(2):224–232.
88. Hrzenjak A, Moinfar F, Tavassoli FA, et al. JAZF1/JJAZ1 gene fusion in endometrial stromal sarcomas: molecular analysis by reverse transcriptase-polymerase chain reaction optimized for paraffin-embedded tissue. J Mol Diagn. 2005;7(3):388–395.
89. Micci F, Panagopoulos I, Bjerkehagen B, Heim S. Consistent rearrangement of chromosomal band 6p21 with generation of fusion genes JAZF1/PHF1 and EPC1/PHF1 in endometrial stromal sarcoma. Cancer Res. 2006;66(1):107–112.
90. Nucci MR, Harburger D, Koontz J, Cin PD. Molecular analysis of the JAZF1-JJAZ1 gene fusion by RT-PCR and fluorescence in situ hybridization in endometrial stromal neoplasms. Am J Surg Pathol. 2007;31:65–70.
91. Oliva E, de Leval L, Soslow RA, Herens C. High frequency of JAZF1-JJAZ1 gene fusion in endometrial stromal tumors with smooth muscle differentiation by interphase FISH detection. Am J Surg Pathol. 2007; 31(8):1277–1284.

Prognostic Factors in Uterine Cancer

Patricia M. Baker and Esther Oliva

Abstract Pathologic staging determines the management of patients with endometrial adenocarcinoma and uterine sarcomas following the initial surgery and it is an essential component of the initial assessment. FIGO stage, tumor subtype, grade of differentiation, myometrial invasion, lymphovascular invasion, and other factors that guide the treatment decisions covered in the subsequent chapters are extensively discussed.

Keywords Stage • Myometrial invasion • Differentiation • Histologic subtype • Lymphovascular invasion

Endometrial Carcinoma

Endometrial carcinoma (EC) ranks as the fourth most common malignancy in women and is the most common malignancy in the female reproductive tract, affecting slightly <150,000 women worldwide, with an estimated 40,000 women dying each year (1). Most women are postmenopausal at diagnosis and have an overall 5-year survival rate of approximately 80% (2). Conventional histopathologic evaluation to determine pathologic stage has remained the cornerstone of prognosis and therapy (3).

While EC has a favorable outcome overall, poor outcome in "low-risk" patients assessed by conventional histologic parameters does occur. Newer therapies recognize the need for adjuvant treatment in high-risk patients with an aggressive tumor type or an advanced stage at presentation. The success of adjuvant therapy has generated much interest and work in finding new markers

P. Baker and E. Oliva (✉)
Department of Pathology, Massachusetts General Hospital, Boston, MA
e-mail: eoliva@partners.org

F. Muggia and E. Oliva (eds.), *Uterine Cancer*, Current Clinical Oncology,
DOI: 10.1007/978-1-60327-044-1_6,
© Humana Press, a Part of Springer Science+Business Media, LLC 2009

Table 1. Clinicopathologic prognostic factors in endometrial carcinoma

Confirmed prognostic factors
1. Pathologic stage
2. Histologic grade
3. Histologic type
4. Myometrial invasion
5. Lymphovascular invasion
6. Lymph node metastases
7. Age
Conflicting-possible prognostic factors
1. Serosal involvement
2. Cervical involvement

that are more accurate prognostic indicators. This work parallels the recent knowledge that the molecular biology of tumors is strongly related to aggressiveness, and therefore to patient outcome. The ability to individualize treatment by accurately separating low-risk from high-risk patients is important to improve outcome and avoid potential complications and morbidity of unnecessary treatment in low-risk groups, many of whom are elderly. Clinicopathologic factors to be considered in prognosis are listed in Table 1.

FIGO Stage

The International Federation of Gynecology and Obstetrics (FIGO) stage is the single most powerful prognostic parameter in EC. In its earlier form, FIGO (1971) was a clinical based staging system, where imaging was used to determine depth of invasion, fractional curettage to assess cervical involvement, and pelvic examination to exclude spread beyond the uterus. The surgico-pathologic FIGO stage replaced the clinically based staging system in 1988 (4). It is based on histopathologic examination of a hysterectomy specimen as well as assessment of the peritoneal cavity and ascitic fluid, adnexa, and pelvic and para-aortic lymph nodes (4, 5). It has been shown that the old clinical staging system frequently underestimated surgical stage as the cervical fraction of the D&C specimen was interpreted as positive for adenocarcinoma even though the tumor was found free floating and not attached to cervical tissue; consequently, the patient was automatically assigned to a stage II (6–10). Besides downstaging clinical stage II tumors to surgico-pathologic stage I tumors, the second biggest change occurred with clinical stage III tumors which frequently became pathologic stage IV tumors (10). Staging should be assigned at the time of definitive surgery and prior to administration of adjuvant treatment and should not be changed based on disease progression, recurrence, or response to adjuvant treatment preceding surgical treatment.

Using the surgico-pathologic FIGO staging system, EC is divided into four main stages (Table 2): (I) tumor is confined to the uterine corpus, (II) tumor involves the cervix, (III) tumor extents to the true pelvis, and (IV) tumor is present beyond the true pelvis. Stage I disease is further subclassified into three categories based on depth of myometrial invasion, the latter closely interrelated to prognosis in stage I tumors (3). Stage IA tumors are confined to the endometrium and carry an excellent prognosis with close to 100% overall survival (Fig. 1). Stage IB and

Table 2. Correlation between TNM and FIGO staging systems in endometrial carcinoma

TNM	FIGO	
Tis	0	Carcinoma in situ
T1	I	Tumor confined to corpus
T1a	IA	Tumor limited to endometrium
T1b	IB	Tumor invades <1/2 myometrium
T1c	IC	Tumor invades ≥1/2 myometrium
T2	II	Tumor invades cervix
T2a	IIA	Tumor limited to endocervical glands
T2b	IIB	Invasion of cervical stroma
T3	III	Local and/or regional spread
T3a	IIIA	Tumor involves serosa and/or adnexa and/or positive ascites or washings
T3b	IIIB	Vaginal involvement
T4	IVA	Tumor involves bladder and or bowel mucosa
NX		Regional LNs cannot be assessed
N0		No regional LNs metastases
N1	IIIC	Regional LNs metastases to pelvic and or para-aortic nodes
MX		Distant metastases cannot be assessed
M0		No distant metastases
M1	IVB	Distant metastases (LN metastases other than pelvic or para-aortic) and excludes metastases to vagina, pelvic serosa, or adnexa

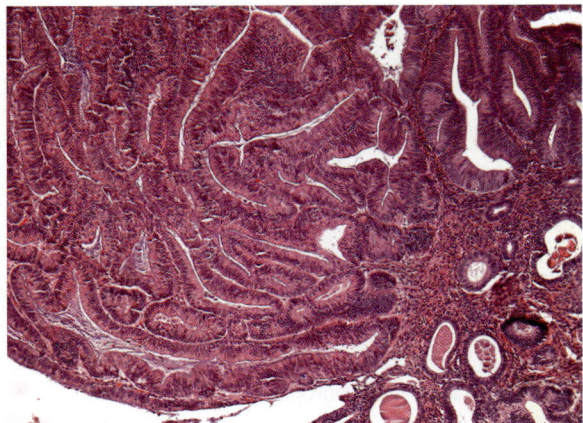

Fig. 1 A well-differentiated endometrioid carcinoma composed of well-formed glands is confined to the endometrium (stage IA).

stage IC tumors show invasion of the inner half or the outer half of the myometrium, respectively. Stage II tumors are divided into two subcategories depending on involvement of the cervical epithelium (IIA) or the cervical stroma (IIB) (Fig. 2). Stage III tumors are further subdivided into three categories; IIIA indicates uterine

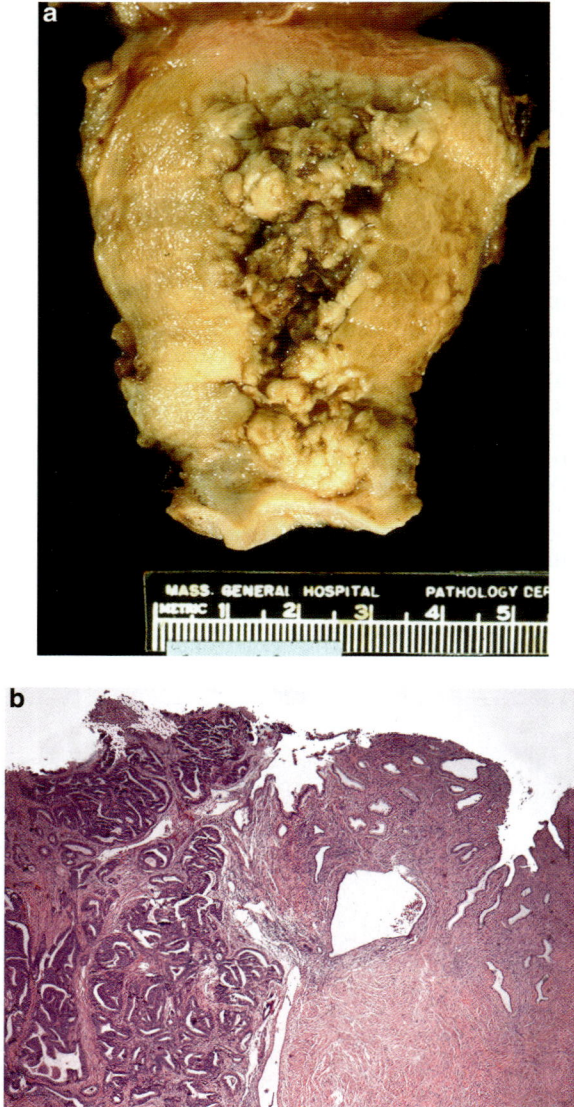

Fig. 2 Secondary involvement by direct extension of the cervix by endometrial carcinoma may be seen grossly (**a**) or only microscopically (**b**) (stage II).

serosal and/or adnexal involvement and/or positive peritoneal cytology (Fig. 3), IIIB tumors involve the vagina either by direct extension or metastases, and IIIC tumors are associated with positive pelvic and/or para-aortic lymph nodes (Fig. 4). Finally, stage IV tumors directly extend to bladder and/or bowel mucosa (IVA) or are associated with distant metastases including intra-abdominal and/or inguinal lymph nodes (IVB) (4). The majority of patients with EC (approximately 70–80%) have stage I tumors at the time of diagnosis, stage II comprises between 5% and 15%, and the remainder have stage III or IV disease (10). Surgico-pathologic staging has proven to be very accurate and has been shown to be the single strongest predictor of survival in multivariate analysis studies (3, 11–16). Even though the overall 5-year survival rate for EC is approximately 75–80%, when stratified by

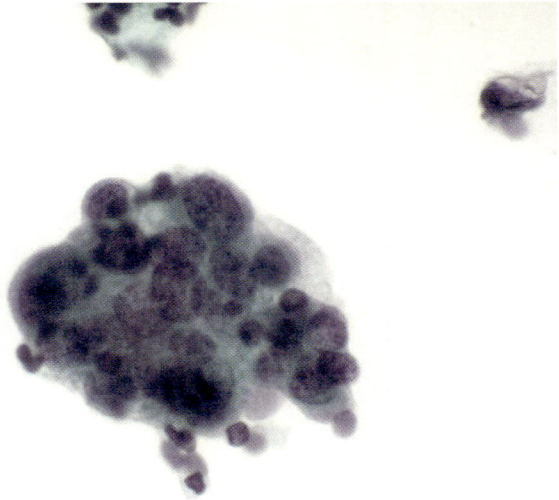

Fig. 3 Malignant epithelial cells forming a large cluster are indicative of a positive ascitic fluid (stage IIIA).

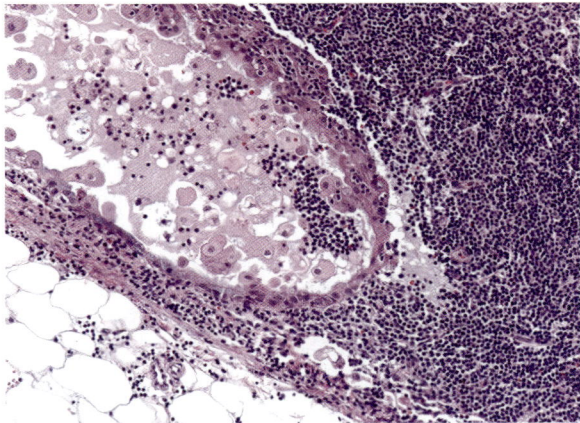

Fig. 4 A neoplastic gland is present in the subcapsular sinus of a lymph node (stage IIIC).

Fig. 5 Moderately differentiated endometrioid carcinoma with solid growth that comprised >5% and <50% of the malignant glandular growth.

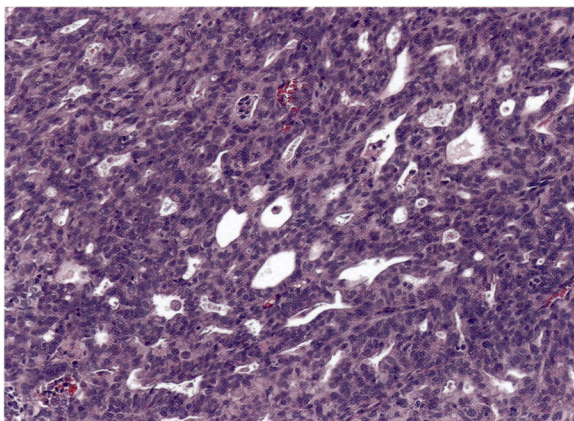

stage, the 5-year survival rate for EC is as follows: 85–90% for stage I tumors, 75% for stage II tumors, and 45% and 25% for stage III and IV tumors, respectively (10, 12, 17). Following this approach, surgically staged patients without extrauterine disease are associated with low recurrence rates, whereas if disease is found outside the uterus, the recurrence rate is close to 50% (18). Although not perfect, this surgico-pathologic staging system allows for the best approach to tailoring treatment of patients with EC.

Histologic Grade

Histologic grade is an important prognostic parameter in EC, especially for endometrioid carcinomas (EECs). However, in some large studies, histologic grade is not as important a prognostic factor as surgico-pathologic stage or myometrial invasion in multivariate analyses, but is closely related to them (3, 12, 19). EECs are graded in a three-tier system based on the amount of solid growth of the glandular component following the FIGO/ISGP surgico-pathologic grading system. EEC grade I shows ≤5% of solid areas (Fig. 1), grade II contains 6–50% of solid areas (Fig. 5), and grade III EEC displays >50% of a solid glandular component (Fig. 6). The squamous component which may be present as keratinizing or morular differentiation should not be taken into account when grading. The 1988 FIGO stage revision incorporated nuclear grade as part of the grading system. However, the definition used at that time was subjective as stated that "notable cytologic atypia, inappropriate for the architectural grade, should raise the grade of a grade I or grade II tumor by one" (Fig. 7) (4). Some investigators have found the interobserver reproducibility acceptable for architectural grade but poor for nuclear grade (20, 21). Only when striking nuclear atypia, defined by large, pleomorphic nuclei with coarse chromatin and large and irregular nucleoli equating nuclear grade 3, is present in a

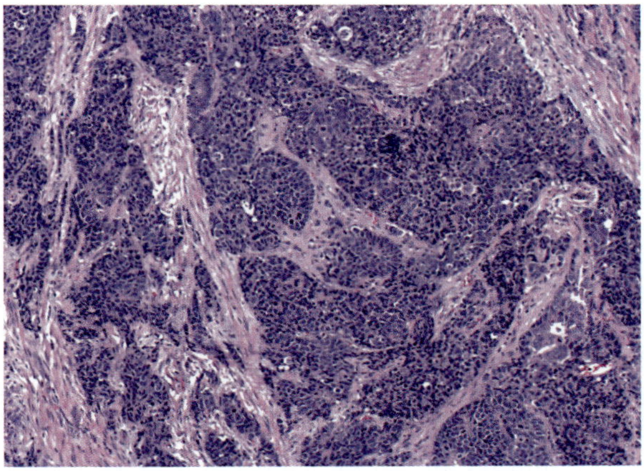

Fig. 6 Poorly differentiated endometrioid carcinoma composed of diffuse solid growth.

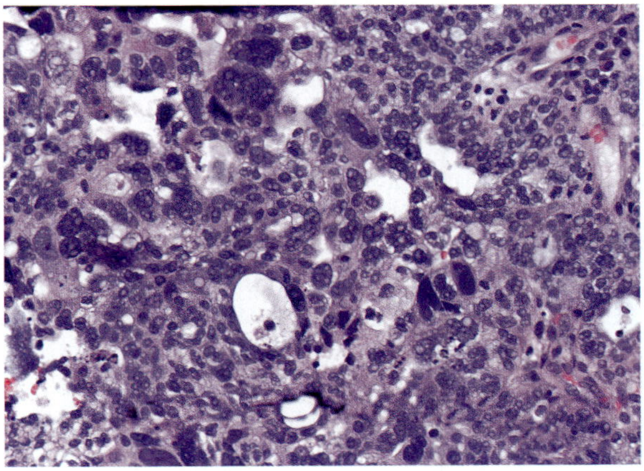

Fig. 7 Endometrioid carcinoma showing marked cytological atypia. The presence of this histologic feature increases the grade of the tumor by one.

grade I or grade II EEC, should the tumor be upgraded to a grade II or III EEC, respectively. Upgrading a grade I EEC when either grade 2 or 3 nuclei are identified results in reassignment of a sizable number of EECs. This may not always be justified, as patients with architectural grade I tumors and grade 2 nuclei have a similar outcome compared with patients with grade I tumors by architecture and cytology (3). The distribution of EEC by grade is approximately as follows: 20–35% grade I, 40–45% grade 2, and 15–30% grade 3 tumors (12, 22, 23). As mentioned earlier, grade is closely related to myometrial invasion, < 10% of grade I tumors invade the outer half of the myometrium while > 40% of grade 3 EECs show invasion of the outer half of the myometrium (12, 19). FIGO grade is also closely related to the risk of lymph node metastases as well as the risk of recurrences (11, 18, 21, 23–25). Grade I EECs are typically associated with a low rate of lymph node metastases and recurrence (2–3% and 4%, respectively) in comparison to grade 3 tumors (23–27% and 40%, respectively) (18, 19). The 5-year survival rate for grade I EEC ranges from 85% to 100% while it decreases to 55% for grade 3 tumors (12, 26, 27). In some studies, the survival rate of grade 3 EEC is comparable to serous papillary and clear cell carcinoma (CCC) (28). Furthermore, in some studies, grade 3 tumors are associated with the highest risk of recurrence among all surgico-pathologic parameters (17).

Recently, two new binary grading systems have been proposed to grade EECs into either low or high grade. The first one uses low-magnification assessment of the amount of solid growth, pattern of invasion, and the presence of necrosis. An EEC is classified as high grade if it has at least two of the following three criteria: (1) > 50% solid growth (without distinction of squamous from nonsquamous epithelium), (2) a diffusely infiltrative, rather than expansive, growth pattern, and (3) tumor cell necrosis. This system separates patients into three prognostically and therapeutically different groups. Patients with stage I low-grade tumors with invasion confined to the inner half of the myometrium (stages IA and IB) have 100% survival rate. Patients with low-grade tumors that invade the outer half of the myometrium (stage IC and stages II–IV) and patients with high-grade tumors with invasion confined to the myometrium (stage IB and IC) have a 5-year survival rate of 67–76% (29). This binary grading system permits greater interobserver and intraobserver reproducibility compared to FIGO and nuclear grading. However, overall, no dramatic differences exist between the two systems (22). A second, more recent system divides EECs into high or low grade based on assessment of the following features: (1) predominantly papillary or solid growth pattern, (2) mitotic index ≥ 6/10 HPFs, and (3) severe nuclear atypia. The presence of at least two of these three criteria results in a tumor being classified as high grade. This system seems more reproducible than FIGO and at the same time is an independent predictor of patient outcome when survival is adjusted for FIGO stage, patient age, and tumor cell type. However, the FIGO grading system is still superior for prognostication in EECs (30). The grading system in serous carcinomas, CCCs, and squamous cell carcinomas is based on nuclear features even though most of these tumors form glands. As these tumors typically display high-grade nuclei, they are classified as grade II or III cancers.

Histologic Type

Cell type is an important prognostic factor in EC (26, 31). A dualistic model to explain the pathogenesis of EC based on cell type was first described by Bockhman (32). Type I tumors represent about 80% of ECs, are typically EECs that develop in pre- or perimenopausal women, are associated with estrogenic stimulation, and frequently coexist or are preceded by endometrial hyperplasia. Most EECs are confined to the uterus at the time of presentation (Fig. 1), display ER positivity, and have a favorable prognosis (33). Squamous differentiation is seen in approximately 25% of EECs. In the past, EECs with squamous differentiation were divided into adenoacanthoma and adenosquamous carcinoma depending on cytologic

Fig. 8 A well-differentiated
endometrioid carcinoma shows
diffuse permeative invasion
(so-called "adenoma maligum").

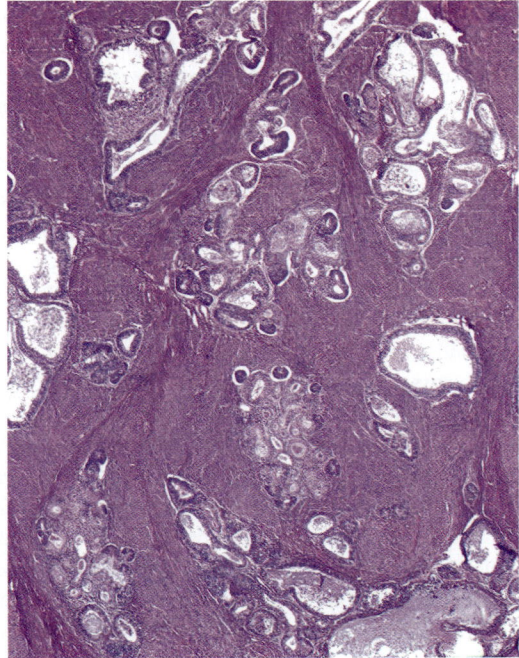

features. Initially it was thought that adenosquamous carcinomas had a poorer
prognosis than adenoacanthomas; however, it has been shown that the degree of
differentiation of the squamous component parallels that of the glandular component in the majority of the cases and that the clinical behavior of EEC with squamous foci is similar to that of conventional EEC (31, 34). There is a subgroup of
EECs that despite being well differentiated show a diffuse infiltrative pattern into
the myometrium (so-called "adenoma malignum") (Fig. 8); in some studies, this
finding is associated with a worse prognosis compared to more well-differentiated
EECs (24, 35–37). Villoglandular adenocarcinoma, considered a variant of EEC,
has been shown by some investigators to behave in a more aggressive manner than
conventional EEC when the papillary component infiltrates into the myometrium.
Higher rates of lymphovascular invasion, lymph node metastases, and a worse
outcome have been found in these type of tumors compared to EEC showing myometrial invasion in the form of glandular or solid patterns (38). However, these
findings have not been corroborated by other investigators who found these
tumors to have a similar behavior to that observed in conventional EEC (39).
Other variants of EECs including those with squamous differentiation, secretory
changes, or ciliated have a similar outcome to that observed in conventional ECC.
Mucinous adenocarcinomas are uncommon and are related to EECs. These are
defined as tumors with > 50% of cells containing mucin (WHO) and have an outcome comparable to conventional EEC (40).

Type II tumors represent about 10% of ECs; this category is largely composed of serous papillary and CCCs. These tumors typically occur in postmenopausal women and are unrelated to estrogen exposure, developing from atrophic endometrium or occurring in endometrial polyps (41) or from the putative precancerous lesion "endometrial intraepithelial carcinoma" (42). They are very aggressive, often with myometrial or lymphovascular invasion, and carry a poor prognosis (43–49). In fact, in a recent series, up to 70% of women have been shown to have extrauterine disease (45). Even patients with stage I serous carcinomas have an overall survival of 30% ranging from 54% to 72% and from 27% to 59% in stage I and stage II tumors, respectively (15, 44, 45, 50). However, some recent studies have shown that patients with stage I serous papillary carcinoma have a better prognosis (51). These tumors are responsible for 50% of all relapses that occur in ECs and surgical staging is extremely important as up to 58% of clinically stage I tumors may be upstaged surgically (46, 52). These tumors are associated with p53 mutations, are ER negative, and show a high degree of chromosomal instability (53). Some investigators have hypothesized that non-EECs may arise from two different pathways: (1) de novo through p53 mutations, LOH at several loci, or by another still unknown gene alterations; or (2) through dedifferentiation of a preexisting EEC (54). This, in fact, may explain EC with endometrioid and serous components, and additionally may explain why high-grade EECs behave more like serous and CCCs, as they may have similar molecular alterations but may not have yet switched phenotypes. It is important to recognize and report any foci of serous carcinoma as it is prognostically significant.

Clear cell carcinoma is also considered a type II carcinoma, associated with an aggressive behavior and poor outcome with an overall 5- and 10-year survival rates of 42% and 31%, respectively (26, 49). Myometrial invasion occurs in approximately 80% and lymphovascular invasion in about 25% of CCCs (15, 55, 56). As reported for serous carcinoma, CCC is associated with a high incidence of extrapelvic disease. In contrast to the peritoneal spread seen in serous carcinoma, the distribution of recurrent disease does not have a distinctive pattern but includes intra-abdominal and retroperitoneal organs as well as distant sites (55). Some studies have also shown that patients with CCC confined to the uterine corpus and without extension to the cervix did significantly better than patients with same stage serous carcinoma (55).

Squamous cell carcinomas and transitional cell carcinomas are rare tumors and their prognosis may be related to tumor stage. Stage II–IV squamous cell carcinomas carry a poor prognosis (57), while transitional cell carcinomas seem not to have a more aggressive behavior than conventional EC (58). Other rare carcinomas, including small cell carcinoma and undifferentiated carcinoma are typically associated with poor outcome (59–61).

Myometrial Invasion

The depth of myometrial invasion often has an inverse relationship to the degree of tumor differentiation and has been shown to be a strong (18, 24, 26, 62, 63) and often independent prognostic risk factor based on multivariate analysis in several studies (3, 10, 12, 23).

In the FIGO (1988) staging system, the presence or absence of myometrial invasion and the depth of the invasion define stage I. The histologic features of myometrial invasion include irregularly shaped endometrial glands that are unaccompanied by stroma, often appearing "naked" within the myometrial smooth muscle, lying below the level of the endomyometrial junction, which is by nature very irregular. On occasion, the infiltrative nature of the glands is recognized by an adjacent desmoplastic appearing stroma containing scattered inflammatory cells (64). Failure to recognize the very irregular, undulating nature of the endomyometrial junction may result in the diagnosis of a noninvasive carcinoma as invasive (Fig. 9). The depth of invasion may be overestimated if carcinoma involving adenomyotic foci, rather than true myometrial invasion, is not recognized. Studies have shown that carcinoma involving adenomyosis does not adversely affect prognosis (65–67). Foci of adenomyosis are felt to represent deep herniation of endometrium into the myometrium with continuity to the surface. Residual benign endometrial glands or stroma and lack of a desmoplastic reaction are helpful in identifying adenomyotic foci involved by carcinoma. Very rarely, carcinoma may arise in adenomyosis in the absence of carcinoma in the endometrium and the prognosis in these cases is the same as carcinoma confined to the endometrium (65).

FIGO (1988) separates stage I myoinvasive tumors into those confined to the inner one-half (1B) and those involving the outer one-half (1C); however, other methods of measuring the depth of myometrial invasion have been suggested. These methods include division of the myometrium into thirds or measurement of the distance of the invasive tumor from the uterine serosa. One study found the tumor-free distance from the serosa to be a more accurate predictor of survival than depth of invasion (68). A recent study confirmed the validity of the FIGO (1988) staging system by showing that myometrial invasion in stage IB, defined as < one-third, compared with invasion > one-third but < one-half, showed no statistical difference in outcome (69). No conclusion or consensus has been reached as to the best method of measuring depth of invasion.

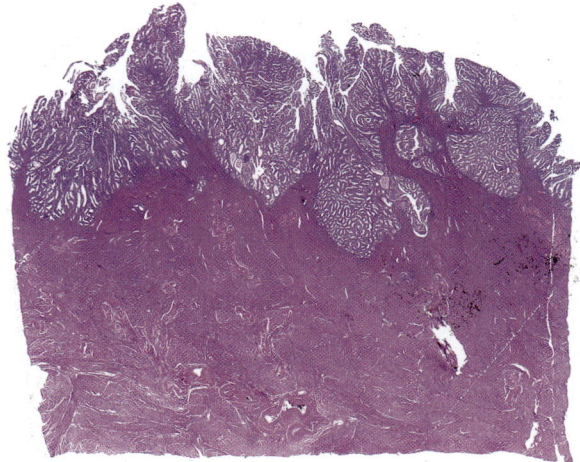

Fig. 9 A well-differentiated endometrioid carcinoma is filling the irregular endomyometrial junction. This phenomenon should not be misinterpreted as myometrial invasion.

A large study of women with EC showed the overall 5-year survival rate to be 94% when tumor was confined to the endometrium, while it decreased to 59% with tumor involving the outer one-third of the myometrium (70). Also, the importance of accurately assessing myometrial invasion is underscored by the fact that pelvic and para-aortic lymph node dissection is in part determined by the degree of invasion. Studies have suggested that the use of intraoperative frozen section to determine depth of invasion (71), particularly in high-grade carcinomas, is more accurate than gross intraoperative assessment alone (71–73). Low-grade carcinomas may be associated with lymph node involvement particularly when deep myometrial invasion is present. The depth of invasion can often be accurately assessed by gross examination, particularly in low-grade tumors (74), while the depth of invasion in high-grade tumors may be difficult to assess grossly. Finally, a recent study involving 80 women with stage I EC determined that the presence of lower uterine segment involvement does not correlate with outcome (75).

Cervical Involvement

Cervical involvement was added to FIGO staging in 1963 based on the results of fractional dilation and curettage. Since then, many authors have commented on the inaccuracy of clinical staging in detecting cervical involvement in EC (8, 76, 77). A 52% false positive rate for predicting cervical invasion by endocervical curettage was found in one series (6), and in another, endocervical curettage was found to have a 50% false positive rate and a 13% false negative rate (8).

Overall, cervical involvement is present in 9–32% of ECs (78, 79). It may be the result of contiguous extension (Fig. 2a, b) or due to lymphovascular spread (76, 79). One study noted that free-floating tumors so-called "tumor migrants" were often seen in association with cervical involvement and this relationship was found to be statistically significant in that "tumor migrants" were found to be more often associated with high-grade tumors such as serous carcinoma (79). Some investigators found a statistically worse outcome for women with cervical stromal invasion compared with those with endocervical glandular involvement (6), while others have suggested no significant difference in outcome between women with stage IIA and IIB EC (76, 80).

Several conflicting reports on the prognostic significance of cervical involvement are found in the literature. This may be due, in part, to the fact that some studies included patients that were clinically rather than surgically staged, had received preoperative radiation therapy, or had stage III or IV disease (6). Others have found cervical involvement to be an independent prognostic indicator on multivariate analysis (81), and due to this controversy, as well as the lack of controlled prospective trials, the optimal management for stage II patients has yet to be determined (82).

Finally, in exceptional cases, an independent, primary endocervical adenocarcinoma may be found in women with EC (83). In cases where this possibility is considered, additional sections to show continuity between the endocervical and endometrial tumors, or immunohistochemical studies to differentiate between the two are usually helpful.

Age

Most ECs occur in females who are postmenopausal and older than 50 years. Several studies support age as an independent, nontumor factor strongly related to prognosis (3, 12, 81, 84, 85). A recent study found age > 70 years to be an independent predictor of local disease recurrence as well as overall survival. This study also found age to be independent of other poor prognostic factors including tumor type or deep myometrial invasion (81). This finding was supported by other investigators who found age to be a significant predictor of poor outcome even in patients with CCC (15). Some investigators have suggested that poor outcome in elderly patients is due to an association with high-grade tumors and less-aggressive therapy (86). It has also been found that poor outcomes in women of advanced age are not due to treatment toxicities (81).

In summary, many studies support the finding that EC is intrinsically more aggressive in older patients and in some studies age seems to be a specific, significant, and independent predictor of outcome (3, 12, 24, 81, 87–89).

Lymphovascular Invasion

Lymphovascular invasion has been reported to occur in approximately one-quarter of ECs (90–92) with a considerable range of frequencies up to 37% (22). This variability may be due in part to differences in the criteria used to diagnose lymphovascular invasion as well as to interobserver variation. Mimics of lymphovascular invasion, such as retraction artifact around invasive tumor nests within the myometrium can be diagnostically challenging, and the use of immunohistochemical studies to highlight vascular endothelium have been found to be of help (24, 93). As well, a greater frequency of lymphovascular invasion has been found in high-grade EECs and tumors of serous and clear cell types in some series. For example, lymphovascular invasion has been noted in 42% of poorly differentiated tumors and in 2% of well-differentiated tumors (94). Several studies have looked at the strength of lymphovascular invasion as a predictor of pelvic lymph node metastasis and/or recurrent disease as well as whether lymphovascular invasion should be used to determine the need for pelvic lymph node sampling or adjuvant therapy. Lymphovascular invasion has been found to be an independent prognostic factor (22, 24, 87, 91–99). Furthermore, investigators have shown that lymphovascular invasion significantly increases the risk of pelvic lymph node metastasis compared to cancers with no lymphovascular invasion for all FIGO grades and depths of myometrial invasion (92).

Finally, perivascular lymphocytic infiltrates and associated changes have been noted to be associated with lymphovascular invasion. In one study, lymphovascular invasion and/or perivascular associated infiltrates were not found to be independent prognostic variables, but proved to be the best predictors of pelvic lymph node metastasis in a multivariate analysis (90). In another study, lymphovascular invasion was found in 12% of cases and perivascular lymphocytic infiltrates in 20%, with the latter being present in 93% of cases with lymphovascular invasion. The authors found this feature to be an independent poor prognostic factor on multivariate analysis (93). It is noteworthy that not all authors have found perivascular lymphocytic infiltrates to be associated with an unfavorable outcome. It can be hypothesized that this finding may reflect a favorable immune response by the host, at least in some cases (24, 100).

Stage IIIA

Stage IIIA combines three very diverse prognostic indicators, namely adnexal involvement, serosal invasion, and positive peritoneal cytology. The number of patients presenting with stage IIIA is small, and studies show conflicting data regarding the prognostic significance of each (101). In stage IIIA, poor outcome appears to be related to coexistent risk factors, such as unfavorable histology, deep myometrial invasion, lymphovascular invasion, or other sites of metastatic disease.

Adnexal involvement occurs in approximately 7% of patients with EC (23). Solitary adnexal involvement, which refers to adnexal metastasis as the only site of extrauterine spread, has been found in 2–3% of patients (102). The exact mechanism of spread has been debated, with several theories emerging. A close association between adnexal involvement and positive peritoneal washings has been recognized, and for this reason, transtubal spread is felt to be responsible for the majority of cases of ovarian or fallopian tube involvement. Direct extension of tumor through the uterine wall or lymphovascular spread likely accounts for a much smaller number of cases (Fig. 10). Finally, a synchronous primary ovarian and uterine carcinoma may occur, and this possibility, should on occasion, be considered. Criteria proposed by Ulbright and Roth suggests that metastasis is typically associated with bilateral ovarian involvement, small ovaries, a multinodular pattern of growth, and lymphovascular invasion (103).

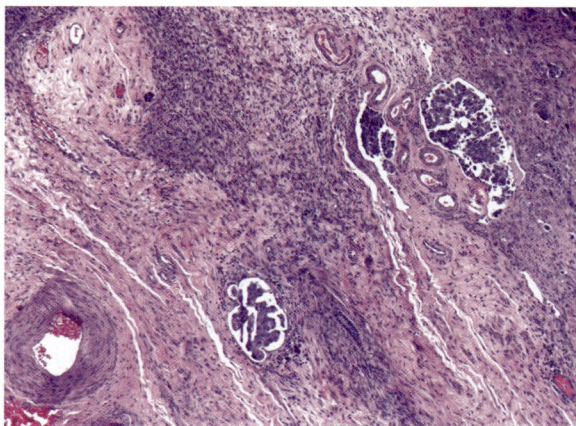

Fig. 10 An endometrial carcinoma shows lymphovascular permeation of the ovary (stage IIIA).

While many studies report that patients with adnexal involvement have a relatively poor prognosis (102, 104–106), the 5-year survival rate is generally more favorable than that expected for stage III disease, if this is the only site of extrauterine spread (17, 102, 105, 107). In fact, some investigators found that the incidence of adnexal involvement increased when other known pathologic risk factors were present; a poor outcome in patients with adnexal involvement seemed to be a result of other coexistent prognostic indicators (102). Adnexal involvement has generally not been found to be an independent prognostic factor on multivariable analysis with the exception of a few studies (106, 108).

Serosal involvement defined as disease extending through the myometrium into the uterine serosa is uncommon, occurring in about 7% of patients (109), with a range of frequencies reported between 3% and 16% (106, 110). When present, it is associated with a significant risk of recurrence and a poor outcome, even if it is the only site of extrauterine disease (26, 109). Solitary serosal involvement, defined as the only site of extrauterine disease, has an outcome that is significantly better than serosal involvement with disease at other extrauterine sites (109). Overall, isolated serosal involvement has a worse outcome than either isolated adnexal involvement (102, 107) or isolated positive peritoneal cytology (111, 112).

Positive peritoneal cytology occurs in approximately 15% of ECs (113) and the prognostic significance of peritoneal cytology is controversial, with variable results in the literature (Fig. 3). Isolated positive peritoneal cytology, defined as the only evidence of extrauterine spread, has not been found to significantly affect survival. A recent study found the 5-year survival rate to be > 90%, even in patients with positive peritoneal cytology (114). This finding is often found in conjunction with other adverse prognostic factors. Most studies have not found peritoneal cytology to be an independent prognostic factor (95, 105, 111–116). However, some investigators found positive peritoneal cytology to be a strong prognostic indicator, while others found it to be an independent prognostic factor by multivariate analysis (85, 117–119). Peritoneal cytology and preoperative serum CA125 have also been found to be independent prognostic factors in stage II–IV disease (119).

In summary, the balance of the literature suggests that positive peritoneal cytology is often associated with other known poor prognostic factors and probably has little or no significant effect on prognosis as an isolated finding of extrauterine disease (101, 120).

Lymph Nodes

Lymph node metastases have a strong (17–19, 23) and often independent (90, 121–123) prognostic significance in patients with EC (Fig. 4). Despite its importance, precise guidelines outlining the type or extent of lymph node assessment required to properly stage a patient have not been provided. Methods of lymph node

assessment have included palpation with biopsy of suspicious nodes, selective
sampling of multiple sites, limited sampling of < four sites or complete, systematic
pelvic and para-aortic lymphadenectomy (123–126). Intraoperative assessment of
lymph nodes by palpation is inaccurate, as < 10% of patients with metastases have
grossly enlarged lymph nodes (19). Larson found 13% of positive lymph nodes to
be normal on palpation (125). Arango found 36% of positive lymph nodes to be
missed on palpation (127), while Chuang and Boronow found approximately 50%
of metastases to be missed by palpation (23, 123).

The practice of routine, systematic pelvic and para-aortic lymphadenectomy
potentially places patients at risk for morbidity, particularly those that are elderly,
obese, or have preexisting medical conditions. In one study, low-risk patients
(grade I histology with or without myometrial invasion or grade II or III tumors
without myometrial invasion and excluding serous and CCC) had < 5% chance
of lymph node metastasis while the high-risk group (grade III tumors with invasion into the outer one-third of the myometrium) had > 10% risk of lymph node
metastasis. The remaining patients, with a few exceptions due to limited experience, including grade II and III tumors and/or tumors having inner or mid muscle
invasion had a moderate risk of lymph node metastasis (19). In the same study
the relative risk of pelvic and para-aortic node involvement increased to 25% and
17%, respectively, for deep muscle invasion (19). In general, pelvic lymph node
metastases have been found to be highly predictive of para-aortic lymph node
involvement (23). Creasman and Mariani found only 2% of para-aortic lymph
nodes to be positive when patients had negative pelvic lymph nodes, while
Yokoyama et al. found a slightly higher rate of 8% positivity in para-aortic lymph
nodes with negative pelvic nodes (19, 126, 128). A significant number of stage I
patients have been found to have pelvic and para-aortic lymph node metastases
(19, 126). In one study, multivariate analysis found only two independent factors
predictive of para-aortic metastasis: positive pelvic lymph nodes and lymphovascular space invasion (129). Some investigators have suggested that surgical evaluation of para-aortic lymph nodes could be limited to those patients with suspicious
nodes on palpation or high-risk factors such as positive pelvic lymph nodes, gross
adnexal involvement, grade II or III tumors, or outer one-third myometrial invasion (17). A range of positivity from 10% to 80% has been found in para-aortic
lymph nodes (17, 19, 125, 126, 128, 129, 130). This variability may in part be
due to the incidence of serous or clear cell tumors in the series as well as to the
extent of sampling.

The need for routine lymph node dissection in the treatment of stage I EC is
controversial. Recently, it has been suggested that lymph node dissection (pelvic
and para-aortic) could safely be avoided in low-risk patients having EEC, either
grade I or II with < 50% invasion, and tumor < 2 cm in maximal dimension (130).
In a study of 607 patients, survival for all patients with retroperitoneal lymph node
dissection (pelvic and/or para-aortic) was 77% at 3 years and 65% at 5 years; however, it did not find survival to be statistically different for patients with positive
para-aortic nodes compared to patients with only positive pelvic lymph nodes.

For patients with para-aortic lymph node involvement, the 3- and 5-year survival rates were 70% and 62%, respectively, versus 87% and 69% for patients with only positive pelvic lymph nodes. When patients with IIIC disease were separated into those with positive peritoneal cytology or adnexal involvement, a marked reduction in survival for patients with nodal and extranodal disease compared to those with nodal disease only was shown (130).

A therapeutic benefit of lymphadenectomy was found in patients both in low-risk and high-risk groups (124, 131). Mariani et al. noted that para-aortic lymphadenectomy may have a therapeutic effect in select patients with positive lymph nodes (128). Similarly, Lutman found that in patients with stage I and II disease, a lymph node count of 12 or greater was an important positive prognostic variable (132). Despite the therapeutic benefit found by these two studies, most investigators have found lymphadenectomy to be of prognostic value only.

Finally, Girardi et al. noted that approximately 37% of metastatic tumors are < 2 cm and have suggested that submission of the entire lymph node for histologic examination with stepwise sectioning improves tumor detection (133), while other investigators have suggested that small metastatic tumor emboli can be better detected by immunohistochemistry, particularly cytokeratin (134, 135). These approaches are time consuming and costly and are not currently recommended.

The role of sentinel lymph node in EC remains controversial as there is limited experience with this technique and lymphatic drainage from the uterus is variable with no anatomically defined lymph node basin. It seems very unlikely based on the present knowledge that sampling of sentinel lymph mode(s) will have a significant impact on clinical management of EC (136).

DNA Ploidy

DNA analysis with either flow cytometry or image cytometry measures the quantity of nuclear DNA present in cells, and can therefore be used to measure the number of copies of DNA present in tumors (137). Differences exist between flow and image cytometry with each having advantages and disadvantages. Both methods can be performed on formalin-fixed paraffin-embedded tissue or on fresh single-cell suspensions. Image cytometry requires a microscopic analysis of Feulgen-stained cells; this technique results in fewer cells being analyzed and a greater ability to separate tumor cells from normal cells. In contrast, flow cytometry can analyze large numbers of cells but does not separate neoplastic from normal cells. This method can also be used to calculate the fraction of cells in the S-phase. While there is an 80% agreement between the two methods, small aneuploid populations detected by image cytometry can be missed by flow cytometry which often measures large numbers of normal cells resulting in diploid DNA patterns. As a general principle, tumors that are diploid are less aggressive than tumors that are nondiploid or aneuploid.

Britton et al. found nondiploid DNA patterns in 13% of patients with EECs compared to 55% in non-EECs, with the corresponding 5-year progression-free survival being 91% and 35%, respectively (138). They also used DNA ploidy to stratify patients with low-grade tumors and found the estimated 5-year survival to be significantly different between diploid (94%) and nondiploid neoplasms (64%). In the same study, patients with favorable endometrioid tumors having diploid patterns versus those with nondiploid patterns had estimated 5-year survivals of 93% and 74%, respectively (138). Several investigators have found DNA ploidy to be an independent prognostic indicator on multivariate analysis (138–143), while the prognostic significance of ploidy has not been supported by other studies (144–146).

The balance of data suggests that DNA ploidy is an independent, objective predictor of outcome in patients with EC. Moreover, its use in stratifying patients considered to be low risk based on more traditional prognostic factors may identify patients at risk of recurrence (138).

Estrogen and Progesterone Receptors

The importance of ER and PR in the pathogenesis and treatment of EC has been recognized for many years. In general, the range of positivity for ER varies from 60% to 100% and for PR from 50% to 88%. Approximately 40–80% of tumors contain both receptors (Fig. 11a, b), while tumors having neither represent the minority (10–36%) (147). Type I EC, which includes endometrioid and mucinous carcinomas, is related to estrogen stimulation unopposed by progesterone; these tumors usually express ER and PR. It has been shown that in patients with stage I EC, receptor status is a significant independent prognostic factor (145, 148–152). Although many studies have shown a relationship between ER/PR status and other prognostic factors, this has not been found to be consistent. In type II EC (serous and clear cell), the levels of ER and PR are usually negative or much lower than those observed in type I EC (153–155). Recurrence in patients with stage I disease is significantly more common in PR or ER negative tumors (156). An important consideration is the inherent problem in evaluating ER and PR status, which is due to the lack of a quantitative standard for the measurement of these receptors by immunohistochemical methods (157). Recent studies have looked at ER isoforms and have found that most EECs express ERα alone or in combination with ERβ. It has been suggested that the ERβ/ERα ratio significantly increases in neoplastic compared to normal endometrium. It has also been found that the ERβ/ERα ratio increases in atypical hyperplasia and adenocarcinoma and decreases in hyperplasia without atypia. The finding that the ERβ/ERα ratio is very high in invasive ECs has led some authors to suggest that ERβ may play an important role in the progression of myometrial invasion (157). Similar results have been found when looking at the A and B PR isoforms, as increasing expression of the B isoform seems to play a role in EC (158).

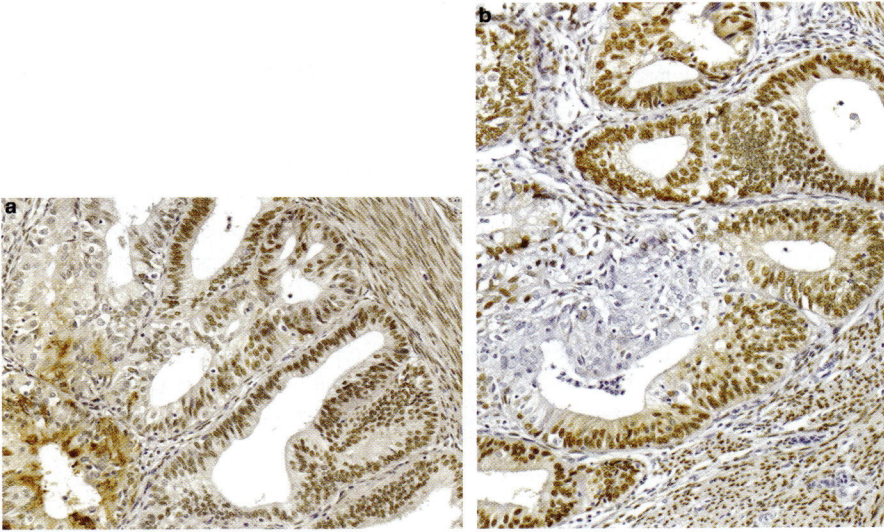

Fig. 11 A well-differentiated endometrioid endometrial carcinoma shows nuclear positivity for *ER* (**a**) and *PR* (**b**).

c-erb-B2 (HER-2/neu)

The human epidermal growth factor receptor-2 (HER-2/neu), also known as c-erb-B2, is located on 17q21 and encodes a transmembrane glycoprotein with tyrosine kinase activity, which is partially homologous to the epidermal growth factor receptor. As such, amplification results in large amounts of receptor on the cell surface with activation of signal transduction pathways, cellular proliferation, and/or neoplastic transformation. Recent interest in this marker is due to its potential role in patient treatment. HER-2/neu amplification has been identified in 10–20% of ECs and tissue overexpression in 10–30% of cases. The role of HER-2/neu overexpression as a prognostic indicator in EC is speculative, with conflicting data, some of which show an association with aggressive biologic behavior and poor survival (159–162). Other studies have shown HER-2/neu expression not to be associated with clinicopathologic factors and in general with prognosis (163–168). HER-2/neu in EC seems to be more frequently observed in CCC, but when correlated with clinical features is not associated with stage or outcome (169, 170).

p53

p53 is a tumor suppressor gene that encodes a nuclear transcription factor involved in cell cycle arrest and apoptosis. It is the most commonly mutated tumor suppressor gene in malignancies. It is felt that mutations in p53 provide fertile soil for additional mutations in the development of tumor. In particular, in type I EC, p53 mutations occur late in tumor development and in a relatively low percentage of tumors (approximately 20%), being more frequently expressed in grade 3 EEC (171). In contrast, p53 is an early event in serous carcinoma and is expressed in the vast majority of these tumors (up to 100%) and in endometrial intraepithelial carcinoma, the putative precursor lesion of serous carcinoma (47, 48, 171). p53 expression is much less frequent in CCCs with only approximately 25% of tumors showing strong positivity (153, 172). p53 has been found to be a strong independent predictor of survival by some investigators (164, 168); however, other studies have not found it to be an independent prognostic parameter (16, 47, 173). In one study, p53 immunostaining was found to be a prognostic indicator independent of patient age and tumor stage; however, when FIGO grade and cell type were included, it lost its predictive value (173). Overall, while p53 overexpression is of prognostic significance in EC, its clinical importance, especially as a single marker, is unclear in patient management.

Bcl-2

Bcl-2 is a proto-oncogene that inhibits programmed cell death or apoptosis. Bcl-2 is normally expressed in the endometrium in a hormone-dependent manner with higher expression in the proliferative phase. Bcl-2 expression is also detected in endometrial hyperplasia but it diminishes in EC. The relationship between the loss of bcl-2 expression and the aggressiveness of EC is a seemingly contradictory one. The mechanism of downregulation of bcl-2 in advanced EC is largely unknown. Loss of bcl-2 expression has been associated with poor prognosis (174–177). Patients with grade 1 or 2 EEC overexpressing bcl-2 are more likely to present with extrauterine disease than those not expressing bcl-2 (178).

Pten

The tumor suppressor gene PTEN (phosphatase and tensin homologue detected from chromosome 10), located on chromosome 10q, plays an important role as a negative regulator of the AKT growth survival pathway (179, 180). PTEN mutations occur almost exclusively in EECs ranging in frequency from 37% to 61%, being only seen in up to 5% of type II ECs (179, 181, 182). In contrast to other tumors where PTEN mutations are associated with poor prognosis, in EC, it is frequently seen in early-stage disease and commonly coexists with endometrial hyperplasia, suggesting that PTEN mutations are an early event in the development of EEC (179, 182). PTEN mutations are frequently present in tumors with microsatellite instability and those lacking p53 overexpression (179–181, 183). Recently, it has been noted that PTEN-positive staining is an indicator of longer survival in patients with advanced EC who received postoperative chemotherapy (184).

K-ras

K-ras encodes a protein (p21) located on the inner plasma cell membranes which has GTPase activity and is involved in cell receptor signal transduction pathways. K-ras mutations occur more frequently in codons 12 and 13 of exon 1 and have been detected in 10–30% of ECs, being quite rare in type II tumors (48). K-ras has been identified in 4–23% of atypical hyperplasias and is also present in nonatypical hyperplasia (185–187). K-ras may correlate with tumor progression and represents an early neoplastic event; however, K-ras mutations are not related to other prognostic factors or survival in most studies (185, 186, 188).

Microsatellite Instability

Microsatellites are short repeat DNA sequences that occur throughout the genome and because of their repetitive sequences are prone to mutations during DNA replication. The majority of these mutations are recognized and fixed by the DNA mismatch repair family of genes. When these genes are mutated, the microsatellites show alterations in size, a phenomenon known as microsatellite instability (MI) which occurs in approximately 20% of ECs (48, 54). MI has been detected in 20–30% of sporadic ECs and in 75% of EC associated with hereditary nonpolyposis colon cancer (HNPCC). In women with HNPCC, EC is often the first manifestation of the disease. These tumors are frequently poorly differentiated, show lymphovascular invasion, and present with high FIGO stage (189). In sporadic ECs, MI has been associated in some studies with a favorable outcome in EECs, even when accounting for other prognostic factors (190). However, in general, MI does not seem to have any definitive association with grade, stage, depth of invasion, hormonal status, or survival (54, 183, 191–197).

β-Catenin

β-catenin is involved in cell to cell adhesion forming complexes with e-cadherin and is important in the maintenance of tissue architecture and cell polarity. β-catenin mutations have been found in approximately 15–40% of low-grade EECs and in atypical hyperplasia, more frequently when squamous differentiation is present (198–200). β-catenin mutations are very rare in type II ECs. In the majority of cases, the presence of β-catenin mutations do not correlate with age, hormonal status, grade, or stage (199). However, a few series have shown an association with early onset (201), low-tumor grade, and the absence of lymph node metastases (202).

Uterine Sarcomas

Malignant mesenchymal tumors of the uterus do not have their own staging system. Thus, the modified FIGO 1988 criteria for EC are used by most pathologists to stage these tumors. In variance to EC, malignant mesenchymal tumors originating in the uterine cervix are considered stage II tumors.

Malignant Smooth Muscle Tumor (Leiomyosarcoma)

Leiomyosarcomas have an overall poor prognosis. Multiple studies have looked at individual prognostic factors and their effects on survival, including age, tumor size, cytologic atypia, mitotic activity, tumor cell necrosis, lymphovascular invasion, type of tumor margin, and extrauterine extension. Only tumor grade (203, 204), mitotic count (205–209), and tumor stage (204, 210–214) have consistently been reported as significant predictors of survival in leiomyosarcomas. In the largest and most recent study of 208 patients with leiomyosarcoma, parameters that were associated with increased overall survival by univariate analysis included age (<51 years), smaller tumor size (≤5 cm), low-grade, and low-stage disease at the time of diagnosis. However, when these parameters were entered into a multivariate analysis, only low grade and low stage remained as independent prognostic factors of survival (203).

Several studies have reported that epithelioid and myxoid leiomyosarcomas are associated with a more aggressive behavior compared to leiomyosarcomas of conventional type (215–217). Because of the rarity of these tumors, criteria predictive of behavior are less well established.

ER and PR expression in leiomyosarcomas is diminished when compared to benign smooth muscle tumors. Approximately 30–50% of uterine leiomyosarcomas express ER and PR. One study has also shown androgen receptor expression in these tumors. Several studies have found tumors positive for steroid receptors to be associated with better prognosis than tumors with negative steroid receptors (204, 214, 218). However, results in the literature are not uniform and some investigators have not found correlation of ER and PR with other prognostic parameters and no influence on disease-free or overall survival (219).

Patients with positive lymph nodes typically also show extrauterine disease. The incidence of lymph node metastases in patients with disease confined to the uterus is 2.5% (207, 220). Therapeutic lymph node sampling does not seem to have a role in increasing the free survival rate in patients with leiomyosarcoma. Only patients with clinically suspicious lymph nodes should undergo lymph node dissection (221).

Several studies have suggested DNA ploidy, S-phase, p53, bcl-2, and c-kit, among others, as potential prognostic parameters (213, 222–230). Further studies are necessary to establish these markers as routine markers for improved prognosis in malignant smooth muscle tumors.

Low-grade Müllerian Adenosarcoma

Myometrial invasion, therefore stage, and sarcomatous overgrowth are the only two independent prognostic parameters that determine survival in these tumors. Several studies have found that among patients with myometrial invasion, those with outer half invasion had a poorer outcome (231–233). In the only study of sarcomatous overgrowth in low-grade müllerian adenosarcomas, this feature was strongly related to postoperative recurrence and metastases and fatal outcome (234). Even though adenosarcomas with heterologous elements were initially thought to be associated with worse prognosis, the presence of this feature was not found to be statistically significant (233).

Malignant Mixed Müllerian Tumor (Carcinosarcoma)

Malignant mixed müllerian tumors are among the most aggressive uterine tumors associated with an overall poor prognosis and a 5-year survival rate ranging from 20% to 35% for all stages despite aggressive treatment (235–237).

Even though initially malignant mixed müllerian tumors were included among sarcomas, more recent data suggests that these tumors behave similarly to high-grade carcinomas (238). In fact, some authors have reported that malignant mixed müllerian tumors have a worse prognosis than high-grade carcinomas (239, 240). Stage is the single and strongest prognostic factor in this malignancy (205, 207, 241–249). In tumors confined to the uterus, survival is related to the degree of myometrial invasion (205, 207, 238, 242, 247–249). In some studies, nuclear grade of the carcinoma component (248, 250), patient age (243), and presence of gross residual disease (243, 247, 249) have also been found to have prognostic significance.

Other histologic variables such as type and grade of the sarcomatous elements (238, 248) do not seem to have any prognostic significance. The prognostic importance of lymphovascular invasion is unclear (207, 238, 243, 247), but it is suggested that it should be documented in the surgical report (238).

Positive peritoneal cytology has been shown to be an indicator of poor outcome in the few studies that have looked at this parameter (251, 252). In particular, in stage I tumors, positive peritoneal cytology seems to be of greater prognostic importance than depth of invasion, as all patients with positive cytology die of disease (251). Patients with a history of previous radiation seem to be associated with more advance stage and carry a worse prognosis (237).

To date, DNA ploidy, proliferation markers, and ER and PR have not been found to be clinically significant (241, 249, 253), although some recent studies suggest that malignant mixed müllerian tumors exhibit decreased ER and PR (254).

Low-Grade Endometrial Stromal Sarcoma

Low-grade endometrial stromal sarcomas which are the most common endometrial stromal tumors are characterized by late recurrences and indolent behavior in most cases. Historically, endometrial stromal sarcomas were stratified on the bases of mitotic activity into low grade (<10/10HPFs) and high grade (≥10/10HPFs) (255, 256). However, in the largest study to date of endometrial stromal sarcomas, mitotic index and cytologic atypia were evaluated and neither were found to be predictive of recurrence in patients with stage I tumors. In the same study, stage was more important than mitotic activity to predict overall survival and recurrences in stage I patients. However, when all patients were considered as a group, stage and mitotic activity were both independent prognostic factors of survival and time to first relapse (257). Other parameters including size of the tumor and grade may have an impact on prognosis (258). A few studies have noted that DNA content may be a useful adjunct to predict behavior in these tumors (245, 259, 260); however, tumor stage is overall still the most influential prognostic factor. Morphologic variations present in these tumors do not alter prognosis (257). ER and PR are expressed in low-grade endometrial stromal sarcomas but not in high-grade tumors; these findings may determine that hormonal treatment should be part of the primary treatment (261–264).

Undifferentiated Endometrial Sarcoma

There are no well-established prognostic parameters for these tumors due to the very limited experience. Note that most of the high-grade endometrial stromal sarcomas referred to in the literature have been diagnosed largely by mitotic activity, a feature that is now known not to be significant. For practical purposes, these are high-grade tumors and some authors consider them as aggressive as malignant mixed müllerian tumors or leiomyosarcomas (265).

Conclusions

- Endometrial carcinoma is the fourth most common malignancy in women. It has an overall favorable prognosis.
- The FIGO surgico-pathologic staging system introduced in 1988 is currently used to stage endometrial cancer.
- The most important prognostic factor in endometrial carcinoma is tumor stage.
- Tumor grade and depth of invasion are the most important factors in tumor stage.
- The FIGO grading system applies only to EECs and is based primarily on the degree of glandular differentiation and secondarily modified by discordant nuclear grade.

- Endometrioid carcinomas are typically estrogen related while serous and clear cell carcinomas are independent of estrogen stimulation.
- Serous and clear cell carcinomas are high-grade aggressive neoplasms regardless of stage.
- Other potential prognostic factors including ER/PR, DNA ploidy, p53, and others have not been shown to have independent prognostic significance on multivariate analysis in EC.
- The FIGO staging, although not ideal, is used to stage pure malignant mesenchymal tumors, low-grade adenosarcomas, and malignant mixed müllerian tumors.
- In uterine leiomyosarcoma, tumor stage and tumor grade are the most important predictors of survival. The role of therapeutic lymph node dissection is limited.
- In low-grade müllerian adenosarcomas, the most important prognostic factors are depth of myometrial invasion and sarcomatous overgrowth.
- The behavior of malignant mixed müllerian tumors parallels that of the epithelial component, with most metastases being composed of epithelial elements.
- Stage is the most important prognostic factor in low-grade endometrial stromal sarcomas, while undifferentiated endometrial sarcomas are associated with poor prognosis even when stage I.

References

1. Amant F, Moerman P, Neven P, Timmerman D, Van Limbergen E, Vergote I. Endometrial cancer. Lancet 2005;366:491–505.
2. Sartori E, Laface B, Gadducci A, et al. Factors influencing survival in endometrial cancer relapsing patients: a Cooperation Task Force (CTF) study. Int J Gynecol Cancer 2003;13: 458–465.
3. Zaino RJ, Kurman RJ, Diana KL, Morrow CP. Pathologic models to predict outcome for women with endometrial adenocarcinoma: the importance of the distinction between surgical stage and clinical stage – a Gynecologic Oncology Group study. Cancer 1996;77:1115–1121.
5. Creasman WT, Odicino F, Maisonneuve P, et al. Carcinoma of the corpus uteri. J Epidemiol Biostat 2001;6:47–86.
6. Fanning J, Alvarez PM, Tsukada Y, Piver MS. Prognostic significance of the extent of cervical involvement by endometrial cancer. Gynecol Oncol 1991;40:46–47.
7. Soothill PW, Alcock CJ, MacKenzie IZ. Discrepancy between curettage and hysterectomy histology in patients with stage 1 uterine malignancy. Br J Obstet Gynaecol 1989;96: 478–481.
8. Cowles TA, Magriña JF, Masterson BJ, Capen CV. Comparison of clinical and surgical staging in patients with endometrial carcinoma. Obstet Gynecol 1985;66:413–416.
9. Chen SS. Extrauterine spread in endometrial carcinoma clinically confined to the uterus. Gynecol Oncol 1985;21:23–31.
10. Wolfson AH, Sightler SE, Markoe AM, et al. The prognostic significance of surgical staging for carcinoma of the endometrium. Gynecol Oncol 1992;45:142–146.
11. Steiner E, Eicher O, Sagemuller J, et al. Multivariate independent prognostic factors in endometrial carcinoma: a clinicopathologic study in 181 patients: 10 years experience at the Department of Obstetrics and Gynecology of the Mainz University. Int J Gynecol Cancer 2003;13:197–203.

12. Abeler VM, Kjorstad KE. Endometrial adenocarcinoma in Norway. A study of a total population. Cancer 1991;67:3093–3103.
13. Gal D, Recio FO, Zamurovic D. The New International Federation of Gynecology and Obstetrics surgical staging and survival rates in early endometrial carcinoma. Cancer 1992;69:200–202.
14. Kosary CL. FIGO stage, histology, histologic grade, age and race as prognostic factors in determining survival for cancers of the female gynecological system: an analysis of 1973–87 SEER cases of cancers of the endometrium, cervix, ovary, vulva, and vagina. Semin Surg Oncol 1994;10:31–46.
15. Abeler VM, Vergote IB, Kjorstad KE, Trope CG. Clear cell carcinoma of the endometrium. Prognosis and metastatic pattern. Cancer 1996;78:1740–1747.
16. Al Kushi A, Lim P, Aquino-Parsons C, Gilks CB. Markers of proliferative activity are predictors of patient outcome for low-grade endometrioid adenocarcinoma but not papillary serous carcinoma of endometrium. Mod Pathol 2002;15:365–371.
17. Morrow CP, Bundy BN, Kurman RJ, et al. Relationship between surgical-pathological risk factors and outcome in clinical stage I and II carcinoma of the endometrium: a Gynecologic Oncology Group study. Gynecol Oncol 1991;40:55–65.
18. DiSaia PJ, Creasman WT, Boronow RC, Blessing JA. Risk factors and recurrent patterns in Stage I endometrial cancer. Am J Obstet Gynecol 1985;151:1009–1015.
19. Creasman WT, Morrow CP, Bundy BN, Homesley HD, Graham JE, Heller PB. Surgical pathologic spread patterns of endometrial cancer. A Gynecologic Oncology Group Study. Cancer 1987;60:2035–2041.
20. Nielsen AL, Thomsen HK, Nyholm HC. Evaluation of the reproducibility of the revised 1988 International Federation of Gynecology and Obstetrics grading system of endometrial cancers with special emphasis on nuclear grading. Cancer 1991;68:2303–2309.
21. Mittal KR, Schwartz PE, Barwick KW. Architectural (FIGO) grading, nuclear grading, and other prognostic indicators in stage I endometrial adenocarcinoma with identification of high-risk and low-risk groups. Cancer 1988;61:538–545.
22. Stefansson IM, Salvesen HB, Immervoll H, Akslen LA. Prognostic impact of histological grade and vascular invasion compared with tumour cell proliferation in endometrial carcinoma of endometrioid type. Histopathology 2004;44:472–479.
23. Boronow RC, Morrow CP, Creasman WT, et al. Surgical staging in endometrial cancer: clinical-pathologic findings of a prospective study. Obstet Gynecol 1984;63:825–832.
24. Lee KR, Vacek PM, Belinson JL. Traditional and nontraditional histopathologic predictors of recurrence in uterine endometrioid adenocarcinoma. Gynecol Oncol 1994;54:10–18.
25. Grigsby PW, Perez CA, Kuten A, et al. Clinical stage I endometrial cancer: prognostic factors for local control and distant metastasis and implications of the new FIGO surgical staging system. Int J Radiat Oncol Biol Phys 1992;22:905–911.
26. Abeler VM, Kjorstad KE, Berle E. Carcinoma of the endometrium in Norway: a histopathological and prognostic survey of a total population. Int J Gynecol Cancer 1992;2:9–22.
27. Konski A, Domenico D, Tyrkus M, et al. Prognostic characteristics of surgical stage I endometrial adenocarcinoma. Int J Radiat Oncol Biol Phys 1996;35:935–940.
28. Alektiar KM, McKee A, Lin O, et al. Is there a difference in outcome between stage I-II endometrial cancer of papillary serous/clear cell and endometrioid FIGO Grade 3 cancer? Int J Radiat Oncol Biol Phys 2002;54:79–85.
29. Lax SF, Kurman RJ, Pizer ES, Wu L, Ronnett BM. A binary architectural grading system for uterine endometrial endometrioid carcinoma has superior reproducibility compared with FIGO grading and identifies subsets of advance-stage tumors with favorable and unfavorable prognosis. Am J Surg Pathol 2000;24:1201–1208.
30. Alkushi A, Abdul-Rahman ZH, Lim P, et al. Description of a novel system for grading of endometrial carcinoma and comparison with existing grading systems. Am J Surg Pathol 2005;29:295–304.
31. Zaino RJ, Kurman R, Herbold D, et al. The significance of squamous differentiation in endometrial carcinoma. Data from a Gynecologic Oncology Group study. Cancer 1991;68:2293–2302.
32. Bockhman JV. Two pathogenetic types of endometrial carcinoma. Gynecol Oncol 1983;15:10–17.

33. Prat J. Prognostic parameters of endometrial carcinoma. Hum Pathol 2004;35:649–662.
34. Abeler VM, Kjorstad KE. Endometrial adenocarcinoma with squamous cell differentiation. Cancer 1992;69:488–495.
35. Longacre TA, Hendrickson MR. Diffusely infiltrative endometrial adenocarcinoma: an adenoma malignum pattern of myoinvasion. Am J Surg Pathol 1999;23:69–78.
36. Mittal KR, Barwick KW. Diffusely infiltrating adenocarcinoma of the endometrium. A subtype with poor prognosis. Am J Surg Pathol 1988;12:754–758.
37. Landry D, Mai KT, Senterman MK, et al. Endometrioid adenocarcinoma of the uterus with a minimal deviation invasive pattern. Histopathology 2003;42:77–82.
38. Ambros RA, Ballouk F, Malfetano JH, Ross JS. Significance of papillary (villoglandular) differentiation in endometrioid carcinoma of the uterus. Am J Surg Pathol 1994;18:569–575.
39. Esteller M, Garcia A, Martinez-Palones JM, Xercavins J, Reventos J. Clinicopathologic features and genetic alterations in endometrioid carcinoma of the uterus with villoglandular differentiation. Am J Clin Pathol 1999;111:336–342.
40. Ross JC, Eifel PJ, Cox RS, Kempson RL, Hendrickson MR. Primary mucinous adenocarcinoma of the endometrium. A clinicopathologic and histochemical study. Am J Surg Pathol 1983;7:715–729.
41. McCluggage WG, Sumathi VP, McManus DT. Uterine serous carcinoma and endometrial intraepithelial carcinoma arising in endometrial polyps: report of 5 cases, including 2 associated with tamoxifen therapy. Hum Pathol 2003;34:939–943.
42. Soslow RA, Pirog E, Isacson C. Endometrial intraepithelial carcinoma with associated peritoneal carcinomatosis. Am J Surg Pathol 2000;24:726–732.
43. Lauchlan SC. Tubal (serous) carcinoma of the endometrium. Arch Pathol Lab Med 1981;105:615–618.
44. Hendrickson M, Ross J, Eifel P, Martinez A, Kempson R. Uterine papillary serous carcinoma: a highly malignant form of endometrial adenocarcinoma. Am J Surg Pathol 1982;6:93–108.
45. Goff BA, Kato D, Schmidt RA, et al. Uterine papillary serous carcinoma: patterns of metastatic spread. Gynecol Oncol 1994;54:264–268.
46. Chambers JT, Merino M, Kohorn EI, Peschel RE, Schwartz PE. Uterine papillary serous carcinoma. Obstet Gynecol 1987;69:109–113.
47. Prat J, Oliva E, Lerma E, Vaquero M, Matias-Guiu X. Uterine papillary serous adenocarcinoma. A 10-case study of p53 and c-erbB-2 expression and DNA content. Cancer 1994;74:1778–1783.
48. Lax SF, Kendall B, Tashiro H, Slebos RJ, Hedrick L. The frequency of p53, K-ras mutations, and microsatellite instability differs in uterine endometrioid and serous carcinoma: evidence of distinct molecular genetic pathways. Cancer 2000;88:814–824.
49. Hamilton CA, Cheung MK, Osann K, et al. Uterine papillary serous and clear cell carcinomas predict for poorer survival compared to grade 3 endometrioid corpus cancers. Br J Cancer 2006;94:642–646.
50. Carcangiu ML, Chambers JT. Uterine papillary serous carcinoma: a study on 108 cases with emphasis on the prognostic significance of associated endometrioid carcinoma, absence of invasion, and concomitant ovarian carcinoma. Gynecol Oncol 1992;47:298–305.
51. Hui P, Kelly M, O'Malley DM, Tavassoli F, Schwartz PE. Minimal uterine serous carcinoma: a clinicopathological study of 40 cases. Mod Pathol 2005;18:75–82.
52. Chan JK, Loizzi V, Youssef M, et al. Significance of comprehensive surgical staging in noninvasive papillary serous carcinoma of the endometrium. Gynecol Oncol 2003;90:181–185.
53. Matias-Guiu X, Catasus L, Bussaglia E, et al. Molecular pathology of endometrial hyperplasia and carcinoma. Hum Pathol 2001;32:569–577.
54. Catasus L, Machin P, Matias-Guiu X, Prat J. Microsatellite instability in endometrial carcinomas: clinicopathologic correlations in a series of 42 cases. Hum Pathol 1998;29:1160–1164.
55. Carcangiu ML, Chambers JT. Early pathologic stage clear cell carcinoma and uterine papillary serous carcinoma of the endometrium: comparison of clinicopathologic features and survival. Int J Gynecol Pathol 1995;14:30–38.
56. Abeler VM, Kjorstad KE. Clear cell carcinoma of the endometrium: a histopathological and clinical study of 97 cases. Gynecol Oncol 1991;40:207–217.

57. Goodman A, Zukerberg LR, Rice LW, Fuller AF, Young RH, Scully RE. Squamous cell carcinoma of the endometrium: a report of eight cases and a review of the literature. Gynecol Oncol 1996;61:54–60.
58. Lininger RA, Ashfaq R, Albores-Saavedra J, Tavassoli FA. Transitional cell carcinoma of the endometrium and endometrial carcinoma with transitional cell differentiation. Cancer 1997;79:1933–1943.
59. Abeler VM, Kjorstad KE, Nesland JM. Undifferentiated carcinoma of the endometrium. A histopathologic and clinical study of 31 cases. Cancer 1991;68:98–105.
60. Huntsman DG, Clement PB, Gilks CB, Scully RE. Small-cell carcinoma of the endometrium. A clinicopathological study of sixteen cases. Am J Surg Pathol 1994;18:364–375.
62. Eifel PJ, Ross J, Hendrickson M, Cox RS, Kempson R, Martinez A. Adenocarcinoma of the endometrium. Analysis of 256 cases with disease limited to the uterine corpus: treatment comparisons. Cancer 1983;52:1026–1031.
63. Mariani A, Webb MJ, Keeney GL, Lesnick TG, Podratz KC. Surgical stage I endometrial cancer: predictors of distant failure and death. Gynecol Oncol 2002;87:274–280.
64. Longacre TA, Chung MH, Jensen DN, Hendrickson MR. Proposed criteria for the diagnosis of well-differentiated endometrial carcinoma. A diagnostic test for myoinvasion. Am J Surg Pathol 1995;19:371–406.
65. Jacques SM, Lawrence WD. Endometrial adenocarcinoma with variable-level myometrial involvement limited to adenomyosis: a clinicopathologic study of 23 cases. Gynecol Oncol 1990;37:401–407.
66. Hall JB, Young RH, Nelson JH, Jr. The prognostic significance of adenomyosis in endometrial carcinoma. Gynecol Oncol 1984;17:32–40.
67. Mittal KR, Barwick KW. Endometrial adenocarcinoma involving adenomyosis without true myometrial invasion is characterized by frequent preceding estrogen therapy, low histologic grades, and excellent prognosis. Gynecol Oncol 1993;49:197–201.
68. Lindauer J, Fowler JM, Manolitsas TP, et al. Is there a prognostic difference between depth of myometrial invasion and the tumor-free distance from the uterine serosa in endometrial cancer? Gynecol Oncol 2003;91:547–551.
69. Gemer O, Uriev L, Harkovsky T, et al. The significance of the degree of myometrial invasion in patients with stage IB endometrial cancer. Eur J Gynaecol Oncol 2004;25:336–338.
70. Zaino RJ. Conventional and novel prognostic factors in endometrial and adenocarcinoma: a critical appraisal. Pathol Case Reviews 2000;5:138–152.
71. Shim JU, Rose PG, Reale FR, Soto H, Tak WK, Hunter RE. Accuracy of frozen-section diagnosis at surgery in clinical stage I and II endometrial carcinoma. Am J Obstet Gynecol 1992;166:1335–1338.
72. Fanning J, Tsukada Y, Piver MS. Intraoperative frozen section diagnosis of depth of myometrial invasion in endometrial adenocarcinoma. Gynecol Oncol 1990;37:47–50.
73. Goff BA, Rice LW. Assessment of depth of myometrial invasion in endometrial adenocarcinoma. Gynecol Oncol 1990;38:46–48.
74. Doering DL, Barnhill DR, Weiser EB, Burke TW, Woodward JE, Park RC. Intraoperative evaluation of depth of myometrial invasion in stage I endometrial adenocarcinoma. Obstet Gynecol 1989;74:930–933.
75. Gemer O, Uriev L, Harkovsky T, et al. Significance of lower uterine segment involvement in women with stage I endometrial adenocarcinoma. J Reprod Med 2004;49:703–706.
76. Kadar NR, Kohorn EI, LiVolsi VA, Kapp DS. Histologic variants of cervical involvement by endometrial carcinoma. Obstet Gynecol 1982;59:85–92.
77. Leminen A, Forss M, Lehtovirta P. Endometrial adenocarcinoma with clinical evidence of cervical involvement: accuracy of diagnostic procedures, clinical course, and prognostic factors. Acta Obstet Gynecol Scand 1995;74:61–66.
78. Weiner J, Bigelow B, Demopoulos RI, Beckman EM, Weiner I. The value of endocervical sampling in the staging of endometrial carcinoma. Diagn Gynecol Obstet 1980;2:265–268.
79. Jordan LB, Al-Nafussi A. Clinicopathological study of the pattern and significance of cervical involvement in cases of endometrial adenocarcinoma. Int J Gynecol Cancer 2002;12:42–48.

80. Eltabbakh GH, Moore AD. Survival of women with surgical stage II endometrial cancer. Gynecol Oncol 1999;74:80–85.
81. Alektiar KM, Venkatraman E, Abu-Rustum N, Barakat RR. Is endometrial carcinoma intrinsically more aggressive in elderly patients? Cancer 2003;98:2368–2377.
82. Menczer J. Management of endometrial carcinoma with cervical involvement. An unsettled issue. Eur J Gynaecol Oncol 2005;26:245–255.
83. Tambouret R, Clement PB, Young RH. Endometrial endometrioid adenocarcinoma with a deceptive pattern of spread to the uterine cervix: a manifestation of stage IIb endometrial carcinoma liable to be misinterpreted as an independent carcinoma or a benign lesion. Am J Surg Pathol 2003;27:1080–1088.
84. Creutzberg CL, van Putten WL, Koper PC, et al. Surgery and postoperative radiotherapy versus surgery alone for patients with stage-1 endometrial carcinoma: multicentre randomised trial. PORTEC Study Group. Post operative radiation therapy in endometrial carcinoma. Lancet 2000;355:1404–1411.
85. Kennedy AW, Webster KD, Nuñez C, Bauer LJ. Pelvic washings for cytologic analysis in endometrial adenocarcinoma. J Reprod Med 1993;38:637–642.
86. Mundt AJ, Waggoner S, Yamada D, Rotmensch J, Connell PP. Age as a prognostic factor for recurrence in patients with endometrial carcinoma. Gynecol Oncol 2000;79:79–85.
87. Pitson G, Colgan T, Levin W, et al. Stage II endometrial carcinoma: prognostic factors and risk classification in 170 patients. Int J Radiat Oncol Biol Phys 2002;53:862–867.
88. Beckner ME, Mori T, Silverberg SG. Endometrial carcinoma: nontumor factors in prognosis. Int J Gynecol Pathol 1985;4:131–145.
89. Farley JH, Nycum LR, Birrer MJ, Park RC, Taylor RR. Age-specific survival of women with endometrioid adenocarcinoma of the uterus. Gynecol Oncol 2000;79:86–89.
90. Yamazawa K, Seki K, Matsui H, Sekiya S. Significance of perivascular lymphocytic infiltrates in endometrial carcinoma. Cancer 2001;91:1777–1784.
91. Briet JM, Hollema H, Reesink N, et al. Lymphvascular space involvement: an independent prognostic factor in endometrial cancer. Gynecol Oncol 2005;96:799–804.
92. Cohn DE, Horowitz NS, Mutch DG, Kim SM, Manolitsas T, Fowler JM. Should the presence of lymphvascular space involvement be used to assign patients to adjuvant therapy following hysterectomy for unstaged endometrial cancer? Gynecol Oncol 2002;87:243–246.
93. Ambros RA, Kurman RJ. Combined assessment of vascular and myometrial invasion as a model to predict prognosis in stage I endometrioid adenocarcinoma of the uterine corpus. Cancer 1992;69:1424–1431.
94. Hanson MB, van Nagell JR, Jr., Powell DE, et al. The prognostic significance of lymphvascular space invasion in stage I endometrial cancer. Cancer 1985;55:1753–1757.
95. Kadar N, Homesley HD, Malfetano JH. Positive peritoneal cytology is an adverse factor in endometrial carcinoma only if there is other evidence of extrauterine disease. Gynecol Oncol 1992;46:145–149.
96. Shah C, Johnson EB, Everett E, et al. Does size matter? Tumor size and morphology as predictors of nodal status and recurrence in endometrial cancer. Gynecol Oncol 2005;99:564–570.
97. Sivridis E, Buckley CH, Fox H. The prognostic significance of lymphatic vascular space invasion in endometrial adenocarcinoma. Br J Obstet Gynaecol 1987;94:991–994.
98. Gal D, Recio FO, Zamurovic D, Tancer ML. Lymphvascular space involvement – a prognostic indicator in endometrial adenocarcinoma. Gynecol Oncol 1991;42:142–145.
99. Watari H, Todo Y, Takeda M, Ebina Y, Yamamoto R, Sakuragi N. Lymph-vascular space invasion and number of positive para-aortic node groups predict survival in node-positive patients with endometrial cancer. Gynecol Oncol 2005;96:651–657.
100. Deligdisch L. Morphologic correlates of host response in endometrial carcinoma. Am J Reprod Immunol 1982;2:54–57.
101. Wong FC, Pang CP, Tang SK, et al. Treatment results of endometrial carcinoma with positive peritoneal washing, adnexal involvement and serosal involvement. Clin Oncol (R Coll Radiol) 2004;16:350–355.

102. Connell PP, Rotmensch J, Waggoner S, Mundt AJ. The significance of adnexal involvement in endometrial carcinoma. Gynecol Oncol 1999;74:74–79.
103. Ulbright TM, Roth LM. Metastatic and independent cancers of the endometrium and ovary: a clinicopathologic study of 34 cases. Hum Pathol 1985;16:28–34.
104. Sutton GP. The significance of positive peritoneal cytology in endometrial cancer. Oncology (Williston Park) 1990;4:21–26; discussion 30–22.
105. Takeshima N, Nishida H, Tabata T, Hirai Y, Hasumi K. Positive peritoneal cytology in endometrial cancer: enhancement of other prognostic indicators. Gynecol Oncol 2001;82:470–473.
106. Schorge JO, Molpus KL, Goodman A, Nikrui N, Fuller AF, Jr. The effect of postsurgical therapy on stage III endometrial carcinoma. Gynecol Oncol 1996;63:34–39.
107. Greven KM, Lanciano RM, Corn B, Case D, Randall ME. Pathologic stage III endometrial carcinoma. Prognostic factors and patterns of recurrence. Cancer 1993;71:3697–3702.
108. Takeshima N, Hirai Y, Yano K, Tanaka N, Yamauchi K, Hasumi K. Ovarian metastasis in endometrial carcinoma. Gynecol Oncol 1998;70:183–187.
109. Ashman JB, Connell PP, Yamada D, Rotmensch J, Waggoner SE, Mundt AJ. Outcome of endometrial carcinoma patients with involvement of the uterine serosa. Gynecol Oncol 2001;82:338–343.
110. Grigsby PW, Perez CA, Kuske RR, Kao MS, Galakatos AE. Results of therapy, analysis of failures, and prognostic factors for clinical and pathologic stage III adenocarcinoma of the endometrium. Gynecol Oncol 1987;27:44–57.
111. Lurain JR. The significance of positive peritoneal cytology in endometrial cancer. Gynecol Oncol 1992;46:143–144.
112. Mariani A, Webb MJ, Keeney GL, Aletti G, Podratz KC. Assessment of prognostic factors in stage IIIA endometrial cancer. Gynecol Oncol 2002;86:38–44.
113. Kashimura M, Sugihara K, Toki N, et al. The significance of peritoneal cytology in uterine cervix and endometrial cancer. Gynecol Oncol 1997;67:285–290.
114. Kasamatsu T, Onda T, Katsumata N, et al. Prognostic significance of positive peritoneal cytology in endometrial carcinoma confined to the uterus. Br J Cancer 2003;88:245–250.
115. Tebeu PM, Popowski Y, Verkooijen HM, et al. Positive peritoneal cytology in early-stage endometrial cancer does not influence prognosis. Br J Cancer 2004;91:720–724.
116. Grimshaw RN, Tupper WC, Fraser RC, Tompkins MG, Jeffrey JF. Prognostic value of peritoneal cytology in endometrial carcinoma. Gynecol Oncol 1990;36:97–100.
117. Ayhan A, Taskiran C, Celik C, Aksu T, Yuce K. Surgical stage III endometrial cancer: analysis of treatment outcomes, prognostic factors and failure patterns. Eur J Gynaecol Oncol 2002;23:553–556.
118. Turner DA, Gershenson DM, Atkinson N, Sneige N, Wharton AT. The prognostic significance of peritoneal cytology for stage I endometrial cancer. Obstet Gynecol 1989;74:775–780.
119. Santala M, Talvensaari-Mattila A, Kauppila A. Peritoneal cytology and preoperative serum CA 125 level are important prognostic indicators of overall survival in advanced endometrial cancer. Anticancer Res 2003;23:3097–3103.
120. Mlyncek M, Uharcek P. Peritoneal cytology in endometrial cancer. Neoplasma 2005;52:103–108.
121. Lampe B, Kurzl R, Hantschmann P. Prognostic factors that predict pelvic lymph node metastasis from endometrial carcinoma. Cancer 1994;74:2502–2508.
122. Ohkouchi T, Sakuragi N, Watari H, et al. Prognostic significance of Bcl-2, p53 overexpression, and lymph node metastasis in surgically staged endometrial carcinoma. Am J Obstet Gynecol 2002;187:353–359.
123. Chuang L, Burke TW, Tornos C, et al. Staging laparotomy for endometrial carcinoma: assessment of retroperitoneal lymph nodes. Gynecol Oncol 1995;58:189–193.
124. Kilgore LC, Partridge EE, Alvarez RD, et al. Adenocarcinoma of the endometrium: survival comparisons of patients with and without pelvic node sampling. Gynecol Oncol 1995;56:29–33.
125. Larson DM, Johnson KK. Pelvic and para-aortic lymphadenectomy for surgical staging of high-risk endometrioid adenocarcinoma of the endometrium. Gynecol Oncol 1993;51: 345–348.

126. Yokoyama Y, Maruyama H, Sato S, Saito Y. Indispensability of pelvic and paraaortic lymphadenectomy in endometrial cancers. Gynecol Oncol 1997;64:411–417.
127. Arango HA, Hoffman MS, Roberts WS, DeCesare SL, Fiorica JV, Drake J. Accuracy of lymph node palpation to determine need for lymphadenectomy in gynecologic malignancies. Obstet Gynecol 2000;95:553–556.
128. Mariani A, Webb MJ, Keeney GL, Haddock MG, Calori G, Podratz KC. Low-risk corpus cancer: is lymphadenectomy or radiotherapy necessary? Am J Obstet Gynecol 2000;182:1506–1519.
129. Mariani A, Keeney GL, Aletti G, Webb MJ, Haddock MG, Podratz KC. Endometrial carcinoma: paraaortic dissemination. Gynecol Oncol 2004;92:833–838.
130. McMeekin DS, Lashbrook D, Gold M, Johnson G, Walker JL, Mannel R. Analysis of FIGO Stage IIIc endometrial cancer patients. Gynecol Oncol 2001;81:273–278.
131. Mohan DS, Samuels MA, Selim MA, et al. Long-term outcomes of therapeutic pelvic lymphadenectomy for stage I endometrial adenocarcinoma. Gynecol Oncol 1998;70:165–171.
132. Lutman CV, Havrilesky LJ, Cragun JM, et al. Pelvic lymph node count is an important prognostic variable for FIGO stage I and II endometrial carcinoma with high-risk histology. Gynecol Oncol 2006;102:92–97.
133. Girardi F, Petru E, Heydarfadai M, Haas J, Winter R. Pelvic lymphadenectomy in the surgical treatment of endometrial cancer. Gynecol Oncol 1993;49:177–180.
134. Yabushita H, Shimazu M, Yamada H, et al. Occult lymph node metastases detected by cytokeratin immunohistochemistry predict recurrence in node-negative endometrial cancer. Gynecol Oncol 2001;80:139–144.
135. Gonzalez Bosquet J, Keeney GL, Mariani A, Webb MJ, Cliby WA. Cytokeratin staining of resected lymph nodes may improve the sensitivity of surgical staging for endometrial cancer. Gynecol Oncol 2003;91:518–525.
136. Bats AS, Clement D, Larousserie F, et al. Is sentinel node biopsy feasible in endometrial cancer? Results in 26 patients. J Gynecol Obstet Biol Reprod (Paris) 2005;34:768–774.
137. Evans MP, Podratz KC. Endometrial neoplasia: prognostic significance of ploidy status. Clin Obstet Gynecol 1996;39:696–706.
138. Britton LC, Wilson TO, Gaffey TA, Lieber MM, Wieand HS, Podratz KC. Flow cytometric DNA analysis of stage I endometrial carcinoma. Gynecol Oncol 1989;34:317–322.
139. Santala M, Talvensaari-Mattila A. DNA ploidy is an independent prognostic indicator of overall survival in stage I endometrial endometrioid carcinoma. Anticancer Res 2003;23:5191–5196.
140. Lundgren C, Auer G, Frankendal B, Moberger B, Nilsson B, Nordstrom B. Nuclear DNA content, proliferative activity, and p53 expression related to clinical and histopathologic features in endometrial carcinoma. Int J Gynecol Cancer 2002;12:110–118.
141. Genest DR, Sheets E, Lage JM. Flow-cytometric analysis of nuclear DNA content in endometrial adenocarcinoma. Atypical mitoses are associated with DNA aneuploidy. Am J Clin Pathol 1994;102:341–348.
142. Mangili G, De Marzi P, Vigano R, et al. Identification of high risk patients with endometrial carcinoma. Prognostic assessment of endometrial cancer. Eur J Gynaecol Oncol 2002;23:216–220.
143. Lukes AS, Kohler MF, Pieper CF, et al. Multivariable analysis of DNA ploidy, p53, and HER-2/neu as prognostic factors in endometrial cancer. Cancer 1994;73:2380–2385.
144. Pfisterer J, Kommoss F, Sauerbrei W, et al. Prognostic value of DNA ploidy and S-phase fraction in stage I endometrial carcinoma. Gynecol Oncol 1995;58:149–156.
145. Geisinger KR, Homesley HD, Morgan TM, Kute TE, Marshall RB. Endometrial adenocarcinoma. A multiparameter clinicopathologic analysis including the DNA profile and the sex steroid hormone receptors. Cancer 1986;58:1518–1525.
146. Sorbe B, Risberg B, Frankendal B. DNA ploidy, morphometry, and nuclear grade as prognostic factors in endometrial carcinoma. Gynecol Oncol 1990;38:22–27.
147. Carcangiu ML, Chambers JT. Sex steroid receptors in gynecologic neoplasms. Pathol Annu 1992;27(Pt 2):121–151.
148. Creasman WT. Prognostic significance of hormone receptors in endometrial cancer. Cancer 1993;71:1467–1470.

149. Chambers JT, MacLusky N, Eisenfield A, Kohorn EI, Lawrence R, Schwartz PE. Estrogen and progestin receptor levels as prognosticators for survival in endometrial cancer. Gynecol Oncol 1988;31:65–81.
150. Hanekamp EE, Gielen SC, Smid-Koopman E, et al. Consequences of loss of progesterone receptor expression in development of invasive endometrial cancer. Clin Cancer Res 2003;9:4190–4199.
151. Kadar N, Malfetano JH, Homesley HD. Steroid receptor concentrations in endometrial carcinoma: effect on survival in surgically staged patients. Gynecol Oncol 1993;50:281–286.
152. Morris PC, Anderson JR, Anderson B, Buller RE. Steroid hormone receptor content and lymph node status in endometrial cancer. Gynecol Oncol 1995;56:406–411.
153. Lax SF, Pizer ES, Ronnett BM, Kurman RJ. Clear cell carcinoma of the endometrium is characterized by a distinctive profile of p53, Ki-67, estrogen, and progesterone receptor expression. Hum Pathol 1998;29:551–558.
154. Carcangiu ML, Chambers JT, Voynick IM, Pirro M, Schwartz PE. Immunohistochemical evaluation of estrogen and progesterone receptor content in 183 patients with endometrial carcinoma. Part I: clinical and histologic correlations. Am J Clin Pathol 1990;94:247–254.
155. Arai T, Watanabe J, Kawaguchi M, et al. Clear cell adenocarcinoma of the endometrium is a biologically distinct entity from endometrioid adenocarcinoma. Int J Gynecol Cancer 2006;16:391–395.
156. Ehrlich CE, Young PC, Stehman FB, Sutton GP, Alford WM. Steroid receptors and clinical outcome in patients with adenocarcinoma of the endometrium. Am J Obstet Gynecol 1988;158:796–807.
157. Hu K, Zhong G, He F. Expression of estrogen receptors ERalpha and ERbeta in endometrial hyperplasia and adenocarcinoma. Int J Gynecol Cancer 2005;15:537–541.
158. De Vivo I, Huggins GS, Hankinson SE, et al. A functional polymorphism in the promoter of the progesterone receptor gene associated with endometrial cancer risk. Proc Natl Acad Sci U S A 2002;99:12263–12268.
159. Hetzel DJ, Wilson TO, Keeney GL, Roche PC, Cha SS, Podratz KC. HER-2/neu expression: a major prognostic factor in endometrial cancer. Gynecol Oncol 1992;47:179–185.
160. Santin AD. HER2/neu overexpression: has the Achilles' heel of uterine serous papillary carcinoma been exposed? Gynecol Oncol 2003;88:263–265.
161. Saffari B, Jones LA, el-Naggar A, Felix JC, George J, Press MF. Amplification and overexpression of HER-2/neu (c-erbB2) in endometrial cancers: correlation with overall survival. Cancer Res 1995;55:5693–5698.
162. Berchuck A, Rodriguez G, Kinney RB, et al. Overexpression of HER-2/neu in endometrial cancer is associated with advanced stage disease. Am J Obstet Gynecol 1991;164:15–21.
163. Peiro G, Mayr D, Hillemanns P, Lohrs U, Diebold J. Analysis of HER-2/neu amplification in endometrial carcinoma by chromogenic in situ hybridization. Correlation with fluorescence in situ hybridization, HER-2/neu, p53 and Ki-67 protein expression, and outcome. Mod Pathol 2004;17:227–287.
164. Pisani AL, Barbuto DA, Chen D, Ramos L, Lagasse LD, Karlan BY. HER-2/neu, p53, and DNA analyses as prognosticators for survival in endometrial carcinoma. Obstet Gynecol 1995;85:729–734.
165. Riben MW, Malfetano JH, Nazeer T, Muraca PJ, Ambros RA, Ross JS. Identification of HER-2/neu oncogene amplification by fluorescence in situ hybridization in stage I endometrial carcinoma. Mod Pathol 1997;10:823–831.
166. Heffner HM, Freedman AN, Asirwatham JE, Lele SB. Prognostic significance of p53, PCNA, and c-erbB-2 in endometrial enocarcinoma. Eur J Gynaecol Oncol 1999;20:8–12.
167. Coronado PJ, Vidart JA, Lopez-Asenjo JA, et al. P53 overexpression predicts endometrial carcinoma recurrence better than HER-2/neu overexpression. Eur J Obstet Gynecol Reprod Biol 2001;98:103–108.
168. Williams JA, Jr., Wang ZR, Parrish RS, Hazlett LJ, Smith ST, Young SR. Fluorescence in situ hybridization analysis of HER-2/neu, c-myc, and p53 in endometrial cancer. Exp Mol Pathol 1999;67:135–143.

169. Rolitsky CD, Theil KS, McGaughy VR, Copeland LJ, Niemann TH. HER-2/neu amplification and overexpression in endometrial carcinoma. Int J Gynecol Pathol 1999;18: 138–143.

170. Khalifa MA, Mannel RS, Haraway SD, Walker J, Min KW. Expression of EGFR, HER-2/neu, P53, and PCNA in endometrioid, serous papillary, and clear cell endometrial adenocarcinomas. Gynecol Oncol 1994;53:84–92.

171. Tashiro H, Isacson C, Levine R, Kurman RJ, Cho KR, Hedrick L. p53 gene mutations are common in uterine serous carcinoma and occur early in their pathogenesis. Am J Pathol 1997;150:177–185.

172. An HJ, Logani S, Isacson C, Ellenson LH. Molecular characterization of uterine clear cell carcinoma. Mod Pathol 2004;17:530–537.

173. Alkushi A, Lim P, Coldman A, Huntsman D, Miller D, Gilks CB. Interpretation of p53 immunoreactivity in endometrial carcinoma: establishing a clinically relevant cut-off level. Int J Gynecol Pathol 2004;23:129–137.

174. Geisler JP, Geisler HE, Wiemann MC, Zhou Z, Miller GA, Crabtree W. Lack of bcl-2 persistence: an independent prognostic indicator of poor prognosis in endometrial carcinoma. Gynecol Oncol 1998;71:305–307.

175. Taskin M, Lallas TA, Barber HR, Shevchuk MM. bcl-2 and p53 in endometrial adenocarcinoma. Mod Pathol 1997;10:728–734.

176. Zheng W, Cao P, Zheng M, Kramer EE, Godwin TA. p53 overexpression and bcl-2 persistence in endometrial carcinoma: comparison of papillary serous and endometrioid subtypes. Gynecol Oncol 1996;61:167–174.

177. Yamauchi N, Sakamoto A, Uozaki H, Iihara K, Machinami R. Immunohistochemical analysis of endometrial adenocarcinoma for bcl-2 and p53 in relation to expression of sex steroid receptor and proliferative activity. Int J Gynecol Pathol 1996;15:202–208.

178. Mariani A, Sebo TJ, Cliby WA, et al. Role of bcl-2 in endometrioid corpus cancer: an experimental study. Anticancer Res 2006;26:823–827.

179. Risinger JI, Hayes K, Maxwell GL, et al. PTEN mutation in endometrial cancers is associated with favorable clinical and pathologic characteristics. Clin Cancer Res 1998;4:3005–3010.

180. Tashiro H, Blazes MS, Wu R, et al. Mutations in PTEN are frequent in endometrial carcinoma but rare in other common gynecological malignancies. Cancer Res 1997;57:3935–3940.

181. Bussaglia E, del Rio E, Matias-Guiu X, Prat J. PTEN mutations in endometrial carcinomas: a molecular and clinicopathologic analysis of 38 cases. Hum Pathol 2000;31:312–317.

182. Levine RL, Cargile CB, Blazes MS, van Rees B, Kurman RJ, Ellenson LH. PTEN mutations and microsatellite instability in complex atypical hyperplasia, a precursor lesion to uterine endometrioid carcinoma. Cancer Res 1998;58:3254–3258.

183. Bilbao C, Rodriguez G, Ramirez R, et al. The relationship between microsatellite instability and PTEN gene mutations in endometrial cancer. Int J Cancer 2006;119:563–570.

184. Terakawa N, Kanamori Y, Yoshida S. Loss of PTEN expression followed by Akt phosphorylation is a poor prognostic factor for patients with endometrial cancer. Endocr Relat Cancer 2003;10:203–208.

185. Lagarda H, Catasus L, Arguelles R, Matias-Guiu X, Prat J. K-ras mutations in endometrial carcinomas with microsatellite instability. J Pathol 2001;193:193–199.

186. Duggan BD, Felix JC, Muderspach LI, Tsao JL, Shibata DK. Early mutational activation of the c-Ki-ras oncogene in endometrial carcinoma. Cancer Res 1994;54:1604–1607.

187. Mutter GL, Wada H, Faquin WC, Enomoto T. K-ras mutations appear in the premalignant phase of both microsatellite stable and unstable endometrial carcinogenesis. Mol Pathol 1999;52:257–262.

188. Caduff RF, Johnston CM, Frank TS. Mutations of the Ki-ras oncogene in carcinoma of the endometrium. Am J Pathol 1995;146:182–188.

189. Parc YR, Halling KC, Burgart LJ, et al. Microsatellite instability and hMLH1/hMSH2 expression in young endometrial carcinoma patients: associations with family history and histopathology. Int J Cancer 2000;86:60–66.

190. Maxwell GL, Risinger JI, Alvarez AA, Barrett JC, Berchuck A. Favorable survival associated with microsatellite instability in endometrioid endometrial cancers. Obstet Gynecol 2001;97:417–422.
191. Caduff RF, Johnston CM, Svoboda-Newman SM, Poy EL, Merajver SD, Frank TS. Clinical and pathological significance of microsatellite instability in sporadic endometrial carcinoma. Am J Pathol 1996;148:1671–1678.
192. Fiumicino S, Ercoli A, Ferrandina G, et al. Microsatellite instability is an independent indicator of recurrence in sporadic stage I–II endometrial adenocarcinoma. J Clin Oncol 2001;19:1008–1014.
193. Orbo A, Eklo K, Kopp M. A semiautomated test for microsatellite instability and its significance for the prognosis of sporadic endometrial cancer in northern Norway. Int J Gynecol Pathol 2002;21:27–33.
194. Kobayashi K, Sagae S, Kudo R, Saito H, Koi S, Nakamura Y. Microsatellite instability in endometrial carcinomas: frequent replication errors in tumors of early onset and/or of poorly differentiated type. Genes Chromosomes Cancer 1995;14:128–132.
195. Tibiletti MG, Furlan D, Taborelli M, et al. Microsatellite instability in endometrial cancer: relation to histological subtypes. Gynecol Oncol 1999;73:247–252.
196. Wong YF, Ip TY, Chung TK, et al. Clinical and pathologic significance of microsatellite instability in endometrial cancer. Int J Gynecol Cancer 1999;9:406–410.
197. MacDonald ND, Salvesen HB, Ryan A, Iversen OE, Akslen LA, Jacobs IJ. Frequency and prognostic impact of microsatellite instability in a large population-based study of endometrial carcinomas. Cancer Res 2000;60:1750–1752.
198. Machin P, Catasus L, Pons C, Muñoz J, Matias-Guiu X, Prat J. CTNNB1 mutations and beta-catenin expression in endometrial carcinomas. Hum Pathol 2002;33:206–212.
199. Moreno-Bueno G, Hardisson D, Sanchez C, et al. Abnormalities of the APC/beta-catenin pathway in endometrial cancer. Oncogene 2002;21:7981–7990.
200. Fukuchi T, Sakamoto M, Tsuda H, Maruyama K, Nozawa S, Hirohashi S. Beta-catenin mutation in carcinoma of the uterine endometrium. Cancer Res 1998;58:3526–3528.
201. Ikeda T, Yoshinaga K, Semba S, Kondo E, Ohmori H, Horii A. Mutational analysis of the CTNNB1 (beta-catenin) gene in human endometrial cancer: frequent mutations at codon 34 that cause nuclear accumulation. Oncol Rep 2000;7:323–326.
202. Saegusa M, Hashimura M, Yoshida T, Okayasu I. Beta-catenin mutations and aberrant nuclear expression during endometrial tumorigenesis. Br J Cancer 2001;84:209–217.
203. Giuntoli RL, Metzinger DS, DiMarco CS, et al. Retrospective review of 208 patients with leiomyosarcoma of the uterus: prognostic indicators, surgical management, and adjuvant therapy. Gynecol Oncol 2003;89:460–469.
204. Bodner K, Bodner-Adler B, Kimberger O, Czerwenka K, Leodolter S, Mayerhofer K. Evaluating prognostic parameters in women with uterine leiomyosarcoma. A clinicopathologic study. J Reprod Med 2003;48:95–100.
205. Pautier P, Genestie C, Rey A, et al. Analysis of clinicopathologic prognostic factors for 157 uterine sarcomas and evaluation of a grading score validated for soft tissue sarcoma. Cancer 2000;88:1425–1431.
206. Jones MW, Norris HJ. Clinicopathologic study of 28 uterine leiomyosarcomas with metastasis. Int J Gynecol Pathol 1995;14:243–249.
207. Major FJ, Blessing JA, Silverberg SG, et al. Prognostic factors in early-stage uterine sarcoma. A Gynecologic Oncology Group study. Cancer 1993;71:1702–1709.
208. Larson B, Silfversward C, Nilsson B, Pettersson F. Prognostic factors in uterine leiomyosarcoma. A clinical and histopathological study of 143 cases. The Radiumhemmet series 1936–1981. Acta Oncol 1990;29:185–191.
209. Dinh TA, Oliva EA, Fuller AF, Jr., Lee H, Goodman A. The treatment of uterine leiomyosarcoma. Results from a 10-year experience (1990–1999) at the Massachusetts General Hospital. Gynecol Oncol 2004;92:648–652.
210. Mayerhofer K, Obermair A, Windbichler G, et al. Leiomyosarcoma of the uterus: a clinicopathologic multicenter study of 71 cases. Gynecol Oncol 1999;74:196–201.

211. Hsieh CH, Lin H, Huang CC, Huang EY, Chang SY, Chang Chien CC. Leiomyosarcoma of the uterus: a clinicopathologic study of 21 cases. Acta Obstet Gynecol Scand 2003;82:74–81.

212. Evans HL, Chawla SP, Simpson C, Finn KP. Smooth muscle neoplasms of the uterus other than ordinary leiomyoma. A study of 46 cases, with emphasis on diagnostic criteria and prognostic factors. Cancer 1988;62:2239–2247.

213. Nordal RR, Kristensen GB, Kaern J, Stenwig AE, Pettersen EO, Trope CG. The prognostic significance of stage, tumor size, cellular atypia and DNA ploidy in uterine leiomyosarcoma. Acta Oncol 1995;34:797–802.

214. Leitao MM, Soslow RA, Nonaka D, et al. Tissue microarray immunohistochemical expression of estrogen, progesterone, and androgen receptors in uterine leiomyomata and leiomyosarcoma. Cancer 2004;101:1455–1462.

215. Kurman RJ, Norris HJ. Mesenchymal tumors of the uterus. VI. Epithelioid smooth muscle tumors including leiomyoblastoma and clear-cell leiomyoma: a clinical and pathologic analysis of 26 cases. Cancer 1976;37:1853–1865.

216. Prayson RA, Goldblum JR, Hart WR. Epithelioid smooth-muscle tumors of the uterus: a clinicopathologic study of 18 patients. Am J Surg Pathol 1997;21:383–391.

217. King ME, Dickersin GR, Scully RE. Myxoid leiomyosarcoma of the uterus. A report of six cases. Am J Surg Pathol 1982;6:589–598.

218. Raspollini MR, Amunni G, Villanucci A, et al. Estrogen and progesterone receptors expression in uterine malignant smooth muscle tumors: correlation with clinical outcome. J Chemother 2003;15:596–602.

219. Bodner K, Bodner-Adler B, Kimberger O, Czerwenka K, Leodolter S, Mayerhofer K. Estrogen and progesterone receptor expression in patients with uterine leiomyosarcoma and correlation with different clinicopathological parameters. Anticancer Res 2003;23:729–732.

220. Goff BA, Rice LW, Fleischhacker D, et al. Uterine leiomyosarcoma and endometrial stromal sarcoma: lymph node metastases and sites of recurrence. Gynecol Oncol 1993;50:105–109.

221. Leitao MM, Sonoda Y, Brennan MF, Barakat RR, Chi DS. Incidence of lymph node and ovarian metastases in leiomyosarcoma of the uterus. Gynecol Oncol 2003;91:209–212.

222. Blom R, Guerrieri C, Stal O, Malmstrom H, Simonsen E. Leiomyosarcoma of the uterus: a clinicopathologic, DNA flow cytometric, p53, and mdm-2 analysis of 49 cases. Gynecol Oncol 1998;68:54–61.

223. Lennart K, Lennart B, Ulf S, Bernard T. Flow cytometric analysis of uterine sarcomas. Gynecol Oncol 1994;55:339–342.

224. Amada S, Nakano H, Tsuneyoshi M. Leiomyosarcoma versus bizarre and cellular leiomyomas of the uterus: a comparative study based on the MIB-1 and proliferating cell nuclear antigen indices, p53 expression, DNA flow cytometry, and muscle specific actins. Int J Gynecol Pathol 1995;14:134–142.

225. Liu FS, Kohler MF, Marks JR, Bast RC, Jr., Boyd J, Berchuck A. Mutation and overexpression of the p53 tumor suppressor gene frequently occurs in uterine and ovarian sarcomas. Obstet Gynecol 1994;83:118–124.

226. Wang L, Felix JC, Lee JL, et al. The proto-oncogene c-kit is expressed in leiomyosarcomas of the uterus. Gynecol Oncol 2003;90:402–406.

227. Rushing RS, Shajahan S, Chendil D, et al. Uterine sarcomas express KIT protein but lack mutation(s) in exon 11 or 17 of c-KIT. Gynecol Oncol 2003;91:9–14.

228. Winter WE, 3rd, Seidman JD, Krivak TC, et al. Clinicopathological analysis of c-kit expression in carcinosarcomas and leiomyosarcomas of the uterine corpus. Gynecol Oncol 2003;91:3–8.

229. Raspollini MR, Paglierani M, Taddei GL, Villanucci A, Amunni G, Taddei A. The protooncogene c-KIT is expressed in leiomyosarcomas of the uterus. Gynecol Oncol 2004;93:718.

230. Raspollini MR, Pinzani P, Simi L, et al. Uterine leiomyosarcomas express KIT protein but lack mutation(s) in exon 9 of c-KIT. Gynecol Oncol 2005;98:334–335.

231. Zaloudek CJ, Norris HJ. Adenofibroma and adenosarcoma of the uterus: a clinicopathologic study of 35 cases. Cancer 1981;48:354–366.

232. Clement PB, Scully RE. Mullerian adenofibroma of the uterus with invasion of myometrium and pelvic veins. Int J Gynecol Pathol 1990;9:363–371.
233. Kaku T, Silverberg SG, Major FJ, Miller A, Fetter B, Brady MF. Adenosarcoma of the uterus: a Gynecologic Oncology Group clinicopathologic study of 31 cases. Int J Gynecol Pathol 1992;11:75–88.
234. Clement PB. Mullerian adenosarcomas of the uterus with sarcomatous overgrowth. A clinicopathological analysis of 10 cases. Am J Surg Pathol 1989;13:28–38.
235. Chuang JT, Van Velden DJ, Graham JB. Carcinosarcoma and mixed mesodermal tumor of the uterine corpus. Review of 49 cases. Obstet Gynecol 1970;35:769–780.
236. DiSaia PJ, Castro JR, Rutledge FN. Mixed mesodermal sarcoma of the uterus. Am J Roentgenol Radium Ther Nucl Med 1973;117:632–636.
237. Dinh TV, Slavin RE, Bhagavan BS, Hannigan EV, Tiamson EM, Yandell RB. Mixed mullerian tumors of the uterus: a clinicopathologic study. Obstet Gynecol 1989;74:388–392.
238. Silverberg SG, Major FJ, Blessing JA, et al. Carcinosarcoma (malignant mixed mesodermal tumor) of the uterus. A Gynecologic Oncology Group pathologic study of 203 cases. Int J Gynecol Pathol 1990;9:1–19.
239. Vaidya AP, Horowitz NS, Oliva E, Halpern EF, Duska LR. Uterine malignant mixed mullerian tumors should not be included in studies of endometrial carcinoma. Gynecol Oncol 2006;103:684–687.
240. Amant F, Cadron I, Fuso L, et al. Endometrial carcinosarcomas have a different prognosis and pattern of spread compared to high-risk epithelial endometrial cancer. Gynecol Oncol 2005;98:274–280.
241. Iwasa Y, Haga H, Konishi I, et al. Prognostic factors in uterine carcinosarcoma: a clinicopathologic study of 25 patients. Cancer 1998;82:512–519.
242. Sartori E, Bazzurini L, Gadducci A, et al. Carcinosarcoma of the uterus: a clinicopathological multicenter CTF study. Gynecol Oncol 1997;67:70–75.
243. Inthasorn P, Carter J, Valmadre S, Beale P, Russell P, Dalrymple C. Analysis of clinicopathologic factors in malignant mixed Mullerian tumors of the uterine corpus. Int J Gynecol Cancer 2002;12:348–353.
244. Larson B, Silfversward C, Nilsson B, Pettersson F. Mixed mullerian tumours of the uterus – prognostic factors: a clinical and histopathologic study of 147 cases. Radiother Oncol 1990;17:123–132.
245. Nola M, Babic D, Ilic J, et al. Prognostic parameters for survival of patients with malignant mesenchymal tumors of the uterus. Cancer 1996;78:2543–2550.
246. Yamada SD, Burger RA, Brewster WR, Anton D, Kohler MF, Monk BJ. Pathologic variables and adjuvant therapy as predictors of recurrence and survival for patients with surgically evaluated carcinosarcoma of the uterus. Cancer 2000;88:2782–2786.
247. Arrastia CD, Fruchter RG, Clark M, et al. Uterine carcinosarcomas: incidence and trends in management and survival. Gynecol Oncol 1997;65:158–163.
248. Gerszten K, Faul C, Kounelis S, Huang Q, Kelley J, Jones MW. The impact of adjuvant radiotherapy on carcinosarcoma of the uterus. Gynecol Oncol 1998;68:8–13.
249. Nordal RR, Kristensen GB, Stenwig AE, Nesland JM, Pettersen EO, Trope CG. An evaluation of prognostic factors in uterine carcinosarcoma. Gynecol Oncol 1997;67:316–321.
250. Barwick KW, LiVolsi VA. Malignant mixed mullerian tumors of the uterus. A clinicopathologic assessment of 34 cases. Am J Surg Pathol 1979;3:125–135.
251. Kanbour AI, Buchsbaum HJ, Hall A. Peritoneal cytology in malignant mixed mullerian tumors of the uterus. Gynecol Oncol 1989;33:91–95.
252. Lotocki R, Rosenshein NB, Grumbine F, Dillon M, Parmley T, Woodruff JD. Mixed Mullerian tumors of the uterus: clinical and pathologic correlations. Int J Gynaecol Obstet 1982;20:237–243.
253. Blom R, Guerrieri C, Stal O, Malmstrom H, Sullivan S, Simonsen E. Malignant mixed Mullerian tumors of the uterus: a clinicopathologic, DNA flow cytometric, p53, and mdm-2 analysis of 44 cases. Gynecol Oncol 1998;68:18–24.

254. Jazaeri AA, Nunes KJ, Dalton MS, Xu M, Shupnik MA, Rice LW. Well-differentiated endometrial adenocarcinomas and poorly differentiated mixed mullerian tumors have altered ER and PR isoform expression. Oncogene 2001;20:6965–6969.

255. Norris HJ, Taylor HB. Mesenchymal tumors of the uterus. I. A clinical and pathological study of 53 endometrial stromal tumors. Cancer 1966;19:755–766.

256. Larson B, Silfversward C, Nilsson B, Pettersson F. Endometrial stromal sarcoma of the uterus. A clinical and histopathological study. The Radiumhemmet series 1936–1981. Eur J Obstet Gynecol Reprod Biol 1990;35:239–249.

257. Chang KL, Crabtree GS, Lim-Tan SK, Kempson RL, Hendrickson MR. Primary uterine endometrial stromal neoplasms. A clinicopathologic study of 117 cases. Am J Surg Pathol 1990;14:415–438.

258. De Fusco PA, Gaffey TA, Malkasian GD, Jr., Long HJ, Cha SS. Endometrial stromal sarcoma: review of Mayo Clinic experience, 1945–1980. Gynecol Oncol 1989;35:8–14.

259. August CZ, Bauer KD, Lurain J, Murad T. Neoplasms of endometrial stroma: histopathologic and flow cytometric analysis with clinical correlation. Hum Pathol 1989;20:232–237.

260. El-Naggar AK, Abdul-Karim FW, Silva EG, McLemore D, Garnsey L. Uterine stromal neoplasms: a clinicopathologic and DNA flow cytometric correlation. Hum Pathol 1991;22:897–903.

261. Spano JP, Soria JC, Kambouchner M, et al. Long-term survival of patients given hormonal therapy for metastatic endometrial stromal sarcoma. Med Oncol 2003;20:87–93.

262. Maluf FC, Sabbatini P, Schwartz L, Xia J, Aghajanian C. Endometrial stromal sarcoma: objective response to letrozole. Gynecol Oncol 2001;82:384–388.

263. Leunen M, Breugelmans M, De Sutter P, Bourgain C, Amy JJ. Low-grade endometrial stromal sarcoma treated with the aromatase inhibitor letrozole. Gynecol Oncol 2004;95:769–771.

264. Balleine RL, Earls PJ, Webster LR, et al. Expression of progesterone receptor A and B isoforms in low-grade endometrial stromal sarcoma. Int J Gynecol Pathol 2004;23:138–144.

265. Gadducci A, Sartori E, Landoni F, et al. Endometrial stromal sarcoma: analysis of treatment failures and survival. Gynecol Oncol 1996;63:247–253.

Primary Hormonal Therapy of Endometrial Cancer

Linda R. Duska

Abstract This chapter discusses the treatment of endometrioid adenocarcinoma of the endometrium with hormonal therapy for the purpose of preserving the corpus and future fertility. This treatment obviously pertains to premenopausal women. An occasional postmenopausal woman who is not a candidate for surgery may benefit from similar approaches.

Keywords Endometrial cancer • Premenopausal • Fertility preservation • Hormonal treatment

Introduction

Endometrial cancer is the most common of the gynecologic malignancies. In 2008, 40,100 cases of endometrial cancer and 7,470 deaths from the disease are estimated in the USA (1). Most cancers occur in women who are postmenopausal, and therefore completed their childbearing. However, some endometrial carcinomas occur in women who perhaps have not yet begun or have not completed their families.

The standard of care for endometrial cancer is surgical treatment. The primary surgery consists of total hysterectomy with removal of both tubes and ovaries. In the USA, this is often associated with staging surgery, including removal of the pelvic and para-aortic lymph nodes. Obviously, this surgical treatment will make future childbearing for the patient impossible. With surgical staging and radiation where appropriate, the cure rate for endometrial cancer confined to the corpus (stage I) is $\geq 80\%$ depending on substage, grade, and histologic subtype.

L.R. Duska (✉)
Division of Gynecologic Oncology, Department of Obstetrics and Gynecology
University of Virginia, Charlottesville, VA
e-mail: lduska@virginia.edu

F. Muggia and E. Oliva (eds.), *Uterine Cancer*, Current Clinical Oncology,
DOI: 10.1007/978-1-60327-044-1_7,
© Humana Press, a Part of Springer Science + Business Media, LLC 2009

This chapter will discuss the alternative treatment of endometrioid adenocarcinoma of the endometrium with hormonal therapy for the purpose of preserving the uterus and therefore future fertility. Since little prospective data exist for this proposed management, mainly retrospective data will be presented. Moreover, the treatment of endometrial cancer with less than hysterectomy at the current time represents a therapy that is outside of the "standard of care", and therefore should be undertaken with caution with a well-informed patient and an experienced physician.

This discussion will also apply to older women with endometrial cancer who are not surgical candidates for medical reasons. However, many of these older women for whom fertility is not an issue may be better served by primary radiation therapy if they cannot undergo surgery.

Epidemiology (see also chapter 1)

Endometrial cancer most often affects postmenopausal women. Over 70% of cases occur in the postmenopause and the mean age of diagnosis was 63.1 years in 1990–1992 (2). However, retrospective reports suggest that between 2–14% of women presenting with endometrial cancer will be ≤40 years old (3–11). This premenopausal group has both similar and different epidemiologic characteristics than the postmenopausal age group that need to be considered. Moreover, because of their young age, the diagnosis of endometrial cancer is not always entertained in these patients when they present with menstrual irregularities.

One of the epidemiologic risk factors shared by young and old women is obesity. Several large retrospective studies have looked at obesity rates in women age ≤40 based on a measurement of BMI >30. The three largest studies that have data regarding BMI are shown in Table 1. If all studies, including those that measure obesity by body weight alone, are included, obesity rates in younger women range from as low as 38% to as high as 62% (12). Interestingly, these obesity rates in young women seem to be higher than those of older women within the same population. For example, in the series from Gallup et al., an obesity rate of 43.8% in women < 40 years with endometrial cancer contrasted

Table 1. Studies of women < 40 years with available BMI data

	Duska et al. (12)	Gitsch et al. (9)	Solimon et al. (11)	Totals
Number of patients	92	17	79	188
BMI > 30	44	6	48	98
Obese (%)	48	35	62	52

with 18% in a group of patients treated at the same institution who were over 40 years of age (6).

All young women with endometrial cancer are not obese; in fact, many of them will present with normal weight. In the series from Massachusetts General Hospital (MGH), 52% of women <40 years with endometrial cancer were of normal weight (BMI < 30), and 43% had a BMI of 25 or less (12). In that study, there was a trend toward higher stage disease and high-risk histology in the normal weight women, though the differences did not reach statistical significance. Schmeler et al. presented a series of women ≤ 50 years and of normal weight seen at the MD Anderson Cancer Center (13). They suggested that hormonal factors, and in particular polycystic ovarian syndrome (PCOS), may be a risk factor for developing endometrial cancer in these women with normal weight. Retrospective data suggests that normal weight younger women are not at higher risk for poor survival, though the numbers are too small in all studies to reach any conclusion.

Obviously, women <40 do not present with postmenopausal bleeding or staining. However, the majority of young women with endometrial cancer will present with some type of menstrual irregularity. In the series from MGH, 29 of 91 women presented with menorrhagia or increasing menorrhagia and 39 of 91 presented with irregular menses or menometrorrhagia (12). Similarly, 26 of 32 women in the Crissman series presented with irregular vaginal bleeding (5). Other studies have also reported high rates of irregular bleeding as the presenting complaint (4, 7, 10). Persistent irregular bleeding, therefore, merits endometrial sampling even in those women age ≤40 to rule out an underlying endometrial carcinoma.

Infertility is also a hallmark of women ≤40 with endometrial cancer, in contrast to their postmenopausal counterparts, who are often characterized as "fertile." In our series, 11 patients (12%) were diagnosed with endometrial cancer incidentally during infertility evaluation (12). In Gallup's study, 44% of women <40 years with endometrial cancer were classified as "infertile," though information is not provided to suggest that infertility was the presenting symptom prompting evaluation (6). Schmeler's study reported a 17% risk of infertility in women under age 50 with endometrial cancer (13). The finding of infertility is a resonable one if we assume that it is a result of anovulation from disorders as Stein-Leventhal syndrome associated with high levels of circulating unopposed estrogen. Unfortunately, all data is retrospective and often limits obtaining hormonal information about patients unless it is specifically documented in the patient's chart.

Genetic disorders, particularly hereditary nonpolyposis colon cancer or Lynch syndrome, are associated with endometrial cancer, usually at a young age. In fact, endometrial cancer is the most common cancer of Lynch syndrome in women and may be the presenting cancer in some patients (14). A detailed family history is instrumental in making this diagnosis, and all young women presenting with endometrial cancer should have a careful family history taken.

Finally, endometrial cancer in a young woman may result from an estrogen-producing ovarian tumor, such as a granulosa cell tumor. Clinically, a very young woman may present with an ovarian mass, irregular bleeding, and/or infertility. Treatment of the ovarian tumor must include dilatation and curettage (D&C) to rule out an underlying endometrial neoplasia.

Complex Atypical Hyperplasia in Women Under 40 Years

The issue of complex atypical hyperplasia (CAH) needs to be addressed, particularly in the setting of a discussion of treating young women with grade 1 endometrial cancer with hormones rather than definitive surgery. While CAH is a precancerous lesion, it cannot reliably be stated that there will be no cancer on the hysterectomy specimen when a preoperative diagnosis of CAH is made. The possibility of an underlying grade 1 adenocarcinoma must be considered when treating CAH with hormones for the purpose of preserving fertility.

Kurman et al. established retrospectively that a preoperative diagnosis of CAH resulted in a postoperative diagnosis of grade 1 adenocarcinoma on the hysterectomy specimen in 29% of cases (15). This study has since been repeated prospectively by the Gynecology Oncology Group (GOG) with somewhat alarming results (16, 17). The study entered women with a preoperative community diagnosis of CAH, all of whom underwent hysterectomy within 12 weeks of diagnosis. All preoperative specimens were reviewed by a panel of "expert" pathologists as were the final hysterectomy specimens. The rate of carcinoma in the final hysterectomy was 43%, much higher than the Kurman's retrospective study. More surprisingly, however, the community diagnosis of CAH was supported by the expert panel in only 38% of cases. In 29% of cases, the expert panel felt that the lesion merited a diagnosis of carcinoma. Finally, there was complete agreement of the experts in only 40% of cases.

From the data presented above, it is clear that CAH needs to be treated as if a grade 1 adenocarcinoma might be present. Care should be taken to exclude carcinoma as a possibility, either via D&C as the "gold standard," slide review by an expert pathologist, or both when considering treatment with hormones and conservation of the uterus. Recurrence risk for CAH will likely be as high as seen in grade 1 adenocarcinoma after treatment with hormonal therapy.

Staging

Endometrial cancer has been surgically staged since 1988, with the publication of the results of the surgical staging study GOG 33 (18). This study demonstrated the importance of lymph node status as well as depth of myometrial invasion as markers of prognosis and recommendations for adjuvant therapy. The GOG defines surgical staging of endometrial cancer as including: exploratory laparotomy, pelvic washings, total abdominal hysterectomy (TAH), bilateral salpingo-oophorectomy (BSO), and sampling of pelvic and para-aortic lymph nodes. Adjuvant therapy recommendations are made based on surgico-pathologic results. GOG 33 also helped clinicians to predict which patients might have positive retroperitoneal lymph nodes based on grade of disease and depth of myometrial invasion.

In GOG 33, women with grade 1 tumors and no myometrial invasion had a 0% rate of positive pelvic or para-aortic retroperitoneal lymph nodes. In fact, the rate of lymph node metastases for noninvasive carcinoma of any grade was ≤3%. However, deeply invasive grade 1 tumors had an 11% rate of positive pelvic lymph nodes and a 6% rate of positive para-aortic lymph nodes, indicating the need for adjuvant therapy after surgery and a poorer prognosis. Therefore, a patient with a grade 1 carcinoma that is (clinically) noninvasive has a theoretical risk of positive retroperitoneal nodes of 0%, making her an ideal candidate for hormonal therapy.

When a clinician is considering managing a patient with hormonal treatment, however, surgical staging is not possible. The determination of clinical staging, then, must be made with the best available data, the limitations of which will be discussed below, with surgical staging considered to be the "gold standard." Since it is generally accepted that only patients with noninvasive endometrial cancer (and grade 1 or at most grade 2 endometrioid histology) should be managed with hormones, the clinician needs to use all possible modalities to assure that the patient has "clinical" stage IA grade 1 disease. For the purposes of the remainder of this discussion, it will be assumed that all histology is endometrioid since hormonal management of any other histology of endometrial cancer is not appropriate.

Grade

Preoperative tumor grade is not always predictive of tumor grade on the final hysterectomy specimen. Cowles et al. demonstrated that preoperative grade 1 tumors were upgraded at the time of hysterectomy in 11% of cases (19), while a larger study by Daniel et al. reported an overall upgrading of 15–20% (20). In combination, the two studies did demonstrate that we do best predicting postoperative grade correctly when the preoperative grade is 1. Most recently, Eltabbakh et al. reviewed 182 patients at their institution who underwent surgical staging for preoperative grade 1 tumors (21). In 30% of cases, the grade was changed on the hysterectomy specimen. In 22% and 6% of cases, the postoperative grade was 2 and 3, respectively. Obviously, then, there is a not insignificant risk that a young woman presenting with a grade 1 tumor will have a higher grade histology discovered if she undergoes hysterectomy, and therefore increased risk of disease outside of the uterus. Since D&C is considered the "gold standard" for preoperative diagnosis, hormonal management of a young patient should always be preceded by a D&C rather than an endometrial biopsy only.

Myometrial Invasion

There is no 100% reliable method to determine depth of muscle invasion short of removing the uterus and examining the myometrium microscopically. Most clinicians will use a combination of MRI, ultrasound, and/or CT scanning to make the diagnosis of clinical Stage Ia disease. None of these modalities are completely reliable, and all are more accurate when diagnosing deep rather than superficial myometrial invasion.

CT scan is useful for identifying large volume extrauterine disease, but fails to detect microscopic lymph node metastases. Accuracy of CT scan in predicting myometrial invasion ranges from 61% to 76%, increasing to 83% with deep invasion (22–24). Zerbe et al. reviewed their experience with preoperative CT scans in predicting the extent of myometrial invasion (25). All patients had a CT scan performed within 10 days of surgery and the results were classified as > or <50% invasion. In this study, CT scan failed to identify 17 of 44 patients (39%) who had myometrial invasion. While this study did not look specifically at grade 1 tumors, it suggests that CT is not useful in determining myometrial invasion. Other authors have confirmed this finding (26).

MRI can be useful for evaluating myometrial invasion as well as pelvic nodes and adnexal masses. In a recent study looking at all grades of endometrial cancer, evaluation of depth of myometrial invasion with MRI had a sensitivity of 79–82% (27), while other authors have reported an accuracy of 58–89% (22, 24). For both CT and MRI, the postmenopausal woman presents a special diagnostic challenge because of the lack of junctional zone between the endo- and myometrium. It is likely that accuracy will be higher in premenopausal women. Tumor grade, however, does not seem to be a factor in predicting myometrial invasion in one meta-analysis (28).

MRI is the most frequently recommended modality for assessing myometrial invasion in the premenopausal woman wishing to preserve her uterus. Contrast-enhanced MRI improves accuracy (29, 30). Transvaginal ultrasound can also be utilized to exclude ovarian lesions. Like CT, MRI will not be able to accurately diagnose microscopically positive retroperitoneal lymph nodes.

Data Supporting Hormonal Therapy

The majority of data supporting hormonal therapy of endometrial cancer is retrospective and, therefore, subject to reporting bias. Most series are small, with numbers of patients reported ranging from 1 to 15. The GOG is currently undertaking a prospective study of women with endometrial cancer (GOG 211) who are given a single dose of intramuscular (IM) progesterone 21–24 days prior to hysterectomy. This study will provide prospective data regarding the action of progesterone, but since most women with endometrial cancer are postmenopausal, it is not clear that the data will also apply to premenopausal women.

Ramirez et al. recently published a literature review of retrospective patients treated with progesterone (31). They identified 27 studies describing 81 patients treated with hormones for endometrial cancer. Overall, the response to progestin therapy was 76%, with a median time of response of 12 weeks. Documentation regarding pregnancy was available for 20 patients, all of whom were able to conceive at least once following treatment. Gottlieb et al. performed a similar and more comprehensive literature review and identified 101 women with a mean age of 29 years treated with hormones for endometrial cancer, with a 71% initial response rate, minimal time to response of 3.6 months, and 56 live births (32).

One of the earliest and largest retrospective studies was that of Bokhman et al., in 1985 (33). It preceded surgical staging, and all patients at that time were clinically staged. Nineteen patients ranging in age from 19 to 37 (mean 28.7) years with endometrial cancer were treated with progesterone, 11 patients with grade 1 tumors, and 8 with grade 2 tumors, all with clinical stage I disease. Seventeen patients had primary infertility and 14 were obese. All patients were treated with 500 mg daily of IM oxyprogesterone caproate. All patients who did not demonstrate response after 3 months underwent hysterectomy. In total, 15 of the 19 patients were cured with hormonal therapy. Data regarding live births following treatment was not reported.

The next consecutive larger series was reported by Randall and Kurman in 1997 (34). It consisted of a retrospective review of cases sent to Johns Hopkins Hospital for pathology consultation. Fourteen women were treated with hormones for grade 1 adenocarcinoma. Most of the patients were described as treated with "high-dose progestins," though the treatments were not standardized as they were in the previous report. In this study, no woman had tumor progression defined as an increase in grade on subsequent sampling. Two women were found to have coexisting ovarian carcinomas following hormonal therapy and underwent surgery; in both cases, a stage Ia grade 1 endometrioid adenocarcinoma was confirmed histologically. Three women had five full-term deliveries. One patient experienced recurrence of her cancer after initial response to therapy. She had another complete regression after reinstitution of progesterone therapy, and ultimately had a full-term delivery.

In 2001, our group presented a retrospective review of 12 patients who underwent hormone therapy of endometrial cancer (12). They ranged in age from 24 to 40 years and 8 presented with infertility. All patients had grade 1 tumors. Two patients eventually underwent hysterectomy for persistent disease, and one of these developed a synchronous ovarian primary tumor. Four women achieved pregnancy with five viable infants delivered.

Gottlieb et al. in 2003 reported 13 patients with ages ranging from 23 to 40 (mean 31) years (32). In six patients, the diagnosis was made during infertility evaluation. Eleven patients had a grade 1 tumor and two had a grade 2 tumor. All patients received treatment for at least 3 months and all responded to therapy with regression of their disease documented by endometrial biopsy. Progestin therapy was not standardized; eight patients were treated with megestrol acetate 160 mg daily. Five patients developed local recurrence. Three patients delivered nine viable infants and two further patients were pregnant at the time of the report.

Wang et al. in 2001 reported a prospective study of hormonal treatment of endometrial cancer (35). In this study, women with clinical stage I grade 1 endometrioid adenocarcinoma were prospectively entered into an IRB-approved trial of hormonal therapy. Nine patients were accrued to the trial over an 8-year period. Despite the prospective nature of the study, all patients did not receive the same therapy, though the majority were treated with megestrol acetate and tamoxifen. Eight of the nine patients achieved complete remission, though one of them did not initially respond to therapy and had to be treated with GnRH agonist and increased dose of megestrol acetate. Two patients had a total of three term pregnancies. However, four of the eight responders developed recurrent disease.

Finally, Niwa et al. presented a prospective study of women <40 years with grade 1 endometrial cancer (36). Ultrasound and MRI were both used to assess myometrial invasion and ovarian involvement. All patients were treated with medroxyprogesterone acetate continuously and all 12 underwent complete remission of disease. Of ten patients attempting pregnancy, five had six full-term deliveries. Eight patients had recurrence of disease, and one of these patients had metastatic disease to the ovary at the time of surgery.

From these and other studies, it can infer that the majority of women will respond to hormonal therapy, though not all, with a response rate of approximately 70%. The presence of ER and PR does not necessarily imply response to hormonal therapy (35) and the recurrence risk is not insignificant, with a range of 8–66%.

Risks of Hormonal Therapy

Progression of Disease

Certainly, there is concern for progression of disease during the delay that occurs during hormonal therapy. It is conceivable that if the cancer being treated is not responsive to hormones and/or more definitive surgical therapy is delayed for 3 months, the stage of disease at the time of ultimate surgery could be higher. Kim et al. reported 3 of 21 initial responders to progesterone who experienced recurrent disease; one of these patients had evidence of metastatic disease at the time of her surgery. The authors raised the possibility of progesterone therapy delaying definitive surgical therapy, possibly resulting in the development of metastatic disease (37). This patient was also the only one in the series with grade 2 disease, prompting the authors to suggest that only patients with grade 1 disease be considered for hormonal management.

Rubatt et al. reported a 40-year-old-obese woman who underwent hormonal therapy for CAH (38). The patient experienced complete regression and was compliant with follow-up. Two years following initial treatment she was diagnosed with a grade 2 endometrial cancer. At the time of surgery, she was found to have a stage IIIC grade 2 endometrial cancer with significant lymphovascular invasion within the myometrium and one positive pelvic lymph node. Kaku et al. reported 12 women with endometrial cancer who underwent hormonal therapy; 2 of 9 responders later developed relapse, and 1 of these had stage IIIC disease, with a positive obturator lymph node (39). Yang et al. reported four patients who were treated with hormones and ultimately at the time of surgery were found to have both ovarian and endometrial tumors; the ovarian tumors were not detected at the time of diagnosis of the endometrial cancer (40). Finally, Ferrandina et al. reported a case of progression of endometrial cancer following successful treatment and pregnancy (41). A 30-year-old woman was treated successfully for her grade 1 clinical stage Ia endometrial cancer as documented by hysteroscopy and D&C. Three months following resolution of her disease she became pregnant and had a cesarean section at 36 weeks. Eight months later, she developed irregular bleeding and underwent definitive surgical therapy. She was diagnosed with stage IV poorly differentiated endometrial cancer and died of her disease.

There is a large number of studies, usually reporting between 1 and 4 cases, of women with endometrial cancer who were treated with hormones and achieved pregnancy (42–51). Most of them had grade 1 tumors that were extensively "clinically" staged with D&C, plus or minus hysteroscopy, CT and/or MRI, and laparoscopy. Many of these women were diagnosed during infertility evaluation and many required artificial reproductive technology (ART) to achieve pregnancy. One must consider when reading these reports the phenomenon of recall bias.

Any patient who chooses hormonal therapy over definitive surgical therapy should be counseled that surgical therapy is almost always curative for stage Ia grade 1 cancers and that hormonal therapy as an alternative poses a theoretical risk of progression of disease to a stage that may expose the patient to an increased risk of recurrence.

Risk of Metastases to the Ovary and/or Synchronous Ovarian Primary Tumors

There is a risk, though small, of endometrial cancer embolizing through the fallopian tube and metastasizing to the ovary. In the GOG staging study of clinical stage I endometrial cancer, this risk was 5% (18). Gross ovarian metastases can be ruled out via pelvic examination and/or pelvic ultrasound, but micrometastases cannot be demonstrated without histologic examination of the ovaries.

Recent literature has raised significant concerns regarding the risk of synchronous ovarian primary tumors in young women with endometrial cancer. The issue was raised by Walsh et al. in the context of considering preserving ovarian function in young women with endometrial cancer, removing the uterus but leaving the ovaries intact (52). The authors reviewed 102 patients age 45 and younger who underwent hysterectomy for endometrial cancer. Twenty-six women in this series (25%) had a coexisting ovarian malignancy, which were felt to be a synchronous ovarian primary in 23 cases. All ovarian tumors were epithelial, and all but one were endometrioid carcinomas. Eighteen of the 26 cases (69%) occurred in women with grade 1 endometrial cancer. Twenty-six patients in this series underwent hormonal treatment for endometrial cancer prior to ultimate surgical management. Four of them (15%) had ovarian involvement with cancer diagnosed at the time of their surgery and one had an ovarian tumor that was felt to be a synchronous ovarian primary.

Other authors have also documented a risk of synchronous ovarian primary cancer in patients with an endometrial cancer (53). Obviously, when considering hormonal therapy, ovarian involvement needs to be carefully ruled out. Pelvic ultrasound may be the most useful modality to evaluate the ovaries for any abnormality and CA-125 can be used preoperatively as well. It has also suggested the use of laparoscopy preoperatively to rule out ovarian involvement (54), though this is not a standard recommendation.

Risk of Tumor Recurrence During Pregnancy

Unfortunately, endometrial cancer recurrence has been documented during pregnancy. In one study, a lesion was interpreted to have been present during pregnancy, despite documentation of resolution of disease after treatment with hormones, and was diagnosed shortly after delivery (55). Intuitively, one would think that high levels of progesterone achieved during pregnancy should be protective against recurrence of endometrial cancer, but this is not always the case.

Method of Treatment

There is no standardized agreed upon method for treating women with endometrial cancer with hormones. Most gynecologic oncologists choose megestrol acetate as a first choice, but doses and schedules are not standardized. Doses as low as 40 mg daily and as high as 160 mg four times daily have been reported. Medroxyprogesterone acetate, depo-medroxyprogesterone acetate, and combinations of tamoxifen and progesterone have also been suggested. While some authors suggest using cyclic therapy to induce a monthly withdrawal bleed, most advocate continuous treatment which ultimately results in an atrophic endometrium. Since progesterone is poorly tolerated by many women, with breast tenderness and weight gain being frequent complaints, it is probably best to use the lowest dose that will also be successful in reversing the neoplastic endometrium, though this lowest dose probably varies from woman to woman and likely its success is dependant on patient's BMI and tumor.

Several authors have suggested the use of a progesterone intrauterine device (IUD) as a means of treating the cancer with high doses of progesterone without the systemic side effects. In the study from Montz et al., women with clinical stage IA grade 1 endometrial cancer underwent hysteroscopy and curettage followed by placement of a progesterone IUD and resampling every 3 months (56). Seven of 11 patients demonstrated complete response at 6 months and six of eight at 12 months.

Dhar et al. performed a similar study using a levonorgestrel containing IUD (57). Four women with grade 1 adenocarcinoma that expressed PR were treated with IUD; only one patient had a complete response within 6 months. However, this study did not exclude myometrial invasion prior to the treatment with IUD. In both studies, the majority of patients were postmenopausal and underwent hormonal treatment because it was felt that they were poor surgical candidates; thus, it is impossible to know whether a similar treatment regimen in premenopausal women would have similar outcome. Moreover, two women were reported to possibly have developed adenocarcinoma in the uterine isthmus while using a levonorgestrel IUD, suggesting that either the uterine cavity does not receive a uniform dose of progesterone, or that the cancer is not uniformly receptive to hormonal treatment (58).

Once the treatment itself is chosen, appropriate follow-up of the patient is also not standardized. How frequently should the endometrium be resampled following treatment? How long should the treating clinician wait for complete response? Once complete response has been established, how should the patient then be followed to rule out recurrence? The appropriate treatment and follow-up course has not been established. It is clear, however, that responses may not be seen at the first 3-month resampling, and that the recurrence risk is high. It seems reasonable to suggest that patients be resampled 3 months after beginning hormonal therapy. If an incomplete response is documented, a further 3-month trial of treatment, perhaps with increased dose or different medication, may be appropriate. Once complete remission is established, pregnancy (if desired) should be aggressively pursued, with ART if required. If pregnancy is not desired, a "maintenance" hormonal treatment must be utilized to prevent recurrence. This maintenance therapy might consist of the birth control pill, monthly withdrawal bleeds with progesterone, or continuous progesterone therapy, either by mouth, intramuscular, or intrauterine.

Many women with endometrial cancer treated with progesterone will require ART to achieve pregnancy. Since ART generates very high serum estradiol levels (which thereby put the patient at risk for recurrence if pregnancy is not achieved), many community in vitro fertility (IVF) programs may feel uncomfortable managing these patients. Moreover, many of these women are in the older range of reproductive age and therefore have lower success rates for IVF, perhaps requiring multiple attempts at ovulation induction to achieve pregnancy. These risks must be considered in the overall counseling of these patients when they are contemplating hormonal management for preservation of fertility.

Mechanisms of Hormone Receptor Action in Endometrial Cancer

The presence of PR in endometrial cancer does not guarantee response to progesterone. The simple notion of a generic progesterone receptor has been replaced over the last 10 years with a better understanding of the complexity of the PR and the mechanism of action of hormones on endometrial cancer. Nevertheless, currently there is no method to predict which cancers will regress with hormonal therapy and which will persist. Moreover, tumors may respond to progesterone therapy only partially, with persistence of disease in some areas of the uterus and response in others. While we have a general clinical sense that many CAH and endometrial cancers will respond to progesterone, the understanding of this response at the molecular level is rudimentary at best.

The GOG is trying to understand the molecular basis of progesterone response in several prospective ongoing studies. In GOG 211, women undergoing hysterectomy for a known diagnosis of endometrioid adenocarcinoma are receiving a single IM dose of depo-medroxyprogesterone acetate 400 mg 21–24 days prior to hysterectomy. Paraffin blocks are being collected from the preoperative biopsy as well as the hysterectomy specimen for scientific study to perhaps obtain a better understanding of the action of this particular formulation of progesterone on all grades of endometrioid adenocarcinoma.

Most endometrioid adenocarcinomas express PR (59). The lower grade tumors express PR more frequently, with a decrease in PR expression with increasing tumor grade (60–62). However, there is a variable response to progesterone treatment within a single tumor and tumors can have both PR-positive and -negative areas (63–66). Therefore, the presence of PR by immunohistochemistry does not reliably predict response to progesterone therapy. Furthermore, we now have more information regarding the complexity of the PR and the interactions between its two isoforms, PRA and PRB. Either the two isoforms have divergent responses or the ratio of the isoforms might be important (67–70). There are also several cofactors and corepressors that can influence PR-mediated action (71–76). The study of Arnett-Mansfield et al. illustrates the difficulty of utilizing immunohistochemistry and the presence or absence of receptor to predict response (77). The authors studied PR isoforms in archived endometrial cancer tissue. Ninety-six percent of tumors expressed PR. Only 30% of tumors expressed PRA alone, 42% expressed both isoforms, and 28% expressed PRB alone. PRB-only tumors had low levels of PR and those tumors that expressed both isoforms tended to express predominantly PRA. Based on their data, the authors hypothesized that loss of PRB resulted in the development of endometrial cancer. The finding of different expression of the isoforms has been supported by other groups (67, 70). Other authors have suggested that it is the ratio of the isoforms that is most important (78). Thus, it is most likely that the ratio of PRA to PRB determines both the development of endometrial cancer and the ultimate response or lack thereof to progesterone treatment.

As the presence of PR alone does not predict response to progesterone therapy, molecular markers of progesterone response that are measurable in paraffin-fixed tissue will be needed in the future to predict response of an individual tumor to progesterone therapy. Moreover, since different areas of each tumor may respond to treatment differently, careful monitoring of response will always be necessary.

Future Directions

As women in the USA continue to delay childbearing and as obesity rates rise, the numbers of women with endometrial cancer who wish to preserve their fertility will continue to increase. Counseling of these women regarding uterine preservation is limited by the lack of data and lack of standardized management schemas. Prospective trials need to be performed to establish a standard drug, dose, and schedule for progesterone therapy, and its appropriate monitoring. In order to establish a new standard of care in this setting, we require a better understanding at the molecular and genetic level of the mechanism of the different progesterone formulations on endometrial cancer at the level of the PR isoforms. It may be that a specific novel progesterone directed at one or the other PR isoforms will be the best treatment in the future, or perhaps directed therapy to each particular tumor depending upon that tumor's expression pattern of PR isoforms.

For the present time, any young woman with endometrial cancer wishing to be treated with progesterone in order to preserve fertility should be managed with the guidance of a gynecologic oncologist wherever possible and should be informed of all of the risks of less than standard of care treatment, including the not insignificant risk of progression of disease and potential development of ovarian synchronous primary tumors or ovarian metastases. Only women with grade 1 endometrioid adenocarcinomas and disease that is clinically felt to be confined to the endometrium with the best available radiologic modality should be considered for therapy. Our own study failed to identify any clinical or immunohistologic factors other than grade that are predictive of stage Ia disease and thus predictive of successful hormonal therapy.

Patients who wish to proceed with progesterone therapy rather than surgery should be counseled that this therapy is not the standard of care treatment for endometrial cancer. Treating with less than the standard of care could potentially result in a young woman dying of a surgically curable disease.

Conclusions

To pursue primary hormonal therapy of endometrial cancer, the following steps are required:

- Confirm that the tumor is endometrioid and grade 1 by pathologic review. If diagnosis was made by endometrial biopsy, perform D&C to ensure complete sampling of the endometrial cavity.
- Obtain a careful medical history and perform physical examination with particular attention to family history. A family history that suggests Lynch syndrome should result in genetic counseling and possible testing as patient is at increased risk for colon and ovarian cancer. Attention should also be paid to medical history that might complicate future pregnancies (obesity, diabetes, hypertension).
- MRI and/or ultrasound should be performed to rule out adnexal metastases and evaluate for myometrial invasion.

If the tumor is well sampled and grade 1 with no evidence of extrauterine disease or myometrial invasion, the patient should undergo:

- Informed counseling, preferably with a gynecologic oncologist.
- Treatment with progesterone, either continuous or cyclic.
- Resampling in 3 months to assess response.
- If resolution of disease: patient should be encouraged to achieve pregnancy quickly. Many of these patients will require ART.
- If incomplete resolution of disease: patient may be retreated with another medication regimen or a higher dose of the same formulation and resample in 3 months.
- Once childbearing is complete or if treatment fails, the patient should be counseled for definitive surgical therapy consisting of TAH–BSO with lymphadenectomy as appropriate.

References

1. Jemal A, Siegel R, Ward E, Murray T, Xu J, Smigal C, et al. Cancer Statistics, 2008. CA Cancer J Clin 2008;58(2):271–296.
2. Creasman W, Odicino F, Maisonneuve P, Benedet J, Shephard J, Sideri M, et al. Carcinoma of the corpus uteri. J Epid Biostats 1998;3(35–61).
3. Peterson EP. Endometrial carcinoma in young women. A clinical profile. Obstet & Gynecol 1968;31(5):702–7.
4. Kempson RL. Adenocarcinoma of the endometrium in women aged forty and younger. Cancer 1968;21(4):650–62.
5. Crissman JD, Azoury RS, Barnes AE, Schellhas HF. Endometrial carcinoma in women 40 years of age or younger. Obstet & Gynecol 1981;57(6):699–704.
6. Gallup DG, Stock RJ. Adenocarcinoma of the endometrium in women 40 years of age or younger. Obstet & Gynecol 1984;64(3):417–20.
7. Farhi DC, Nosanchuk J, Silverberg SG. Endometrial adenocarcinoma in women under 25 years of age. Obstet & Gynecol 1986;68(6):741–5.
8. Jeffery JD, Taylor R, Robertson DI, Stuart GC. Endometrial carcinoma occurring in patients under the age of 45 years. Am J Obstet & Gynecol 1987;156(2):366–70.
9. Gitsch G, Hanzal E, Jensen D, Hacker NF. Endometrial cancer in premenopausal women 45 years and younger. Obstet & Gynecol 1995;85(4):504–8.
10. Evans-Metcalf ER, Brooks SE, Reale FR, Baker SP. Profile of women 45 years of age and younger with endometrial cancer. Obst & Gynecol 1998;91(3):349–54.
11. Soliman PT, Oh JC, Schmeler KM, Sun CC, Slomovitz BM, Gershenson DM, et al. Risk factors for young premenopausal women with endometrial cancer. Obstet Gynecol 2005;105(3):575–80.
12. Duska LR, Garrett A, Rueda BR, Haas J, Chang Y, Fuller AF. Endometrial Cancer in Women 40 Years Old or Younger. Gynecol Oncol 2001;83(2):388–93.
13. Schmeler KM, Soliman PT, Sun CC, Slomovitz BM, Gershenson DM, Lu KH. Endometrial cancer in young, normal-weight women. Gynecol Oncol 2005;99(2):388–92.
14. Lu KH, Dinh M, Kohlmann W, et al. Gynecologic cancer as a "sentinel cancer" for women with hereditary nonpolyposis colorectal cancer syndrome. Obstet Gynecol 2005;105(3):569–74.
15. Kurman RJ, Norris HJ. Evaluation of criteria for distinguishing atypical endometrial hyperplasia from well-differentiated carcinoma. Cancer 1982;49(12):2547–59.

16. Zaino RJ, Kauderer J, Trimble CL, et al. Reproducibility of the diagnosis of atypical endometrial hyperplasia: a Gynecologic Oncology Group study. Cancer 2006;106(4):804–11.
17. Trimble CL, Kauderer J, Zaino R, Silverberg S, Lim PC, Burke JJ, 2nd, et al. Concurrent endometrial carcinoma in women with a biopsy diagnosis of atypical endometrial hyperplasia: a Gynecologic Oncology Group study. Cancer 2006;106(4):812–9.
18. Creasman WT, Morrow CP, Bundy BN, Homesley HD, Graham JE, Heller PB. Surgical pathologic spread patterns of endometrial cancer. A Gynecologic Oncology Group Study. Cancer 1987;60(8 Suppl):2035–41.
19. Cowles TA, Magriña JF, Masterson BJ, Capen CV. Comparison of clinical and surgical-staging in patients with endometrial carcinoma. Obstet Gynecol 1985;66(3):413–6.
20. Daniel AG, Peters WA, 3rd. Accuracy of office and operating room curettage in the grading of endometrial carcinoma. Obstet Gynecol 1988;71(4):612–4.
21. Eltabbakh GH, Shamonki J, Mount SL. Surgical stage, final grade, and survival of women with endometrial carcinoma whose preoperative endometrial biopsy shows well-differentiated tumors. Gynecol Oncol 2005;99(2):309–12.
22. Del Maschio A, Vanzulli A, Sironi S, Spagnolo D, Belloni C, Garancini P, et al. Estimating the depth of myometrial involvement by endometrial carcinoma: efficacy of transvaginal sonography vs MR imaging. Am J Roentgenol 1993;160(3):533–8.
23. Gordon AN, Fleischer AC, Dudley BS, Drolshagan LF, Kalemeris GC, Partain CL, et al. Preoperative assessment of myometrial invasion of endometrial adenocarcinoma by sonography (US) and magnetic resonance imaging (MRI). Gynecol Oncol 1989;34(2):175–9.
24. Kim SH. Detection of deep myometrial invasion in endometrial carcinoma: comparison of transvaginal ultrasound, CT, and MRI. J Cell Biol 1995;130(5):1127–36.
25. Zerbe MJ, Bristow R, Grumbine FC, Montz FJ. Inability of preoperative computed tomography scans to accurately predict the extent of myometrial invasion and extracorporal spread in endometrial cancer. Gynecol Oncol 2000;78(1):67–70.
26. Hardesty LA, Sumkin JH, Hakim C, Johns C, Nath M. The ability of helical CT to preoperatively stage endometrial carcinoma. Am J Roentgenol 2001;176(3):603–6.
27. Sanjuan A, Cobo T, Pahisa J, Escaramis G, Ordi J, Ayuso JR, et al. Preoperative and intraoperative assessment of myometrial invasion and histologic grade in endometrial cancer: role of magnetic resonance imaging and frozen section. Int J Gynecol Cancer 2006;16(1):385–90.
28. Frei KA, Kinkel K, Bonel HM, Lu Y, Zaloudek C, Hricak H. Prediction of deep myometrial invasion in patients with endometrial cancer: clinical utility of contrast-enhanced MR imaging-a meta-analysis and Bayesian analysis. Radiology 2000;216(2):444–9.
29. Kinkel K, Kaji Y, Yu KK, et al. Radiologic staging in patients with endometrial cancer: a meta-analysis. Radiology 1999;212(3):711–8.
30. Saez F, Urresola A, Larena JA, et al. Endometrial carcinoma: assessment of myometrial invasion with plain and gadolinium-enhanced MR imaging. J Magn Reson Imaging 2000; 12(3):460–6.
31. Ramirez PT, Frumovitz M, Bodurka DC, Sun CC, Levenback C. Hormonal therapy for the management of grade 1 endometrial adenocarcinoma: a literature review. Gynecol Oncol 2004; 95(1):133–8.
32. Gottlieb WH, Beiner ME, Shalmon B, et al. Outcome of fertility-sparing treatment with progestins in young patients with endometrial cancer. Obstet Gynecol 2003;102(4):718–25.
33. Bokhman JV, Chepick OF, Volkova AT, Vishnevsky AS. Can primary endometrial carcinoma stage I be cured without surgery and radiation therapy? Gynecol Oncol 1985; 20(2): 139–55.
34. Randall TC, Kurman RJ. Progestin treatment of atypical hyperplasia and well-differentiated carcinoma of the endometrium in women under age 40. Obstet Gynecol 1997; 90(3): 434–40.
35. Wang CB, Wang CJ, Huang HJ, et al. Fertility-preserving treatment in young patients with endometrial adenocarcinoma. Cancer 2002; 94(8):2192–8.
36. Niwa K, Tagami K, Lian Z, Onogi K, Mori H, Tamaya T. Outcome of fertility-preserving treatment in young women with endometrial carcinomas. BJOG 2005;112(3):317–20.

37. Kim YB, Holschneider CH, Ghosh K, Nieberg RK, Montz FJ. Progestin alone as primary treatment of endometrial carcinoma in premenopausal women. Report of seven cases and review of the literature. Cancer 1997;79(2):320–7.
38. Rubatt JM, Slomovitz BM, Burke TW, Broaddus RR. Development of metastatic endometrial endometrioid adenocarcinoma while on progestin therapy for endometrial hyperplasia. Gynecol Oncol 2005;99(2): 472–6.
39. Kaku T, Yoshikawa H, Tsuda A, et al. Conservative therapy for adenocarcinoma and atypical endometrial hyperplasia of the endometrium in young women: central pathologic review and treatment outcome. Cancer Lett 2001;167(1):39–48.
40. Yang YC, Wu CC, Chen CP, Chang CL, Wang KL. Reevaluating the safety of fertility-sparing hormonal therapy for early endometrial cancer. Gynecol Oncol 2005;99(2):287–93.
41. Ferrandina G, Zannoni GF, Gallotta V, Foti E, Mancuso S, Scambia G. Progression of conservatively treated endometrial carcinoma after full term pregnancy: a case report. Gynecol Oncol 2005;99(1):215–7.
42. Ogawa S, Koike T, Shibahara H, et al. Assisted reproductive technologies in conjunction with conservatively treated endometrial adenocarcinoma. A case report. Gynecol & Obstet Investigation 2001;51(3):214–6.
43. Jobo T, Imai M, Kawaguchi M, Kenmochi M, Kuramoto H. Successful conservative treatment of endometrial carcinoma permitting subsequent pregnancy: report of two cases. Eur J Gynaecol Oncol 2000;21(2):119–22.
44. Sardi J. Primary hormonal treatment for early endometrial carcinoma. Hum Reprod 1997;12(8):1649–53.
45. Shibahara H. Successful pregnancy in an infertile patient with conservatively treated endometrial adenocarcinoma after transfer of embryos obtained by intracytoplasmic sperm injection. Cancer Letters 2001;167(1):39–48.
46. Kung FT, Chen WJ, Chou HH, Ko SF, Chang SY. Conservative management of early endometrial adenocarcinoma with repeat curettage and hormone therapy under assistance of hysteroscopy and laparoscopy. Hum Reproduct 1997;12(8):1649–53.
47. Mazzon I, Corrado G, Morricone D, Scambia G. Reproductive preservation for treatment of stage IA endometrial cancer in a young woman: hysteroscopic resection. Int J Gynecol Cancer 2005;15(5):974–8.
48. Yarali H, Bozdag G, Aksu T, Ayhan A. A successful pregnancy after intracytoplasmic sperm injection and embryo transfer in a patient with endometrial cancer who was treated conservatively. Fertil Steril 2004;81(1):214–6.
49. Nakao Y, Nomiyama M, Kojima K, Matsumoto Y, Yamasaki F, Iwasaka T. Successful pregnancies in 2 infertile patients with endometrial adenocarcinoma. Gynecol Obstet Invest 2004;58(2):68–71.
50. Pinto AB. Successful in vitro fertilization pregnancy after conservative management of endometrial cancer. Obstet & Gynecol 1981;57(6):699–704.
51. Kimmig R, Strowitzki T, Muller-Hocker J, Kurzl R, Korell M, Hepp H. Conservative treatment of endometrial cancer permitting subsequent triplet pregnancy. Gynecol Oncol 1995;58(2):255–7.
52. Walsh C, Holschneider C, Hoang Y, Tieu K, Karlan B, Cass I. Coexisting ovarian malignancy in young women with endometrial cancer. Obstet Gynecol 2005;106(4):693–9.
53. Zaino R, Whitney C, Brady MF, DeGeest K, Burger RA, Buller RE. Simultaneously detected endometrial and ovarian carcinomas--a prospective clinicopathologic study of 74 cases: a gynecologic oncology group study. Gynecol Oncol 2001;83(2):355–62.
54. Morice P, Fourchotte V, Sideris L, Gariel C, Duvillard P, Castaigne D. A need for laparoscopic evaluation of patients with endometrial carcinoma selected for conservative treatment. Gynecol Oncol 2005;96(1):245–8.
55. Mitsushita J, Toki T, Kato K, Fujii S, Konishi I. Endometrial carcinoma remaining after term pregnancy following conservative treatment with medroxyprogesterone acetate. Gynecol Oncol 2000;79(1):129–32.

56. Montz FJ, Bristow RE, Bovicelli A, Tomacruz R, Kurman RJ. Intrauterine progesterone treatment of early endometrial cancer. Am J Obstet Gynecol 2002;186(4):651–7.
57. Dhar KK, NeedhiRajan T, Koslowski M, Woolas RP. Is levonorgestrel intrauterine system effective for treatment of early endometrial cancer? Report of four cases and review of the literature. Gynecol Oncol 2005;97(3):924–7.
58. Jones K, Georgiou M, Hyatt D, Spencer T, Thomas H. Endometrial adenocarcinoma following the insertion of a Mirena IUCD. Gynecol Oncol 2002;87(2):216–8.
59. Jeon YT, Park IA, Kim YB, et al. Steroid receptor expressions in endometrial cancer: clinical significance and epidemiological implication. Cancer Lett 2006;239(2):198–204.
60. Ehrlich CE, Young PC, Cleary RE. Cytoplasmic progesterone and estradiol receptors in normal, hyperplastic, and carcinomatous endometria: therapeutic implications. Am J Obstet & Gynecol 1981;141(5):539–46.
61. Ehrlich CE, Young PC, Stehman FB, Sutton GP, Alford WM. Steroid receptors and clinical outcome in patients with adenocarcinoma of the endometrium. Am J Obstet & Gynecol 1988;158(4):796–807.
62. Creasman WT, Soper JT, McCarty KS, Hinshaw W, Clarke-Pearson DL. Influence of cytoplasmic steroid receptor content on prognosis of early stage endometrial carcinoma. Am J Obstet & Gynecol 1985;151(7):922–32.
63. Benraad TJ, Friberg LG, Koenders AJ, Kullander S. Do estrogen and progesterone receptors (E2R and PR) in metastasizing endometrial cancers predict the response to gestagen therapy? Acta Obstetricia et Gynecologica Scandinavica 1980;59(2):155–9.
64. Creasman WT, McCarty KS, Sr., Barton TK, McCarty KS, Jr. Clinical correlates of estrogen- and progesterone-binding proteins in human endometrial adenocarcinoma. Obstet & Gynecol 1980;55(3):363–70.
65. Martin PM, Rolland PH, Gammerre M, Serment H, Toga M. Estradiol and progesterone receptors in normal and neoplastic endometrium: correlations between receptors, histopathological examinations and clinical responses under progestin therapy. Int J Cancer 1979;23(3):321–9.
66. Kauppila A, Kujansuu E, Vihko R. Cytosol estrogen and progestin receptors in endometrial carcinoma of patients treated with surgery, radiotherapy, and progestin. Clinical correlates. Cancer 1982;50(10):2157–62.
67. Smid-Koopman E, Kuhne LC, Hanekamp EE, et al. Progesterone-induced inhibition of growth and differential regulation of gene expression in PRA- and/or PRB-expressing endometrial cancer cell lines. J Soc Gynecol Investig 2005;12(4):285–92.
68. Hanekamp EE, Gielen SC, Smid-Koopman E, et al. Consequences of loss of progesterone receptor expression in development of invasive endometrial cancer. Clin Cancer Res 2003;9(11):4190–9.
69. Smid-Koopman E, Blok LJ, Kuhne LC, et al. Distinct functional differences of human progesterone receptors A and B on gene expression and growth regulation in two endometrial carcinoma cell lines. J Soc Gynecol Investig 2003;10(1):49–57.
70. Miyamoto T, Watanabe J, Hata H, et al. Significance of progesterone receptor-A and -B expressions in endometrial adenocarcinoma. J Steroid Biochem Mol Biol 2004;92(3):111–8.
71. Conneely OM. Progesterone receptors in reproduction: functional impact of the A and B isoforms. Science 2000;289(5485):1751–4.
72. Conneely OM, Mulac-Jericevic B, Lydon JP, De Mayo FJ. Reproductive functions of the progesterone receptor isoforms: lessons from knock-out mice. Mol Cell Endocrinol 2001;179(1-2):97–103.
73. Conneely OM. Perspective: female steroid hormone action. Arthritis & Rheumatism 2001;44(4):782–93.
74. Rowan BG, Bai W. Progesterone receptor coactivators. Differential phosphorylation of chicken progesterone receptor in hormone-dependent and ligand-independent activation. Steroids 2000;65(10-11):545–9.
75. Spitz IM. Progesterone receptor modulators at the start of a new millennium. Steroids 2000;65(10-11):817–23.

76. Bouchard P. Progesterone and the progesterone receptor. J Reprod Med 1999;44(2 Suppl):153–7.
77. Arnett-Mansfield RL, deFazio A, Wain GV, et al. Relative expression of progesterone receptors A and B in endometrioid cancers of the endometrium. Cancer Res 2001; 61(11):4576–82.
78. Dai D, Kumar NS, Wolf DM, Leslie KK. Molecular tools to reestablish progestin control of endometrial cancer cell proliferation. Am J Obstet Gynecol 2001;184(5):790–7.

Early-Stage Endometrial Cancer: Surgery

Yukio Sonoda

Abstract Endometrial cancer typically presents at an early stage and surgery alone can be curative in many of these cases. Traditionally, surgery for early-stage disease has been carried out using an open approach; however, the use of minimally invasive surgery has rapidly grown in the field of gynecologic oncology. Multiple studies have demonstrated its feasibility and oncologic outcomes continue to be validated.

Keywords Endometrial cancer • Surgery • Laparoscopy

Introduction

Endometrial cancer consistently remains the most common gynecologic malignancy in the USA, and it ranks as the fourth most common cancer of the American female population. There will be an estimated 40,100 new cancers of the uterine corpus and 7,470 deaths from this disease in 2008 (1). Fortunately, the vast majority of endometrial cancers will be detected in the early stages: approximately 75% of these cancers are limited to the uterus at time of discovery. This is in large part due to the early warning sign of abnormal uterine bleeding present in the early stages of the disease.

Endometrial cancer is classified into two types (2). Type I cancers are the more common form and are associated with increased levels of circulating estrogen. These tumors usually begin as endometrial hyperplasia and progress to cancer. They tend to occur at a younger age and are less aggressive (typically grade I and

Y. Sonoda (✉)
Gynecology Service, Department of Surgery, Memorial Sloan-Ketering Cancer Center,
New York, NY
e-mail: sonoday@mskcc.org

F. Muggia and E. Oliva (eds.), *Uterine Cancer*, Current Clinical Oncology,
DOI: 10.1007/978-1-60327-044-1_8,
© Humana Press, a Part of Springer Science+Business Media, LLC 2009

II endometrioid adenocarcinomas). Type II cancers are higher-grade, more aggressive, and tend to arise in a background of atrophic endometrium. Histologically, they encompass serous, clear-cell, and grade 3 endometrioid adenocarcinomas. They occur in older patients and do not have an estrogen-related precursor.

Fortunately, early-stage Type I endometrial cancers comprise the vast majority of cases and can be cured. The surgical treatment of early-stage Type I cancers will be the subject of this chapter.

Surgical Therapy

With the change of the staging system for this disease from a clinical to a surgical evaluation, primary treatment for women with endometrial cancer begins with surgery. Prior to undergoing a major surgical procedure, and given that this disease is associated with surgical risk factors such as obesity, hypertension, and diabetes, all patients should undergo a thorough history and physical examination. Physical examination should include areas of potential tumor spread: enlarged supraclavicular and inguinal lymph nodes, signs of intra-abdominal disease or ascites, and close inspection of the cervix and vagina. Chest radiography should be obtained to rule out any pulmonary spread. Other imaging modalities such as computed tomography or magnetic resonance imaging should not be routinely obtained unless there are findings on history and physical examination that warrant further investigation. Serum CA-125 has been shown to be elevated in patients with advanced disease, and this may provide additional information if intra-abdominal spread is suspected (3).

The standard surgical approach to the patient with endometrial cancer clinically confined to the uterus comprises an exploratory laparotomy, exploration of the peritoneal cavity, peritoneal washings, biopsies of any suspicious lesions, TAH, BSO, and selected para-aortic and pelvic lymph node sampling.

After entering the abdomen, a thorough exploration of the peritoneal cavity is performed. Any suspicious lesions should be biopsied. Peritoneal washings are obtained by instilling approximately 100 cc of saline into the pelvis and aspirating for cytological analysis. The fallopian tubes, the round and the utero-ovarian ligaments are occluded by placing a large clamp across them. This serves to prevent retrograde tumor dissemination during uterine manipulation and helps provide uterine traction. An extrafascial hysterectomy with BSO can then be performed.

Once the primary specimen has been removed, the pelvic and para-aortic lymph nodes should be sampled. This is an area that remains controversial in the management of endometrial cancer. The basis for lymph node sampling arose from the Gynecologic Oncology Group (GOG) protocol 33 (4). This study demonstrated that the incidence of pelvic and para-aortic lymph node metastasis was greater for patients with high-grade and deeply invasive tumors. Low-grade tumors with no or only superficial myometrial invasion had a very small incidence of lymph node spread.

Intraoperative Management

In the absence of obvious extrauterine spread, some have advocated using a combination of preoperative tumor grade, intraoperative assessment of myometrial invasion, and clinical evaluation of the lymph nodes to determine if lymph node assessment should be undertaken. However, this approach relies on several uncertainties. Tumor grade can not be accurately determined using office biopsy or curettage. In a retrospective study by Obermair et al. (5), the preoperative histologic grade of the curettage specimen was compared with that of the final specimen. Only 78% of well-differentiated tumors diagnosed on curettage maintained the same histologic grade on final analysis. Similar results of the inaccuracy of preoperative grade assessment have been demonstrated by other authors (6–8).

Accurately assessing depth of myometrial invasion by either intraoperative visual inspection or frozen section analysis can be difficult. Intraoperative visual examination can correctly predict the degree of myometrial invasion in 87% of grade 1 tumors, 65% of grade 2 tumors, and 31% of grade 3 tumors (9). The use of frozen section analysis to assess myometrial invasion has been advocated by some (10). In a recent study of 153 patients with grade 1 or 2 endometrial endometrioid cancer, Frumovitz et al. (11) compared preoperative grade and intraoperative myometrial invasion with final pathology. There were 49 patients (32%) who had a discrepancy between preoperative and final histology. Thirty seven (27%) had their lesions upgraded to a higher grade or were found to be a histology other than endometrioid adenocarcinoma. Twenty-six percent of Pipelle biopsies and 23% of curettage specimens were upgraded on final pathology. The authors concluded that a clinically significant number of patients will be found to have more advanced disease than can be predicted using preoperative and intraoperative prognostic factors, and these should not be relied upon for staging. Palpation of the retroperitoneal nodes can be inaccurate even in experienced hands. In one study of 126 women, assessment by palpation alone would have missed 36% of positive nodes (12). Others have also demonstrated this inaccuracy (13). Additionally, over one-third of lymph nodes may have only microscopic metastasis (14).

Routine Staging

Since intraoperative assessment of pathologic risk factors for extrauterine spread is not perfect, many have advocated the routine use of surgical staging for all patients. In a large population-based study of over 10,000 patients, Trimble et al. (15) demonstrated the impact of lymph node sampling on survival in women with International Federation of Gynecology and Obstetrics (FIGO) stage I and II endometrial adenocarcinoma. Five-year relative survival was not significantly improved in stage I patients who underwent lymph node sampling. When stage I patients were stratified by histologic grade, lymph node sampling was associated with an increased survival in patients with grade 3 tumors but not grade 1 or 2. This may have been due to the identification of women with more advanced disease. The American College of Obstetricians and Gynecologists recently published its clinical management guidelines for endometrial cancer and recommended systemic surgical staging for most women with endometrial cancer. Exceptions mentioned were young or perimenopausal women with grade 1 tumors associated with CAH or women deemed at increased risk secondary to comorbid conditions (16).

Lymph Node Evaluation

The extent of the lymph node sampling is another controversial aspect of this topic. Improved outcomes have been associated with increased number of nodes removed. Kilgore et al. (17) reviewed their experience on 649 patients with adenocarcinoma of the endometrium. Patients were categorized into one of three groups: multiple-site pelvic node sampling, limited pelvic node sampling, and no sampling. Patients in whom multiple-site sampling, which was defined as having at least four sites sampled, was performed had a significantly better survival than patients who had no sampling. Patients with limited or less than four sites sampled did not have a significantly better survival when compared with those patients who did not have sampling. Cragun et al. (18) recently published a single institution series on selective lymphadenectomy in apparent early-stage endometrial cancer. An improvement in overall and progression-free survival was seen in patients with poorly differentiated tumors and greater than 11 nodes removed. This survival advantage was not seen in patients with grade 1 or 2 tumors. These data suggest a therapeutic value to performing a lymphadenectomy, and some advocated the routine use of lymphadenectomy in the management of these patients. Complete lymphadenectomy can provide excellent local control (Table 1) (19–24).

One potential explanation for the therapeutic benefits of lymphadenectomy may be the removal of any subclinically involved nodes. Girardi et al. (14) reported on their experience with systematic pelvic lymphadenectomy in the treatment of

Table 1. Recurrences in moderate and high-risk patients treated with lymphadenectomy without whole-pelvic radiation

Author	Number of patients	Mean number of pelvic nodes	Mean follow-up (months)	Post operative brachy-therapy	Number of local recur-rences	Number of distant recurrences
Fanning et al. (19)	22	28	34	Yes	0	1
Orr et al. (20)	115	24	39	Yes	0	7
Larson et al. (21)	105	N/A	43	No	4	4
Mohan et al. (22)	63	33	96	Yes	0	5 (1 site unknown)
Seago et al. (23)	23	N/A	26	Yes	0	2
Berclaz et al. (24)	19	18	54	Yes	1	0

endometrial cancer. A mean of 37 pelvic nodes were removed, and 27 of 76 (36%) patients were upstaged based on lymph node metastases. Thirty-seven percent of lymph node metastases were ≤2 mm in diameter. Additionally, Yabushita et al. (25) demonstrated that up to 38% of patients with stage I endometrial cancers were found to have metastatic disease detectable by immunostain only. Removal of this otherwise undetectable disease can be performed with low morbidity (20, 26) and may explain the potential therapeutic benefit to lymphadenectomy in early-stage endometrial cancer.

Alternatively, inadequate evaluation of the lymph nodes may lead to miss metastasis and undertreatment of more advanced disease (27). Inadequate nodal evaluation may account for the difference in survival observed in cases that are at higher risk for spread. In a retrospective study of 467 patients with FIGO stage I and II endometrial cancers, a pelvic lymph node count of ≥12 nodes was associated with an improved survival only in cases with high-risk histology. The authors suggested that this observation was a result of improved staging in patients with higher node counts who were at higher risk for spread (28). A more targeted approach to lymph node evaluation may eventually do away with the need to perform lymph node sampling to any degree. Sentinel lymph node mapping was first reported in 1996 (29), and gradually, feasibility studies have begun to appear in the literature (30–33). The concept is promising and would undoubtedly be useful; however, its utility remains to be proven before it is routinely employed in the treatment of endometrial cancer.

Surgery is the mainstay of the treatment of this disease. Yet, surgeons specifically trained for the surgical management of this disease, gynecologic oncologists, are only involved in the care of 40% of women with this disease (34). Thus, a significant portion of patients diagnosed with endometrial cancer will not have appropriate surgery, as gynecologic oncologists are 2.5 times more likely to perform complete surgical staging when compared with general obstetrician/gynecologists (34). Such figures have led the Society of Gynecologic Oncologists to issue statements advising that patients with a primary diagnosis of endometrial cancer or recurrent disease be referred to a gynecologic oncologist to assist in determining the most appropriate surgical approach as well as extent of surgery and the potential benefits of adjuvant therapy (35).

Laparoscopic Surgery and Endometrial Cancer

Minimally invasive surgery has become increasingly popular in the management of gynecologic malignancies. Vaginal hysterectomy has been used in the management of endometrial cancers in certain situations (36). However, the vaginal route does not allow for the evaluation of the peritoneal cavity or the retroperitoneal lymph nodes. With the development of improved instruments and surgeons' skills, laparoscopic surgeons began to perform more complicated procedures including sampling of the retroperitoneal lymph nodes.

Childers et al. (37) first reported on the combined use of laparoscopy with vaginal hysterectomy for the treatment of early-stage endometrial cancer. This group later reported on a series of 59 patients with clinical stage I endometrial cancer who were staged by this new procedure. Their technique included an inspection of the peritoneal cavity, intraperitoneal washings, and a laparoscopically assisted vaginal hysterectomy (LVAH). Patients with preoperative grade 2 or 3 tumors or grade 1 tumors with >50% myometrial invasion underwent laparoscopic pelvic and para-aortic lymphadenectomy. Six patients had intraperitoneal disease. Two patients could not undergo laparoscopic lymphadenectomy secondary to obesity, and two patients required conversion to laparotomy for intraoperative complications.

While surgical staging performed through an open approach remains the standard of care, advances in minimally invasive surgical techniques have allowed the use of laparoscopy in endometrial cancer surgery. Many studies have described the use of a combined laparoscopic and vaginal approach to perform all of the procedures involved in endometrial cancer staging, including a complete assessment of peritoneal surfaces and retroperitoneum (37–41). Total laparoscopic hysterectomy (TLH) has also been well-described as a technique that eliminates the need for vaginal surgery during the procedure (42).

Potential benefits of laparoscopy are numerous and include decreased postoperative morbidity, pain, recovery time, operative time, and complications as well as increased patient satisfaction and quality of life. Gemignani et al. (43) performed a retrospective review of 320 patients with early-stage endometrial cancer treated by LAVH or TAH. They found that LAVH was associated with a decrease in hospital stay, fewer complications, and lower overall hospital charges. Several other authors have reported similar findings. Cost comparisons have had mixed results with similar or even increased cost associated with the laparoscopic approach (38, 44, 45).

While benefits such as decreased pain and recovery time are historically well described in patients with benign disease, questions of feasibility as well as outcomes and equivalency of open versus laparoscopic procedures have been raised in patients with malignancy. General feasibility of minimally invasive approaches has been described in several studies. Eltabbakh et al. (38) reported the results of a prospective series of 86 women with clinical stage I disease who underwent laparoscopic staging. Pelvic and/or para-aortic lymph node dissection were performed based on risk assessment due to myometrial invasion, tumor grade, or high-risk histologic type, such as papillary serous or clear-cell tumors (pelvic lymph node dissection in patients with myometrial invasion, grade >1, or high-risk histology; para-aortic lymph node dissection in patients with grade 3 disease and myometrial invasion, invasion > half depth, or high-risk histology). Mean operating time was 190 min, mean estimated blood loss (EBL) was 278.3 ml, and conversion to laparotomy occurred in 5 (5.8%) of 86 patients. When compared with their own historical controls of patients undergoing open staging, they found an increase in mean pelvic lymph nodes harvested (10.8 with laparoscopy vs 4.9 with open surgery), while para-aortic lymph node count was not significantly different (2.7 with laparoscopy versus 4.2 with open surgery). Laparoscopy was associated with longer surgical time, no significant difference in major complications, and decreases in EBL, pain medication, and hospitalization.

The equivalency of lymph node dissection was also addressed by Kohler et al. (46) in an analysis of 650 laparoscopic pelvic and/or para-aortic transperitoneal lymphadenectomies in patients with gynecologic malignancies. Of the 112 patients with endometrial cancer, 66 presented for primary surgery with LAVH, BSO, and complete pelvic and para-aortic lymph node dissection. A mean of 26.7 lymph nodes (pelvic, 15.4; para-aortic, 9.6) was harvested, with mean durations of 56 and 63 min for pelvic and para-aortic lymph node dissections, respectively. These minimally invasive techniques can also be applied in situations where inadequate staging has been performed. Since the majority of patients with endometrial cancer are not treated by specifically trained surgeons, many will not have had complete staging. Laparoscopic restaging can be performed with low morbidity and short hospitalization while performing valuable prognostic information (47).

Several authors have retrospectively studied outcomes and survival of laparoscopic surgery for endometrial cancer and found comparable results. Eltabbakh (48) found similar 2- and 5-year overall survival rates with no difference in sites of recurrence in 100 patients undergoing laparoscopy compared with patients undergoing laparotomy. In a review of 45 patients with stage I disease with a mean follow-up of 6.4 years, Magriña et al. (49) found a 5-year recurrence rate of 4.9% and a 5-year cause-specific survival rate of 94.7% – rates similar to those achieved with laparotomy. Reporting on TLH specifically, Obermair (42) compared TLH (226 patients) and TAH (284 patients) with or without staging and found that intention to treat (TLH versus TAH) did not influence disease-free survival or overall survival. Patterns of recurrence in the two groups were similar as well.

Smaller prospective randomized controlled trials have also compared the combined laparoscopic and vaginal approach to abdominal approach in the management of endometrial cancer. Malur et al. (50) compared 37 patients treated by laparoscopically assisted approach with 33 patients treated by laparotomy. Pelvic and aortic lymph node dissections were performed, except in patients with well-differentiated tumors that invaded to < the inner third of the myometrium. While there was no difference in mean number of lymph nodes and mean operation time, patients who underwent laparoscopic staging had less blood loss, fewer transfusions, and a shorter hospital stay. With a mean follow-up of 16.5 months (range, 2–43 months) and 21.6 months (range, 2–48 months) for laparoscopic and laparotomy groups, respectively, the recurrence-free and overall survival rates were not significantly different (97.3% versus 93.3% and 83.9% versus 90.9%, respectively). Fram (51) reported on 61 clinical stage I patients randomized to laparoscopic versus open staging. Laparoscopy was associated with a significant decrease in EBL (145 vs 501 ml) and hospitalization (2.3 versus 5.5 days), and there was not much difference in the number of lymph nodes removed (21.3 versus 21.9). Currently, the GOG is conducting a large prospective trial (GOG LAP 2) to determine the equivalency of LAVH with laparoscopic staging compared with the traditional laparotomy approach in terms of cancer outcome.

A recent prospective study on quality of life in patients with endometrial cancer treated with laparoscopy or laparotomy was published by Zullo et al. (52).

Eighty-four patients were enrolled and randomized to either surgical approach. There was a control group of 40 patients with matched demographic characteristics who did not have cancer. Subjects were surveyed prior to and until 6 months after surgery. At entry, both treatment groups demonstrated significantly worse quality of life compared to controls. Comparing the two treatment groups, those treated with laparoscopic surgery had a significantly higher quality of life compared with subjects managed with laparotomy. A quality-of-life instrument is included in the GOG LAP 2 study which should provide more information on this subject.

A theoretical concern specific to laparoscopy is the potential for retrograde seeding with the use of a uterine manipulator. In a retrospective study of 377 patients with early-stage endometrial cancer treated with either LAVH or TAH, the authors found that patients in the LAVH group had a significantly higher incidence of positive peritoneal washings (10.3% versus 2.8%, $P = 0.002$) (53). As no difference in known prognostic factors was identified, the authors hypothesized that this finding may have been caused by the use of an intrauterine manipulator during the LAVH procedure in this series. Supporting this hypothesis, other authors found no difference in positive peritoneal cytology in series in which a manipulator was not used (54). However, in a recently published prospective series of 42 patients undergoing laparoscopic surgery for clinical stage I endometrial cancer, peritoneal washings were obtained before and after the insertion of a uterine manipulator. The overall incidence of positive peritoneal cytology was 14.3%, but no patient had positive peritoneal washings after the insertion of the manipulator if the washings were negative before insertion. The authors felt that use of a uterine manipulator did not increase the incidence of positive peritoneal cytology (55).

Surgery for Stage II Disease

Extrafascial hysterectomy is usually employed in the surgical management of endometrial cancer. However, when there is known or suspected cervical involvement, radical hysterectomy can be used to effectively control local disease. In a retrospective series of 202 patients with cervical involvement from endometrial cancer, Boente et al. (56) defined five treatment groups: radical hysterectomy ± radiation, TAH/BSO, radiation therapy alone, radiation therapy followed by TAH/BSO, and TAH/BSO followed by radiation therapy. Despite having more frequent adverse prognostic factors, patients treated with radical hysterectomy had an 86% 5-year actuarial survival. This was in contrast to 5-year survival rates of 38% and 19% in the radiation group followed by TAH/BSO and TAH/BSO ± radiotherapy groups, respectively. Although formal statistical comparisons were not made, the authors supported the use of radical hysterectomy in patients with stage II endometrial cancer.

Improved outcomes with radical hysterectomy were described by Mariani et al. (57) in a review of 82 patients with cervical involvement. Although this study included both stage II and III patients, a subgroup analysis of only patients with stage II disease treated with radical hysterectomy demonstrated superior results.

Both disease-related and recurrence-free survival were 100% in patients treated with radical hysterectomy compared to 80% and 73%, respectively, in patients treated with simple hysterectomy. Thus, treatment of patients that have known cervical extension using radical hysterectomy appears to be a reasonable approach.

Surgery in the Morbidly Obese Patient

Obesity is a major risk factor for the development of endometrial cancer and many patients will present with a high BMI [also described as Quetelet Index (QI)]. Patients classified as morbidly obese can be technically challenging to operate on. This sub-classification of patients may comprise over one-quarter of patients with endometrial cancer (58). These patients require longer operating times and experience greater blood loss when compared to patients with BMIs < 30 kg/m^2. However, hospital stay and perioperative complications do not appear to be greater.

Consideration may be given to performing a panniculectomy in these patients. In a retrospective series of patients undergoing panniculectomy for endometrial neoplasms, it was associated with a higher para-aortic node count when compared with matched controls (59). The procedure was not associated with an increase in perioperative morbidity. Although pelvic node count was not higher, the authors suggested that panniculectomy may enhance operative exposure and facilitate the staging procedure.

While technically challenging, obesity may not be an absolute contraindication to performing a laparoscopic staging procedure. Scribner et al. (60) reported on their experience of laparoscopic pelvic and para-aortic lymphadenectomy in obese patients. In 55 patients, laparoscopic staging was completed in 82% of them with a QI < 35 compared with only 44% in patients with a QI ≥ 35 (P= 0.004). Despite this difference, these authors and others concluded that obesity is not an absolute contraindication to laparoscopic staging (60, 61). In contrast, Kohler et al. (46) found no significant difference in lymph node yield according to BMI in patients undergoing laparoscopic para-aortic lymphadenectomy, although they reported a significant increase in duration of right-sided para-aortic lymph node dissections in patients with a BMI > 30. They attribute this finding to increased difficulty with exposure in the para-aortic region – a problem they did not encounter in the pelvis.

Conclusions

- Early-stage endometrial cancer is surgically treated, yielding valuable information for diagnostic and therapeutic purposes.
- The potential variability between preoperative and final histologic grade, depth of invasion, and other prognostic factors mandates that surgical staging be performed in the majority of patients with early-stage cancer.

- Advances in minimally invasive techniques, skills, and instrumentation offer many potential benefits to patients undergoing surgical management. Some anatomic barriers, however, such as large fibroid uteri, are contraindications to laparoscopic surgery in the presence of endometrial cancer.
- The equivalency of outcome with the abdominal approach, when applying such laparoscopic procedures is being sought in a Gynecologic Oncology Group trial. However, initial reports of feasibility as well as improved patient satisfaction with decreased morbidity are promising.
- Data suggest that laparoscopic surgery may become the main treatment option in patients with early-stage endometrial cancer.

References

1. Jemal A, Siegel R, Ward E, Hao Y, Xu J, Murray T, Thun MJ. Cancer statistics, 2008. CA Caner J Clin. 2008;58(2):271–296.
2. Kurman RJ, Zaino RJ, Norris HJ. Endometrial carcinoma. In: Kurman RJ (ed.). Blaustein's Pathology of the Female Genital Tract (4th Edn). Springer-Verlag. New York, p 439–486 (1994).
3. Sood AK, Buller RE, Burger RA, Dawson JD, Sorosky JI, Berman M. Value of preoperative CA 125 level in the management of uterine cancer and prediction of clinical outcome. Obstet Gynecol. 1997;90(3):441–447.
4. Creasman WT, Morrow CP, Bundy BN, Homesley HD, Graham JE, Heller PB. Surgical pathologic spread patterns of endometrial cancer. A Gynecologic Oncology Group study. Cancer. 1987;60(8 Suppl):2035–2041.
5. Obermair A, Geramou M, Gucer F, et al. Endometrial cancer: accuracy of the finding of a well differentiated tumor at dilatation and curettage compared to the findings at subsequent hysterectomy. Int J Gynecol Cancer. 1999;9(5):383–386.
6. Daniel AG, Peters WA 3rd. Accuracy of office and operating room curettage in the grading of endometrial carcinoma. Obstet Gynecol. 1988;71(4):612–614.
7. Ben-Shachar I, Pavelka J, Cohn DE, et al. Surgical staging for patients presenting with grade 1 endometrial carcinoma. Obstet Gynecol. 2005;105(3):487–493.
8. Larson DM, Johnson KK, Broste SK, Krawisz BR, Kresl JJ. Comparison of D&C and office endometrial biopsy in predicting final histopathologic grade in endometrial cancer. Obstet Gynecol. 1995;86(1):38–42.
9. Goff BA, Rice LW. Assessment of depth of myometrial invasion in endometrial adenocarcinoma. Gynecol Oncol. 1990;38(1):46–48.
10. Fanning J, Tsukada Y, Piver MS. Intraoperative frozen section diagnosis of depth of myometrial invasion in endometrial adenocarcinoma. Gynecol Oncol. 1990;37(1):47–50.
11. Frumovitz M, Singh DK, Meyer L, et al. Predictors of final histology in patients with endometrial cancer. Gynecol Oncol. 2004;95(3):463–468.
12. Arango HA, Hoffman MS, Roberts WS, DeCesare SL, Fiorica JV, Drake J. Accuracy of lymph node palpation to determine need for lymphadenectomy in gynecologic malignancies. Obstet Gynecol. 2000;95(4):553–556.
13. Eltabbakh GH. Intraoperative clinical evaluation of lymph nodes in women with gynecologic cancer. Am J Obstet Gynecol. 2001;184(6):1177–1181.
14. Girardi F, Petru E, Heydarfadai M, Haas J, Winter R. Pelvic lymphadenectomy in the surgical treatment of endometrial cancer. Gynecol Oncol. 1993;49(2):177–180.
15. Trimble EL, Kosary C, Park RC. Lymph node sampling and survival in endometrial cancer. Gynecol Oncol. 1998;71(3):340–343.

16. ACOG Practice Bulletin #65. Management of endometrial cancer. Obstet Gynecol. 2005; 106(2):413–425.
17. Kilgore LC, Partridge EE, Alvarez RD et al. Adenocarcinoma of the endometrium: survival comparisons of patients with and without pelvic node sampling. Gynecol Oncol. 1995;56(1):29–33.
18. Cragun JM, Havrilesky LJ, Calingaert B, et al. Retrospective analysis of selective lymphadenectomy in apparent early-stage endometrial cancer. J Clin Oncol. 2005;23(16):3668–3675.
19. Fanning J, Nanavati PJ, Hilgers RD. Surgical staging and high dose rate brachytherapy for endometrial cancer: limiting external radiotherapy to node-positive tumors. Obstet Gynecol. 1996;87(6):1041–1044.
20. Orr JW Jr, Holimon JL, Orr PF. Stage I corpus cancer: is teletherapy necessary? Am J Obstet Gynecol. 1997;176(4):777–788.
21. Larson DM, Broste SK, Krawisz BR. Surgery without radiotherapy for primary treatment of endometrial cancer. Obstet Gynecol. 1998;91(3):355–359.
22. Mohan DS, Samuels MA, Selim MA, et al. Long-term outcomes of therapeutic pelvic lymphadenectomy for stage I endometrial adenocarcinoma. Gynecol Oncol. 1998;70(2): 165–171.
23. Seago DP, Raman A, Lele S. Potential benefit of lymphadenectomy for the treatment of node-negative locally advanced uterine cancers. Gynecol Oncol. 2001;83(2):282–285.
24. Berclaz G, Hanggi W, Kratzer-Berger A, Altermatt HJ, Greiner RH, Dreher E. Lymphadenectomy in high risk endometrial carcinoma stage I and II: no more morbidity and no need for external pelvic radiation. Int J Gynecol Cancer. 1999;9(4):322–328.
25. Yabushita H, Shimazu M, Yamada H et al. Occult lymph node metastases detected by cytokeratin immunohistochemistry predict recurrence in node-negative endometrial cancer. Gynecol Oncol. 2001;80(2):139–144.
26. Fanning S, Firestein S. Prospective evaluation of the morbidity of complete lymphadenectomy in endometrial cancer. Int J Gynecol Cancer. 1998;8:270–273.
27. Benedetti-Panici P, Maneschi F, Cutillo G, et al. Anatomical and pathological study of retroperitoneal nodes in endometrial cancer. Int J Gynecol Cancer. 1998;8:322–327.
28. Lutman CV, Havrilesky LJ, Cragun JM, et al. Pelvic lymph node count is an important prognostic variable for FIGO stage I and II endometrial carcinoma with high-risk histology. Gynecol Oncol. 2006; 5;102(1):92–97.
29. Burke TW, Levenback C, Tornos C, Morris M, Wharton JT, Gershenson DM. Intraabdominal lymphatic mapping to direct selective pelvic and paraaortic lymphadenectomy in women with high-risk endometrial cancer: results of a pilot study. Gynecol Oncol. 1996;62(2):169–173.
30. Holub Z, Kliment L, Lukac J, Voracek J. Laparoscopically-assisted intraoperative lymphatic mapping in endometrial cancer: preliminary results. Eur J Gynaecol Oncol. 2001;22(2):118–121.
31. Pelosi E, Arena V, Baudino B, et al. Pre-operative lymphatic mapping and intra-operative sentinel lymph node detection in early stage endometrial cancer. Nucl Med Commun. 2003;24(9):971–975.
32. Niikura H, Okamura C, Utsunomiya H, et al. Sentinel lymph node detection in patients with endometrial cancer. Gynecol Oncol. 2004;92(2):669–674.
33. Raspagliesi F, Ditto A, Kusamura S, et al. Hysteroscopic injection of tracers in sentinel node detection of endometrial cancer: a feasibility study. Am J Obstet Gynecol. 2004;191(2):435–439.
34. Partridge EE, Jessup JM, Donaldson ES, et al. 1996 Patient Care Evaluation Study (PCE) of Cancer of the Corpus Uteri. National Cancer Database (NCDB), American College of Surgery. Gynecol Oncol. 1999;72(3):445.
35. Society of Gynecologic Oncologists. Referral Guidelines in Gynecologic Oncology. Gynecol Oncol. 2000;78:S1–S13.
36. Chan JK, Lin YG, Monk BJ, Tewari K, Bloss JD, Berman ML. Vaginal hysterectomy as primary treatment of endometrial cancer in medically compromised women. Obstet Gynecol. 2001;97:707–711.

37. Childers JM, Brzechffa PR, Hatch KD, Surwit EA. Laparoscopically assisted surgical staging (LASS) of endometrial cancer. Gynecol Oncol. 1993;51(1):33–38.
38. Eltabbakh GH, Shamonki MI, Moody JM, Garafano LL. Laparoscopy as the primary modality for the treatment of women with endometrial carcinoma. Cancer. 2001;91(2):378–387.
39. Homesley HD, Boike G, Spiegel GW. Feasibility of laparoscopic management of presumed stage I endometrial carcinoma and assessment of accuracy of myoinvasion estimates by frozen section: a gynecologic oncology group study. Int J Gynecol Cancer. 2004;14(2):341–347.
40. Magriña JF, Mutone NF, Weaver AL, Magtibay PM, Fowler RS, Cornella JL. Laparoscopic lymphadenectomy and vaginal or laparoscopic hysterectomy with bilateral salpingo-oophorectomy for endometrial cancer: morbidity and survival. Am J Obstet Gynecol. 1999;181(2):376–381.
41. Gil-Moreno A, Diaz-Feijoo B, Morchon S, Xercavins J. Analysis of survival after laparoscopic-assisted vaginal hysterectomy compared with the conventional abdominal approach for early-stage endometrial carcinoma: A review of the literature. J Minim Invasive Gynecol. 2006;13(1):26–35.
42. Obermair A, Manolitsas TP, Leung Y, Hammond IG, McCartney AJ. Total laparoscopic hysterectomy for endometrial cancer: patterns of recurrence and survival. Gynecol Oncol. 2004;92(3):789–793.
43. Gemignani ML, Curtin JP, Zelmanovich J, Patel DA, Venkatraman E, Barakat RR. Laparoscopic-assisted vaginal hysterectomy for endometrial cancer: clinical outcomes and hospital charges. Gynecol Oncol. 1999;73(1):5–11.
44. Spirtos NM, Schlaerth JB, Gross GM, Spirtos TW, Schlaerth AC, Ballon SC. Cost and quality-of-life analyses of surgery for early endometrial cancer: laparotomy versus laparoscopy. Am J Obstet Gynecol. 1996;174(6):1795–1799.
45. Scribner DR, Jr., Mannel RS, Walker JL, Johnson GA. Cost analysis of laparoscopy versus laparotomy for early endometrial cancer. Gynecol Oncol. 1999;75(3):460–463.
46. Kohler C, Klemm P, Schau A, et al. Introduction of transperitoneal lymphadenectomy in a gynecologic oncology center: analysis of 650 laparoscopic pelvic and/or paraaortic transperitoneal lymphadenectomies. Gynecol Oncol. 2004;95(1):52–61.
47. Childers JM, Spirtos NM, Brainard P, Surwit EA. Laparoscopic staging of the patient with incompletely staged early adenocarcinoma of the endometrium. Obstet Gynecol. 1994;83(4):597–600.
48. Eltabbakh GH. Analysis of survival after laparoscopy in women with endometrial carcinoma. Cancer. 2002;95(9):1894–1901.
49. Magriña JF, Weaver AL. Laparoscopic treatment of endometrial cancer: five-year recurrence and survival rates. Eur J Gynaecol Oncol. 2004;25(4):439–441.
50. Malur S, Possover M, Michels W, Schneider A. Laparoscopic-assisted vaginal versus abdominal surgery in patients with endometrial cancer – a prospective randomized trial. Gynecol Oncol. 2001;80(2):239–244.
51. Fram KM. Laparoscopically assisted vaginal hysterectomy versus abdominal hysterectomy in stage I endometrial cancer. Int J Gynecol Cancer. 2002;12(1):57–61.
52. Zullo F, Palomba S, Russo T, et al. A prospective randomized comparison between laparoscopic and laparotomic approaches in women with early stage endometrial cancer: a focus on the quality of life. Am J Obstet Gynecol. 2005;193(4):1344–1352.
53. Sonoda Y, Zerbe M, Smith A, Lin O, Barakat RR, Hoskins WJ. High incidence of positive peritoneal cytology in low-risk endometrial cancer treated by laparoscopically assisted vaginal hysterectomy. Gynecol Oncol. 2001;80(3):378–382.
54. Vergote I, De Smet I, Amant F. Incidence of positive peritoneal cytology in low-risk endometrial cancer treated by laparoscopically assisted vaginal hysterectomy. Gynecol Oncol. 2002;84(3):537–538.
55. Eltabbakh GH, Mount SL. Laparoscopic surgery does not increase the positive peritoneal cytology among women with endometrial carcinoma. Gynecol Oncol. 2006;100(2):361–364.

56. Boente MP, Yordan EL, Jr, McIntosh DG, et al. Prognostic factors and long-term survival in endometrial adenocarcinoma with cervical involvement. Gynecol Oncol. 1993;51(3):316–322.
57. Mariani A, Webb MJ, Keeney GL, Calori G, Podratz KC. Role of wide/radical hysterectomy and pelvic lymph node dissection in endometrial cancer with cervical involvement. Gynecol Oncol. 2001;83(1):72–80.
58. Everett E, Tamimi H, Greer B, et al. The effect of body mass index on clinical/pathologic features, surgical morbidity, and outcome in patients with endometrial cancer. Gynecol Oncol. 2003;90(1):150–157.
59. Wright JD, Powell MA, Herzog TJ, et al. Panniculectomy: improving lymph node yield in morbidly obese patients with endometrial neoplasms. Gynecol Oncol. 2004;94(2):436–441.
60. Scribner DR, Jr, Walker JL, Johnson GA, McMeekin DS, Gold MA, Mannel RS. Laparoscopic pelvic and paraaortic lymph node dissection in the obese. Gynecol Oncol. 2002;84(3):426–430.
61. Obermair A, Manolitsas TP, Leung Y, Hammond IG, McCartney AJ. Total laparoscopic hysterectomy versus total abdominal hysterectomy for obese women with endometrial cancer. Int J Gynecol Cancer. 2005;15(2):319–324.

Early-Stage Endometrial Cancer: Radiation

Lea Baer, A. Gabriella Wernicke, and Silvia Formenti

Abstract Radiotherapy has been used as an adjunct to surgical intervention for the last five decades, in view of documented effect on local control and reduced rates of vaginal vault recurrences. As surgical staging became established as part of the initial approach, a reassessment of the role of radiation in well-staged patients with low and intermediate risks of recurrence is ongoing. Intracavitary brachytherapy has low morbidity and is often used to reduce vaginal vault recurrences. External beam radiotherapy, on the other hand, achieves local control at the cost of some morbidity, and its impact on survival is uncertain.

Keywords Endometrial cancer • Brachytherapy • External beam

Introduction

In the USA, endometrial cancer (EC) is the most common cancer of the female genital tracts (1). Seventy percent of patients have localized disease, heralded by the characteristic sign of abnormal vaginal bleeding. Radiotherapy (RT) has been used as an adjunct to surgical intervention for the last five decades, following seminal reports of improved local control and reduced rates of vaginal recurrences (2, 3). The type of RT used is based on the estimated risk of locoregional recurrence and it ranges from a brief course of intracavitary brachytherapy (BT), external beam radiotherapy (EBRT), or a combination of both. The role of adjuvant RT in the treatment of patients in low- or intermediate-risk groups has been repeatedly revisited in the era of surgical staging, with the emerging understanding that the criteria inspiring the original classification of risk based on depth of myometrial invasion and tumor grade are

L. Baer (✉), A.G. Wernicke, and S. Formenti
Department of Radiation Oncology, NYU Cancer Institute, NYU Medical Center,
New York, NY
e-mail: Lea.n.baer@gmail.com

F. Muggia and E. Oliva (eds.), *Uterine Cancer*, Current Clinical Oncology,
DOI: 10.1007/978-1-60327-044-1_9,

surrogates of extrauterine disease spread. The benefit derived from adjuvant radiation treatment by properly staged patients is a matter of ongoing debate, with some advocating omission of RT in all low- to intermediate-risk early-stage EC, and others supporting a better patient selection based on more elaborate prognostication.

Definition of Low and Intermediate Risk

Women with stage I EC are considered to be at low risk of recurrence if surgico-pathologic staging reveals a grade 1–2 tumor, with invasion of < one-half of the myometrium (stages IA–IB) or a grade 3 tumor with no myometrial invasion (stage IA). Additionally, the tumor has to be confined to the uterine fundus with no evidence of lymphovascular involvement (LVSI) or lymph node involvement. Women are considered to be at intermediate risk for disease recurrence if diagnosed with a grade 1–2 EC with invasion >50% of the myometrial thickness (stage IC) or with disease extension to cervix (stage II). Additionally, no evidence of LVSI or distant metastases is required to be included in the intermediate-risk subset.

Conservative Management

The locoregional relapse rate found in the control arm of prospective studies evaluating adjuvant therapy for early-stage EC ranges from 14% in trials without surgical staging (4) to 7% in those requiring surgical staging (5). Two-thirds of the recurrences involve the vagina and specifically the vaginal vault. However, distant relapse rates are similar, regardless of the extent of lymph node dissection, with 7% in the absence of surgical staging and 8% following surgical staging. While the salvage rate of isolated vaginal recurrence in previously unirradiated patients ranges from 40% to 81%, the salvage rate after a pelvic or distant relapse is dismal (4, 6–9).

Pelvic lymph node metastases are found in clinical stage I grades 1, 2, and 3 EC in 2.8%, 8.7%, and 18.3% of women, respectively. The risk of aortic lymph node involvement is reported to be 1.6%, 4.9%, and 11.1%, respectively (10). Some authors recommend routine lymph node sampling in patients with clinical low- or intermediate-risk early-stage disease due to reports of significant rates of both histologic and stage upgrades, warranting a surgical approach that includes lymph node evaluation (10–13). Mariani et al. reported on 328 patients with clinical low-risk EC (endometrioid histology, stages IA–IB and grades 1–2). One hundred and eighty-seven patients were assessed for pelvic node involvement by either sampling or full dissection, with nine patients diagnosed with positive nodes (5%), all of them with tumors > 2 cm in diameter. Twenty-three women out of 308 were assessed for peritoneal cytology and 23 had positive cytology (7%). Altogether, 10% of patients were upgraded to stage III disease following surgical staging (12).

A complete surgical staging results in significant upstaging of clinical stage II as well. Creasman et al. analyzed 148 patients with clinical stage II accrued to Gynecology Oncology Group (GOG) clinical trials that underwent surgical staging. Only 66 (45%) patients were found to have pathologic involvement of the cervix. However, 31 of 66 (46%) were found to have extrauterine disease with lymph node or adnexal involvement, therefore, the patients were upstaged to stage III (13).

Straughn et al. reported on 617 women treated with surgery alone for early-stage EC (14). All women underwent complete surgical staging including peritoneal cytology, bilateral pelvic lymphadenectomy, and para-aoric lymphadenectomy. No recurrences were reported in women with stage IA grades 1–2 tumors. In the 296 patients with stage IB grades 1–2 EC, 11 recurrences were recorded. Five of them were in patients with adenosquamous carcinomas. In the six patients with endometrioid EC, four had vaginal recurrence, one had distant metastases, and one was diagnosed with both vaginal and distant relapses. Other surgical series have reported vaginal failure rates of 1–3% and recurrence rates of 4–7% (15–17). Kilgore et al. found that patients undergoing multiple-site pelvic node sampling had significantly better survival than patients without node sampling ($p = 0.0002$). Sampling conveyed a survival advantage even in patients categorized as low risk defined as carrier of EC confined to the corpus ($p = 0.026$) and the effect persisted even in the absence of adjuvant radiation (17).

Adjuvant Radiotherapy

The value of adjuvant RT after surgical treatment of early-stage EC has been evaluated in several retrospective series and in two population-based analyses from the National Cancer Institute of Surveillance, Epidemiology, and End Results (SEER) database and the American College of Surgeons National Cancer Database (Table 1). While most series suggested an improvement in locoregional control, a survival benefit was not evident. Such retrospective analyses are obviously greatly limited by selection biases (preferential assignment of patients with high-risk features to adjuvant radiation), inconsistent surgical staging (lymph node sampling versus formal dissection, with or without peritoneal washing), and the use of a variety of radiation regimens and modalities.

Adjuvant Pelvic External Beam Radiotherapy

Two large prospective randomized trials studied the effect of adjuvant pelvic external beam radiation. The multicenter prospective clinical trial – Post Operative Radiation Therapy in Endometrial Carcinoma (PORTEC) evaluated the benefit of adjuvant radiation in stage I EC (4). A total of 715 patients were accrued and randomized to postoperative 46 Gy of pelvic EBRT or no further treatment, control arm. Patients

Table 1. Retrospective series evaluating adjuvant RT in early-stage EC

	Number of patients	Adjuvant therapy	Relapse rate	Treatment-related complication rate	Type of recurrence
Carey et al., 1995 (18)	384 total	–	5-year relapse-free rate		60% local recurrence
Stage I (endometroid or adenosquamous histology)	227 low risk	–	95%	–	60% local recurrence
	157 high risk (either grade 3 or MI > 50% or adenosquamous histology or cervical involvement)	Pelvic EBRT 40–45 Gy	81%	5%	66% distant recurrence
Elliott et al., 1994 (19)	811 total low risk (stage I with grade 1–2 and with MI < 1/3 of thickness)	No adjuvant RT		3.4% serious treatment-related complications in the vaginal vault BT arm	3% local recurrence
	308	Vaginal vault RT		1.6% serious treatment-related complications in the total vaginal irradiation arm	5% local recurrence
	40	Whole vaginal RT			0% local recurrence
	163	No adjuvant RT			11.9% local recurrence
	High risk (stage I grade 3 and/or MI > 1/3 of thickness or stage II)	Vaginal vault RT			4.7% local recurrence
	184 105 127	Whole vaginal RT			0.7% local recurrence

	Number of patients	Adjuvant therapy	Relapse rate	Treatment-related complication rate	Type of recurrence
Straughn et al., 2003 (20)	220 total	56/99 BT 21–40 Gy	Mean follow-up 53 months		7/14 local recurrences
Stage Ic, endometroid or adenosquamous histology, following surgical staging	121 no adjuvant RT	19/99 whole pelvis RT	12% recurrence rate, mean follow-up 30 months		5/6 distant recurrences
	99 adjuvant RT	40–50.4 Gy 24/99 both	6% recurrence rate		Adjuvant RT associated with a statistically significant improvement in overall survival in patients with stage IC grades 1, 3, and 4. HR 0.44 and 0.72, respectively
Lee et al., 2006 (21); stage I SEER data	21,249 total, 17,169 no adjuvant RT (80.8%), 4,080 adjuvant RT (19.2%), 2,551 EBRT, 732 BT, 1078 both				
Straughn et al., 2005 (22); American College Surgeons National Cancer Database	Stage I: 5,121 patients – surgery alone; 1,447 patients – adjuvant RT		5-year recurrence rate		Adjuvant RT in clinical stage IC – a trend toward improved 5-year relative survival (81.2% vs 92.5%) when compared to surgery alone. No such trend detected in clinical stages IIA–B. In surgically staged patients, no improvement in 5-year relative survival was detected in patients receiving adjuvant RT compared to surgery alone

Table 1. (continued)

Number of patients	Adjuvant therapy	Relapse rate	Treatment-related complication rate	Type of recurrence
Stage II: 225 patients – surgery alone; 400 patients – adjuvant RT		Stage IC: Clinical: 11.4% vs 9.7%; Surgical: 11.4% vs 11.6%		Stage IC: 91.7% vs 93.9%
		Stage IIA: Clinical: 14.9% vs 20.6%; Surgical: 27.6% in RT arm		Stage IIA: 83.7% vs 98%
		Stage IIB: Clinical: 27.6% in RT arm; Surgical: 14.8% vs 14%		Stage IIB: 82.3% vs. 81.8%
Macdonald et al., 2006 (23); multi-institutional analysis 608 women with stage IA–IIA, patients underwent lymph node sampling or dissection		No significant differences observed in the 5-year rates of vaginal relapse (2% vs 3%, $p = 0.68$), local relapse (4% vs 7%, $p = 0.54$)		Median follow-up 5.2 years. There were no significant differences observed in the 5-year rates of DFS (84% vs 81%, $p = 0.59$), and OS (88% vs 86%, $p = 0.92$) between the surgery and surgery + RT groups. Kaplan–Meier analysis of DFS and OS stratified by stage (stage IA–IB vs stage IC–IIA) revealed that women with stage IC–IIA disease (79% were surgically staged) experienced a significant improvement in OS at 5 years with the addition of RT (83% vs 60%, $p = 0.04$), but no significant benefit in DFS ($p = 0.22$)

	Number of patients	Adjuvant therapy	Relapse rate	Treatment-related complication rate	Type of recurrence
Irwin et al., 1998 (24)	228 surgery alone	EBRT – 40 Gy in 20 fractions to 94% of patients with EC showing >50% MI and to 89% of patients with FIGO grade 3 EC	5-year local control rates	12 patients grade 3–4 complications; all treated with S + EXT + IC	5-year overall survival rates
550 women with pathological stage I	97 surgery + EBRT	Colpostats in 40% of patients, the majority with lower uterine segment involvement	Surgery alone – 93%		Surgery alone 5-year OS 90%, 5-year DFS 84%
	217 surgery + EBRT + colpostats; 8 surgery + colpostats		Surgery + EBRT – 94%; Surgery + EBRT + colpostats – 95%		Surgery + EBRT 5-year OS 79%, 5-year DFS 77%; Surgery + EBRT + colpostats 5-year OS 82%, 5-year DFS 77%
Greven et al., 1997 (25); 294 women with pathologic stage I and II					Pathologic stage I 5-year; pelvic control rate: BT alone 100%, EBRT alone 96%, BT + EBRT 96%
All women underwent TAH + BSO. 49% had LN sampling and 48% peritoneal washing					5-year DFS; BT alone 94%, EBRT alone 89%, BT + EBRT 89%

Table 1. (continued)

	Number of patients	Adjuvant therapy	Relapse rate	Treatment-related complication rate	Type of recurrence
Calvin et al., 1999 (26)	44 patients stage II	22 (50%) WPRT	13 patients (30%) with recurrence	No severe chronic RT sequelae	5-year actuarial DFS 72.4% (entire group)
All patients TAH + BSO and peritoneal washing	9 (20%) – evidence of microscopic cervical involvement on endocervical curettage and/or cervical biopsy before surgery	8 (18%) VBT	1 pelvic recurrence		
77% patients pelvic and para-aortic lymph node sampling	35(80%) had occult involvement noted only in the pathology specimen	14 (32%) WPRT+ VB	1 pelvic + distant recurrence		
			11 distant recurrences		

EC endometrial cancer, BT brachytherapy, EBRT external beam radiotherapy, MI myometrial invasion, TAH total abdominal hysterectomy, BSO bilateral salpingo-oophorectomy, VBT vaginal brachytherapy, WPRT whole pelvic RT

with stage IC grade 3 or stage IB grade 1 were excluded as risk was considered too high or too low, respectively. Patients underwent TAH + BSO but no lymph node sampling or dissection. Following a median follow-up of 52 months, 714 patients were evaluated. The 5-year actuarial locoregional recurrence rates were 4% in the treatment arm and 14% in the control arm ($p < 0.001$). Actuarial 5-year overall survival rates were not statistically different being 81% in the treatment arm and 85% in the control arm ($p = 0.31$). EC-specific death rates were 9% in the radiation arm and 6% in the control arm ($p = 0.37$). Twenty-five percent of the patients in the radiation arm experienced treatment-related complications, two-thirds were grade 1. Eight patients experienced grade 3–4 complications, seven of them in the treatment arm. Multivariate analysis showed that for locoregional recurrence, RT and age < 60 years were statistically significant favorable prognostic factors. Whether patients found to be at low risk after complete surgical staging derive any benefit from adjuvant therapy remains controversial. In GOG 99, a randomized trial comparing adjuvant pelvic RT to no additional therapy, 392 women underwent surgical staging with TAH + BSO, peritoneal cytology, and bilateral pelvic and para-aortic lymphadenectomy (5). While the study was aimed at patients with intermediate risk of recurrence, two-thirds of the patients accrued were actually at low-risk (58.9% stage IB, >70% grades 1–2, 75% with endometrioid histology, and most patients with myometrial invasion < inner two-thirds) with only a 6% recurrence rate in control arm. The relative hazard reduction following RT was similar in the intermediate-risk group and the low-risk group (58% and 54%, respectively), but the absolute difference was more pronounced in the higher risk group (recurrence rate reduced from 27% to 13% in the higher risk group versus 6% to 2% in the low risk group). No survival difference was detected. It is worth noting that grade 3–4 gastrointestinal complications were more common in the RT arm in this study than other studies utilizing similar radiation regimens, 8% in the GOG 99 versus 3% in the PORTEC trial (4), arguably due to the extensive node dissection.

An additional study has assessed the role of EBRT, after initial intracavitary procedure. Aalders et al. reported on 540 patients with surgical stage I EC (27) that underwent TAH and BSO. Postoperatively, all patients were treated with intravaginal BT, delivering 60 Gy to the surface of the vaginal mucosa. Subsequently, patients were randomized to no further treatment or to an additional 40 Gy to the pelvis by EBRT. A significant reduction in locoregional recurrence was observed, 1.9% in the BT plus EBRT arm compared with 6.9% in BT only arm ($p < 0.01$). No improvement was documented in survival (5-year survival 89% vs 91% and 9-year survival 87% vs 90%, respectively). A nonplanned subset analysis demonstrated that EBRT conferred a clear benefit in the subgroup of patients with myometrial invasion > half the thickness and grade 3 tumors (corresponding to the high-risk group), resulting in a reduction in both local recurrence (4.5% versus 19.6%) and cancer-specific death (18.2% vs 27.5%).

Several ongoing randomized phase III trials aim to further define the benefit offered by the various modalities of adjuvant RT in early stage. The NSGO EC-9501/EORTC-55991 accrued 382 patients with stages I–IIIA ECs. Patients underwent TAH and BSO but comprehensive staging was not mandatory. The majority of patients were stage II, with grade 3 tumors and with endometroid histology. All patients received adjuvant radiation and were then randomized to either a treatment arm receiving adjuvant chemotherapy or a control arm receiving no further treatment. While 92% completed radiation therapy, 27% of the patients in the treatment arm did not complete the scheduled chemotherapy. Initial results were reported at the American Society of Clinical Oncology meeting in 2007. The estimated 5-year overall survival Hazard Ratio (HR) was 0.65 with an absolute improvement of 8% observed in patients receiving adjuvant chemotherapy. The cancer-specific survival was improved by 10% (78–88%, HR 0.51).

Another trial recently completed is the MRC ASTEC – EN5. A total of 905 patients with stages I–III ECs were randomized to adjuvant pelvic external beam irradiation (EBI) with or without vaginal brachytherapy (VBT), or to an arm without adjuvant EBI, with or without VBT. Patients for the most part were not surgically staged. The VBT was not uniform and ranged between surface doses of 40 and 46 Gy. The results are awaiting publication. PORTEC-2, a multicentre randomized phase III trial, compares EBRT alone versus VBT alone in patients with EC. Patients with one of the following combinations of postoperative FIGO stage and age have been included: 1) stage IC, grade 1 or 2 and age 60 or over; 2) stage IB, grade 3 and age 60 or over; 3) stage IIA, any age, grade 1 or 2; 4) stage IIA, any age, grade 3 with < half myometrial invasion. The study objectives are 5-year cancer-specific survival, overall survival, locoregional relapse free survival, and distant metastases free survival, complication rate and quality of life, but results are not available yet.

Adjuvant Brachytherapy

The limited benefit in preventing local recurrence, which does not translate into survival benefit, especially in view of the risk of severe treatment related complications, led many investigators to believe that pelvic RT has no role in the management of low-risk patients. Some have explored the use of intracavitary BT to prevent the more common vaginal failure (28–30). In a prospective series, Piver et al. reported on 92 low-risk patients (defined as stage I, grade 1 or 2 EC, < 50% myometrial invasion, and no evidence of disease outside the corpus) treated by hysterectomy and BSO and postoperative vaginal intracavitary BT (28). No recurrences were documented and the 5-year estimated disease-free survival rate was 99%. In another prospective series, Eltabbakh et al. reported on 303 low-risk patients treated with postoperative VBT (31). With a follow-up of 8.1 years, no vaginal recurrences had occurred and the 10-year disease-free survival was 97.8%. Each of the six patients with distant relapse died of disease (1.8%).

With regard to intermediate-risk patients, Alektiar et al. reported on 382 patients treated with postoperative high-dose rate (HDR) BT (32). Comprehensive surgical staging with lymph node sampling and peritoneal washing was preformed in only

20% of the patients. The indications for surgical staging were based on depth of myometrial invasion and tumor grade. Following a median follow-up of 48 months, the 5-year local control rate was 96% with a minimal incidence of grade 3–4 complications (1%).

Pearcey et al. reviewed 13 publications on HDR BT in low- to intermediate-risk EC (33). The vaginal control rates ranged from 98% to 100% corresponding to a reduction in relative risk of recurrence of 80–85%.

High Dose Rate Brachytherapy

Brachytherapy, traditionally delivered by low-dose rate (LDR) techniques, is increasingly being replaced worldwide by high-dose rate (HDR) techniques. HDR offers several advantages over LDR BT, especially in the treatment of EC, including minimization of radiation exposure of the professional staff, elimination of hospitalization, anesthesia and bed immobilization that can lead to thromboembolism, and minimization of patient discomfort. A report by Orton et al. suggested a radiobiologic advantage to HDR owing to the slow repair of late-responding normal tissue (34). The two intracavitary radiation techniques were compared in three retrospective studies (35–37). In a large review, Fayed et al. reported on 1,179 patients with stages I–III ECs treated with postoperative brachytherapy (35). Around 1,004 patients were treated with LDR, 695 diagnosed with stage I (69.2%). One hundred and seventy-five patients were treated with HDR, 74 with stage I (42.3%), 47 with stage II (26.8%), and 54 with stage III tumors (30.9%). The median follow-up was 50 months in the LDR group and 28 months in the HDR group. Overall survival for all stages at 5 years was 70% in the LDR group and 68% in the HDR group ($p= 0.44$). Subgroup analysis revealed statistically significant differences only in the stage II patients' subset. The actuarial overall survival at 5 years for patients with stage II EC was 53% in the LDR group and 74% in the HDR group ($p= 0.026$) and the actuarial 5-year disease-free survival of stage II patients was 50% for the LDR group and 75% for the HDR group ($p= 0.009$). Actuarial 5-year local control for stage II patients was 65% in the LDR group and 90% in the HDR group ($p= 0.016$), with the rate of grade 3–4 complications being comparable in both LDR and HDR.

In 2005, an American Brachytherapy Society (ABS) survey regarding practice patterns of postoperative irradiation of EC reported that HDR had become an increasingly popular method, though with no standardized treatment approach (38). Compelled by the lack of standardized treatment recommendations, a panel of the ABS members with clinical experience in HDR endometrial BT performed a literature review, supplemented their clinical experience with biomathematical modeling, and formulated recommendations for HDR-BT for EC (39). They included intravaginal BT typically delivered about 4–6 weeks postoperatively or a week after completion of EBRT and administered in three fractions every 1–2 weeks.

Selection of High-Dose Rate Applicators

Cylinders

Selection of HDR applicators largely depends on patient anatomy. Postoperatively, the vagina displays a cylindrical shape and can be adequately treated by a vaginal cylinder (Fig.1). Since cylinders are available in various lengths, they can treat not only the vaginal cuff but also the entire vaginal canal, including the introitus, if necessary. Furthermore, due to the range of diameters (1.5 to 4.0 cm), vaginal cylinders can accommodate a narrow as well as a wide vaginal canal. The disadvantage of the use of vaginal cylinders is delivery of higher doses to the bladder and rectum for a given vaginal dose.

Most commonly, vaginal cylinders have a single central channel through which the radioactive sources deliver RT. However, there are other variations to this construct such as a multichannel vaginal applicator (Fig. 4). The latter renders differential loading of the channels that allows shaping of the isodose distributions to various clinical presentations (40–42). Other vaginal cylinders are described, including shielded ones that selectively decrease the absorbed dose to adjacent normal structures. Upon insertion of the vaginal cylinder, it is imperative for the vaginal mucosa to be in contact with the applicator surface to achieve the desired

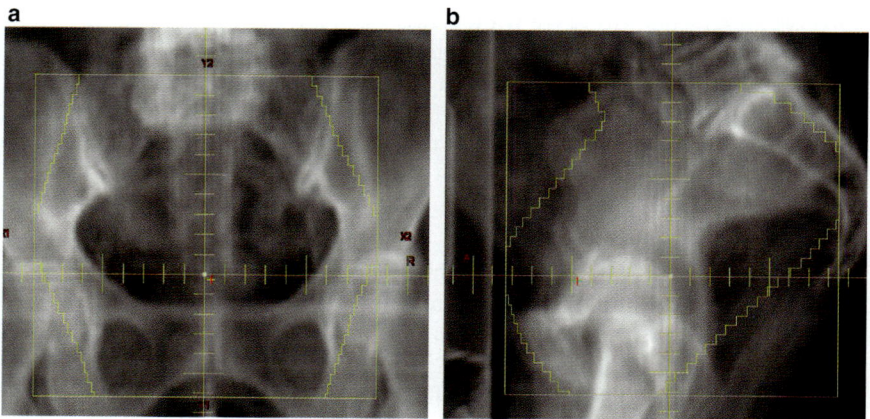

Fig. 1 Images of anterior–posterior (**a**) and lateral radiation portals (**b**) of a patient treated with external beam radiotherapy for endometrial cancer.

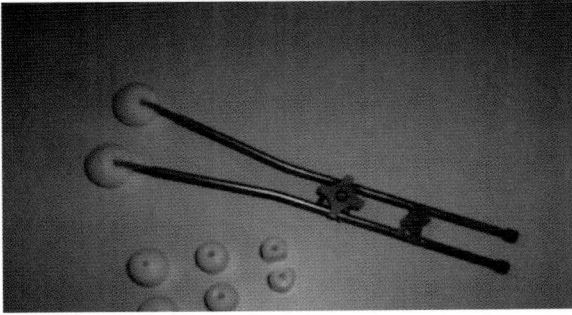

Fig. 2 Colpostats or ovoids used for brachytherapy. Different sizes of caps are used based on patient's vagina anatomy in the postoperative setting.

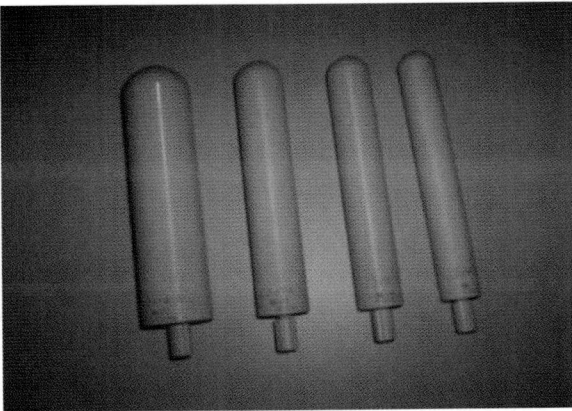

Fig. 3 Stump vaginal cylinders of various sizes used in brachytherapy.

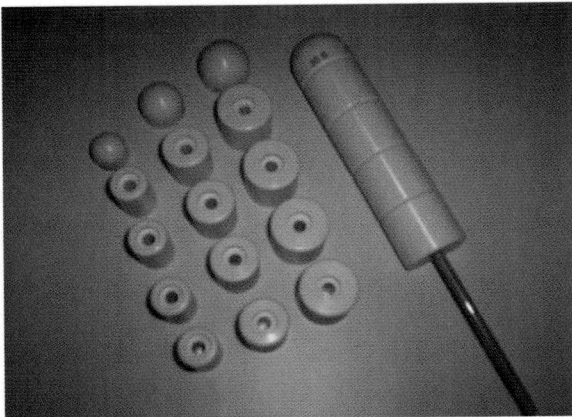

Fig. 4 Segmented vaginal cylinders of various sizes used in brachytherapy.

dose distribution. The ABS recommends the use of the largest diameter cylinder (or ovoids) that can comfortably fit in the vagina (2). The applicator should be positioned in the midline of the patient and secured with an external immobilizing device to minimize movement between planning and treatment.

Ovoids

Postoperatively, the vagina may display a "dog-ear" configuration which is best treated with vaginal ovoids. These applicators, whether shielded or unshielded, are available in various diameters, ranging from 2 to 3 cm. ABS deems the choice of applicators to be a personal and institutional preference as long as the desired segment of vagina is adequately covered with radiation (39). Upon insertion of the largest ovoids, comfortably fitted in vagina, their proper position should be verified, and their medial aspects should touch (Fig. 1). A rectal displacement should be attained with the use of either a radio-opaque packing or a rectal retractor. Radio-opaque packing should be used to displace the bladder.

External Beam Radiotherapy to the Pelvis

With no evidence of gross residual disease after hysterectomy, the majority of patients are treated with adjuvant EBRT to the pelvis to encompass areas at risk: pelvic lymph node stations (lower common iliac, external, and internal) and proximal two-thirds of the vagina. A conventional four-field pelvic box technique (Fig. 1) is employed along with the use of high-energy linear accelerators to deliver the designated therapy. The use of multiple fields and higher energy photons allows normal tissue sparing and reduction in radiation-related complications (43). The long-term severe complication rates associated with pelvic radiation following hysterectomy range between 2% and 5%, with reduced toxicity using modern radiotherapeutic techniques (4, 18, 43, 44). All fields are treated daily with a minimum dose of 1.8 Gy to the target. When EBRT is used alone, a total dose of 50.4 is typically used, but when used in combination with intravaginal BT, it is lowered to 45 Gy.

Sequelae of Radiotherapy

External Beam Radiotherapy to the Pelvis

Acutely, pelvic irradiation may cause self-limiting diarrhea, cystitis, and abdominal bloating. Late toxicities are uncommon (< 5%) and are related to small bowel adhesions and/or obstruction (a result of combined treatment with surgery and RT), proctitis, and cystitis. The overall rate of late complications reported in the

PORTEC trial was 26% in the irradiated group as compared to 4% in the control group ($p < 0.0001$) (4). While the majority of complications (22%) were 1–2, 3% of patients experimented grade 3–4 toxicity (45).

Vaginal Brachytherapy

Vaginal brachytherapy affords delivering high doses of RT to the vagina while sparing other normal close structures such as bowel and bladder. This ability of VBT translates into a low rate of long-term sequelae (0–1%) (46–48). In a recent publication, Alektiar et al. reported a 1% grade 3 late toxicity at 5 years with the use of VBT alone (32). None of the patients developed grade 3 or worse gastrointestinal toxicity. Yet, vaginal stenosis is a long-term side effect of vaginal HDR with reported frequencies as high as 15% (49). Despite low rates of complications, a radiation oncologist should pay special attention to dose per fraction, prescription point, length of vagina irradiated, and the diameter of the vaginal cylinder utilized.

Conclusions

- Current treatment of early-stage endometrial cancer with radiation is based on surgicopathologic risk factors such as stage, grade, age, tumor size and location, and the presence of lymphovascular space involvement.
- Vaginal brachytherapy is often used for stage IA tumors in the presence of adverse factors such as high grade, age >60 years, lower uterine segment involvement, or presence of lymphovascular space involvement.
- Whole pelvic radiation therapy is usually omitted in these IA patients because its morbidity outweighs any possible benefit with relatively low risk of recurrence.
- In stage IB patients, vaginal brachytherapy is the suggested treatment, with whole pelvic radiation therapy being considered in patients with adverse factors.
- Whole pelvic radiation therapy with or without vaginal brachytherapy is recommended in most patients with stages IC (with grade 3 and/or other adverse factors) to IIB since this treatment results in a significant reduction of recurrence rates.
- Future clinical trials need to address the relative benefit of these treatments in combination with chemotherapy in subsets of patients using clearly defined modern prognostication parameters and surgical staging.

References

1. Jemal, A., Siegel, R., Ward, E., Murray, T., Xu, J., Thun, M.J. Cancer statistics, 2007. CA Cancer J Clin. 2007;57:43–66.
2. Stander, R.W. Vaginal metastastases following treatment of endometrial carcinoma. Am J Obstet Gynecol. 1956;71:776–9.

3. Price, J.J., Hahn, G.A., Rominger, C.J. Vaginal Involvement in Endometrial Carcinoma. Am J Obstet Gynecol. 1965;91:1060–5.

4. Creutzberg, C.L., van Putten, W.l., Koper, P.C., Lybeert, M.L., Jobsen, J.J., Warlam-Rodenhuis, C.C., et al. Surgery and postoperative radiotherapy versus surgery alone for patients with stage-1 endometrial carcinoma: multicentre randomized trial. PORTEC Study Group. Post Operative Radiation Therapy in Endometrial Carcinoma. Lancet. 2000;355:1404–11.

5. Keys, H.M., Roberts, J.A., Brunetto, V.L., Zaino, R.J., Spirtos, N.M., Bloss, J.D., et al. A phase III trial of surgery with or without adjunctive external pelvic radiation therapy in intermediate risk endometrial adenocarcinoma: a Gynecologic Oncology Group study. Gynecol Oncol. 2004;92:744–51.

6. Nag, S., Yacoub, S., Copeland, L.J., Fowler, J.M. Interstitial brachtherapy for salvage treatment of vaginal recurrences in previously unirradiated endometrial cancer patients. Int J Radiat Oncol Biol Phys. 2002;54:1153–9.

7. Jereczek-Fossa, B., Badzio, A., Jassem, J. Recurrent endometrial cancer after surgery alone: results of salvage radiotherapy. Int J Radiat Oncol Biol Phys. 2000;48:405–13.

8. Petignat, P., Jolocoeur, M., Alobaid, A., Drouin, P., Gauthier, P., Provencher, D., et al. Salvage treatment with high-dose-rate brachytherapy for isolated veginal endometrial cancer recurrence. Gynecol Oncol. 2006;101:445–9.

9. Huh, W.K., Straughn, J.M., Jr., Mariani, A., Podratz, K.C., Havrilesky, L.J., Alvarez-Secord, A., et al. Salvage of isolated vaginal recurrences in women with surgical stage I endometrial cancer: a multiinstitutional experience. Int J Gyenecol Cancer. 2007;17:886–9.

10. Creasman, W.T., Morrow, C.P., Bundy, B.N., Homesley, H.D., Graham, J.E., Heller, P.B. Surgical pathologic spread patterns of endometrial cancer. A Gynecologic Oncology Group Study. Cancer. 1987;60:2035–41.

11. Ben-Shacher, I., Pavelka, J., Cohn, D.E., Copeland, L.J., Ramirez, N., Manolotsas, T., et al. Surgical staging for patients presenting presenting with grade 1 endometrial carcinoma. Obstetrics and gynecology. 2005;105:487–93.

12. Mariani, A., Webb, M.J., Keeney, G.L., Haddock, M.G., Calori, G., Podratz, K.C. Low-risk corpus cancer: is lymphadenectomy or radiotherapy necessary? Am J Obstet Gynecol. 2000;182:1506–19.

13. Creasman, W.T., DeGeest, K., DiSaia, P.J., Zaino, R.J. Significance of true surgical pathologic staging: a Gynecologic Oncology Group Study. Am J Obstet Gynecol. 1999; 181:31–4.

14. Straughn, J.M., Jr., Huh, W.K., Kelly, F.J., Leath, C.A., 3rd, Kleinberg, M.J., Hyde, J., Jr., et al. Conservative management of stage I endometrial carcinoma after surgical staging. Gynecol Oncol. 2002;84:194–200.

15. Shumsky, A.G., Brasher, P.M., Stuart, G.C., Nation, J.G. Risk-specific follow-up for endometrial carcinoma patients. Gynecol Oncol. 1997;65:379–82.

16. DiSaia, P.J., Creasman, W.T., Boronow, R.C., Blessing, J.A. Risk factors and recurrent patterns in Stage I endometrial cancer. Am J Obstet Gynecol. 1985;151:1009–15.

17. Kilgore, L.C., Partidge, E.E., Alvarez, R.D., Austin, J.M., Shingleton, H.M., Noojin, F., 3rd, et al. Adenocarcinoma of the endometrium: survival comparisons of patients with and without pelvicnode sampling. Gynecol Oncol. 1995;56:29–33.

18. Carey, M.S., O'Connell, G.J., Johansson, C.R., Goodyear, M.D., Murphy, K.J., Daya, D.M., et al. Good outcome associated with a standardized treatment protocol using selective postoperative radiation in patients with clinical stage I adenocarcinoma of the endometrium. Gynecol Oncol. 1995;57:138–44.

19. Elliott, P., Green, D., Coates, A., Krieger, M., Russell, P., Coppleson, M., et al. The efficacy of postoperative vaginal irradiation in preventing vaginal recurrence in endometrial cancer. Int J Gynecol Cancer. 1994;4:84–93.

20. Straughn, I.M., Huh, W.K., Orr, J.W., Jr., Kell, F.J., Roland, P.Y., Gold, M.A., et al. Stage IC adenocarcinoma of the endometrium: survival comparisons of surgically staged patients with and without adjuvant radiation therapy. Gynecol Oncol. 2003;89:295–300.

21. Lee, C.M., Szabo, A., Shrieve, D.C., Macdonald, O.K., Gaffney, D.K. Frequency and effect of adjuvant radiation therapy among women with stage | endometrial adenocarcinoma. Jama. 2006;295:389–97.

22. Straughn, J.M., Jr., Numnum, T.M., Kilgore, L.C., Partridge, E.E., Phillips, J.L., Markman, M., et al. The use of adjuvant radiation therapy in patients with intermediate-risk Stages IC and II uterine corpus cancer: a patient care evaluation study from the American College of Surgeons National Cancer Data Base. Gynecol Oncol. 2005;99:530–5.

23. Macdonald, O.K., Sause, W.T., Lee, R.J., Lee, C.M., Dodson, M.K., Zempolich, K., et al. Adjuvant radiotherapy and survival outcomes in early-stage endometrial cancer: a multi-institutional analysis of 608 women. Gynecol Oncol. 2006;103:661–6.

24. Irwin, C., Levin, W., Fyles, A., Pintilie, M., Manchul, L., Kirkbride, P. The role of adjuvant radiotherapy in carcinoma of the endometrium-results in 550 patients with pathologic stage I disease. Gynecol Oncol. 1998;70:247–54.

25. Greven, K.M., Corn, B.W., Case, D., Purser, P., Lanciano, R.M. Which prognostic factors influence the outcome of patients with surgically staged endometrial cancer treated with adjuvant radiation? Int J Radiat Oncol Biol Phys. 1997;39:413–8.

26. Calvin, D.P., Connell, P.P., Rotmensch, J., Waggoner, S., Mundt, A.J. Surgery and postoperative radiation therapy in stage II endometrial carcinoma. Am J Clin Oncol. 1999;22:338–43.

27. Aalders, J., Abeler, V., Kolstad, P., Onsrud, M. Postoperative external irradiation and prognostic parameters in stage I endometrial carcinoma: clinical and histopathologic study of 540 patients. Obstetrics and gynecology. 1980;56:419–27.

28. Piver, M.S., Hempling, R.E. A prospective trial of postoperative vaginal radium/cesium for grade 1–2 less than 50% myometrial invasion and pelvic radiation therapy for grade 3 or deep myometrial invasion in surgical stage I endometrial adenocarcinoma. Cancer. 1990;66:1133–8.

29. Chadha, M., Nanavati, P.J., Liu, P., Fanning, J., Jacobs, A. Patterns of failure in endometrial carcinoma stage IB grade 3 and IC patients treated with postoperative vaginal vault brachytherapy. Gynecol Oncol. 1999;75:103–7.

30. Chong, I.Y., Hoskin, P.J. Vaginal vault brachytherapy for low risk endometrial carcinoma. Clin Oncol (R Coll Radiol). 2007;19:S8.

31. Eltabbakh, G.H., Piver, M.S., Hempling, R.E., Shin, K.H. Excellent long-term survival and absence of vaginal recurrences in 332 patients with low-risk stage I endometrial adenocarcinoma treated with hysterectomy and vaginal brachytherapy without formal staging lymph node sampling: report of a prospective trail. Int J Radiat Oncol Biol Phys. 1997;38:373–80.

32. Alektiar, K.M., Venkatraman, E., Chi, D.S., Barakat, R.R. Intravaginal brachytherapy alone for intermediate-risk endometrial cancer. Int J Radiat Oncol Biol Phys. 2005;62:111–7.

33. Pearcey, R.G., Petereit, D.G. Post-operative high dose rate brachytherapy in patients with low to intermediate risk endometrial cancer. Radiother Oncol. 2000;56:17–22.

34. Orton, C.G. High-dose-rate brachytherapy may be radiobiologically superior to low-dose rate due to slow repair of late-responding normal tissue cells. Int J Radiat Oncol Biol Phys. 2001;49:183–9.

35. Fayed, A., Mutch, D.G., Rader, J.S., Gibb, R.K., Powell, M.A., Wright, J.D., et al. Comparison of high-dose-rate and low-dose-rate brachytherapy in the treatment of endometrial carcinoma. Int J Radiat Oncol Biol Phys. 2007;67:480–4.

36. Bekerus, M., Durbaba, M., Frim, O., Vujnic, V. comparison of HDR and LDR results in endometrium cancer. Sonderb Strahlenther Onkol. 1988;82:222–7.

37. Rauthe, G., Vahrson, H., Giers, G. Five-year results and complications in endometrium cancer: HDR afterloading vs. conventional radium therapy. Sonderb Strahlenther Onkol. 1988;82:240–5.

38. Small, W., Jr., Erickson, B., Kwakwa, F. American Brachytherapy Society survey regarding practice patterns of postoperative irradiation for endometrial cancer: current status of vaginal brachytherapy. Int J Radiat Oncol Biol Phys. 2005;63:1502–7.

39. Nag, S., Erickson, B., Thomadsen, B., Orton, C., Demanes, J.D., Petereit, D. The American Brachytherapy Society recommendations for high-dose-rate brachytherapy for carcinoma of the cervix. Int J Radiat Oncol Biol Phys. 2000;48:201–11.

40. Houdek, P.V., Schwade, J.G., Abitbol, A.A., Pisciotta, V., Wu, X.D., Serago, C.F., et al. Optimization of high dose-rate cervix brachytherapy; Part I: Dose distribution. Int J Radiat Oncol Biol Phys. 1991;21:1621–5.
41. Maruyama, Y., Ezzell, G., Porter, A.T. Afterloading high dose rate intracavitary vaginal cylinder. Int J Radiat Oncol Biol Phys. 1994;30:473–6.
42. Demanes, D.J., Rege, S., Rodriquez, R.R., Schutz, K.L., Altieri, G.A., Wong, T. The use and advantages of a multichannel vaginal cyclinder in high-dose-rate brachytherapy. Int J Radiat Oncol Biol Phys. 1999;44:211–9.
43. Corn, B.W., Lanciano, R.M., Greven, K.M., Noumoff, J., Schultz, D., Hanks, G.E., et al. Impact of improved irradiation technique, age, and lymph node sampling on the severe complication rate of surgically staged endometrial cancer patients: a multivariate analysis. J Clin Oncol. 1994;12:510–5.
44. Algan, O., Tabesh, T., Hanlon, A., Hogan, W.M., Boente, M., Lanciano, R.M. Improved outcome in patients treated with postoperative radiation therapy for pathologic stage I/II endometrial cancer. Int J Radiat Oncol Biol Phys. 1996;35:925–33.
45. Creutzberg, C.L., van Putten, W.L., Koper, P.C., Lybeert, M.L., Jobsen, J.J., Warlam-Rodenhuis, C.C., et al. The morbidity of treatment for patients with Stage I endometrial cancer; results from a randomized trial. Int J Radiat Oncol Biol Phys. 2001;51:1246–55.
46. Horowitz, N.S., Peters, W.A., 3rd, Smith, M.R., Drescher, C.W., Atwood, M., Mate, T.P. Adjuvant high dose rate vaginal brachytherapy as treatment of stage I and II endomentrial carcinoma. Obstetrics and gynecology. 2002;99:235–40.
47. Alektiar, K.M., McKee, A., Venkatraman, E., Mckee, B., Zelefsky, M.J., Mychalczak, B.R., et al. Intravaginal high-dose-rate brachytherapy for Stage IB (FIGO Grade 1, 2) endometrial cancer. Int J Radiat Oncol Biol Phys. 2002;53:707–13.
48. Petereit, D.G., Tannehill, S.P., Grosen, E.A., Hartenbach, E.M., Schink, J.C. Outpatient vaginal cuff brachytherapy for endometrial cancer. Int J Gynecol Cancer. 1999;9:456–62.
49. Sorbe, B.G., Smeds, A.C. Postoperative vaginal irradiation with high dose rate afterloading technique in endometrial carcinoma stage I. Int J Radiat Oncol Biol Phys. 1990;18:305–14.

Therapeutic Modalities in Early-Stage Uterine Papillary Serous Carcinomas, Carcinosarcomas, Clear-Cell and Mixed Histology Carcinomas: Building a Case for Combined Chemotherapy and Radiation

Nicholas P. Taylor and Matthew A. Powell

Abstract The entities covered in this chapter are uterine papillary serous carcinoma (UPSC), carcinosarcoma, and clear-cell carcinoma together with tumors of mixed histology. Overall, these represent 3–5% of all endometrial cancers but they are responsible for a significant percentage of endometrial cancer mortality. Recent strides in chemotherapy of some of these cancers offer hope that their addition, either alone or as part of combined modality treatment including radiation, will lead to improvements in survival.

Keywords Papillary serous • Carcinosarcoma • Clear cell • Chemotherapy • Chemo-radiation

Introduction

Endometrial cancer is the most common gynecologic malignancy being responsible for more than 7000 deaths in 2008 in USA (1). The high-risk histologic subtypes of endometrial cancer, carcinosarcoma, papillary serous carcinoma (UPSC), and clear-cell carcinoma individually represent 3–5% of all cancers of the uterine corpus. Although rare, these subtypes have a high risk of local and distant recurrence even when diagnosed at an early stage. Rosenberg and colleagues examined 841 patients with endometrial cancer, UPSC represented 5% of the cohort, and 52% of these patients died of disease (2). Treatment schemes for early stage (FIGO I and II), high-risk histologic subtypes of endometrial cancer are variable and include radiotherapy, chemotherapy, or a combination of both. This chapter will focus on therapy for FIGO stage I and II

N.P. Taylor and M.A. Powell (✉)
Division of Gynecologic Oncology, Department of Obstetrics and Gynecology, Washington University School of Medicine, St. Louis, MO
e-mail: mpowell@wustl.edu

F. Muggia and E. Oliva (eds.), *Uterine Cancer*, Current Clinical Oncology,
DOI: 10.1007/978-1-60327-044-1_10,
© Humana Press, a Part of Springer Science+Business Media, LLC 2009

uterine carcinosarcomas, UPSC, clear-cell, and mixed histology carcinomas. Given the low frequency of these malignancies, current treatment recommendations are based on multiple retrospective series. There is clearly a growing need for randomized controlled therapeutic trials for early stage, high-risk histology carcinomas of the uterine corpus.

Papillary Serous Carcinoma

Epidemiology and Natural History

Papillary serous carcinoma was first described as a distinct pathologic entity by two different groups in 1982 (3, 4). It represents approximately 2.2–9% of all endometrial cancers (5–7). Histologically, it resembles serous carcinoma of the ovary and fallopian tube and behaves like them as it commonly spreads to peritoneal surfaces. In one of the original reports, the relapse rate among stage I tumors was 50% (4). Table 1 summarizes the most common clinical findings. The median age at diagnosis is 67 years (5, 7), older than the median age (63 years) of endometrioid endometrial cancer (8). In one study, UPSC was significantly more common in African American compared to Caucasian (34% versus 15%, $P < 0.001$) (7). Postmenopausal bleeding is the most common presenting symptom, occurring in up to 80% of patients (5, 9). Preoperative endometrial sampling demonstrates a papillary serous component in 50–89% of cases (5, 9–12). Abnormal cervical cytology (AGUS or worse) is present in approximately 50% of patients (9, 11). One study examining all stages of UPSC found that 13 of 16 (81%) patients had an elevated serum CA-125 level prior to therapy and that 57% experienced a reduction or normalization of CA-125 following therapy (13). A diagnosis of UPSC should be suspected if >10% of the preoperative endometrial biopsy specimen contains papillary architecture associated with high-grade cytology. It has been shown that even when 10% of a mixed tumor contains UPSC, there is a trend toward decreased overall survival when compared to grade 3 endometrioid adenocarcinomas (14).

As stated previously, UPSC is a biologically aggressive form of endometrial cancer. It has a different spectrum of genetic alterations than endometrioid-type

Table 1. Uterine papillary serous carcinoma: Clinical features

Median age at diagnosis = 67 years
More common in African American women
Postmenopausal bleeding common (80%)
CA-125 frequently elevated
Endometrial sampling establishes the diagnosis in 50–89%
AGUS or worse cervical cytology in 50%

AGUS abnormal glands of undetermined significance

cancers that contribute to its tumorigenesis. Mutations in p53 and e-cadherin are more common in UPSC, whereas PTEN inactivation, K-ras mutations, and microsatellite instability are more common in endometrioid endometrial cancers (15). These molecular differences have translated into significant clinical differences between UPSC and endometrioid adenocarcinoma. Extrauterine disease is common in clinical stage I and II UPSC. All patients with a suspicion of UPSC should therefore undergo a surgical staging procedure similar to that employed for early-stage ovarian cancer including TAH, BSO, pelvic and para-aortic lymph node dissection, infracolic omentectomy or omental biopsy, pelvic washings, and diaphragmatic cytology. Goff et al. (10) reviewed 50 cases of UPSC and found extrauterine disease in 72% of them. A large retrospective, single-institution analysis found that among patients without myometrial invasion, 37% had stage III or IV disease (16). Chan et al. (17) reported on 12 surgically staged patients (including omentectomy) with UPSC limited to the endometrium and 50% were found to have disease outside the uterus (3 of 6 had omental disease). In that series, 1 of 6 (16.7%) patients with stage IA disease had a distant recurrence. Another study demonstrated that 42% of patients with clinical stage I UPSC had advanced-stage (III and IV) disease. A similar trend was observed by Cirisano in clinical stage II tumors with 64% of patients being upstaged at laparotomy (7). Kato et al. (5) found that when patients had an omentectomy or omental biopsy as part of their initial staging laparotomy, seven of eight (88%) were positive for malignancy. Several series have documented a high frequency of retroperitoneal lymph node involvement ranging from 13 to 33% (10, 18). Not surprisingly, one retrospective study identified a 2-year and 5-year overall survival advantage in patients who had complete surgical staging ($N = 21$) versus patients who did not ($N = 17$). The 5-year overall survival (OS) with combined modality was 95% in the surgically staged group compared to 45% in the unstaged group (6).

The contribution of pathologic variables such as lymphovascular space invasion (LVSI), myometrial invasion, and admixture of endometrioid features to overall survival in UPSC is controversial. One study of 47 patients found that myometrial invasion, LVSI, or presence of an endometrioid component did not contribute to overall survival (19). The 5-year overall survival of stage I patients in this series was only 44%, suggesting that many of these patients were understaged. Goff et al. found that histologic grade and presence of mixed histologic subtypes were not predictive of extrauterine disease (10). Tumors with LVSI, however, were more likely to have extrauterine disease (85%), but even without it, extrauterine disease was common (58%). Kato et al. did not demonstrate an association between myometrial invasion and overall survival (5). Slomovitz et al., found that among patients with all stages, LVSI and depth of myometrial invasion were pathologic features that were predictive of overall survival in UPSC (16). Another study found that age >60, advanced stage, LVSI, and >50% myometrial invasion were prognostic factors associated with decreased overall survival (7). As will be demonstrated later, the clinical utility of these pathologic variables is limited. Based on recent data (20), it is likely that all patients with UPSC will receive some form of adjuvant therapy.

The overall survival (5 year) of UPSC limited to the uterus varies from 34–81% depending on completeness of surgical staging as well as substage (5, 12, 16, 19, 21–23). In one of the largest series to date, the 5-year OS was 81.5% for patients with stage IA, 58.6% for stage IB, and 34.3% for patients with stage IC tumors (16). In contrast, stage I and II (occult) endometrial adenocarcinomas had 5-year survivals in the 90% range (24).

One of the contributors to poorer overall survival in UPSC is the high frequency of recurrence in patients with early-stage disease. Recurrence rates in UPSC limited to the uterus can be as high as 20–50% (4, 5, 7, 12, 22). Thus, successful therapy for UPSC should address both local and distant failures.

Treatment

The aggressive intrinsic biology of UPSC as well as its high relapse rate in patients with disease clinically (and pathologically) confined to the uterus have led many investigators to suggest the addition of some form of adjuvant therapy regardless of stage. Given the pattern of local as well as distant relapse in stage I and II UPSC, it appears that combined modality therapy with radiation and chemotherapy would be efficacious. Radiation therapy theoretically would provide local control while chemotherapy would provide distant control. UPSC has been excluded from prospective, randomized therapeutic trials of early-stage endometrial cancer because of its uniformly poor prognosis. Therefore, currently, there are no published randomized-controlled trials demonstrating the efficacy of radiotherapy, chemotherapy, or a combined approach. Additionally, much of the published literature has focused on small numbers of early-stage (I and II) UPSC and many of these series did not require stringent surgical staging. Therefore, perceived treatment benefits may actually reflect more advanced disease. Despite these limitations, available data have suggested a therapeutic benefit to adjuvant treatment in early-stage UPSC.

Radiotherapy

The role of radiotherapy in controlling local disease and improving overall survival is controversial. The type of treatment modality (whole abdominal radiotherapy, whole pelvic radiation, brachytherapy, or some combination thereof) that is best suited for UPSC is also controversial. For early-stage patients who have had complete surgical staging (TAH, BSO, retroperitoneal lymph node dissection, washings, and omentectomy/omental biopsy), radiotherapy is employed to control local recurrence. Therefore, vaginal brachytherapy or intensity-modulated radiotherapy to the pelvis will carry the most benefit with the least morbidity. Table 2 illustrates a review of irradiation treatment types, recurrence rates, and sites of failure.

Grice et al. (9) examined 14 patients with surgically staged I and II UPSC. Six patients received adjuvant whole pelvic radiation (WPRT), two whole abdominal

Table 2. Stage I and II UPSC radiation treatment failures

Reference	Modality	Recurrence rate (%)	Failures
Grice et al. (9)	WPRT/WART	25	Local and distant
Turner et al. (6)	HDR/LDR +/− chemotherapy	0	N/A
Bristow et al. (12)	BT/WPRT	16.7	Local
Sood et al. (22)	WPRT/BT	29	Local and distant
Huh et al. (25)	WPRT/BT/WART	16.7	Distant
Hamilton et al. (26)	WPRT/WART	15.4	Local and distant

Local recurrences are defined as vaginal and pelvic. Distant failures are either abdominal or extraabdominal
WPRT whole pelvic radiotherapy; WART whole abdominal radiotherapy; BT brachytherapy
N/A not applicable

radiotherapy (WART), and six patients did not receive adjuvant treatment (although one patient had preoperative brachytherapy). Among patients who received radiation, three had additional vaginal brachytherapy. Two of eight (25%) patients in the radiation group recurred (1 distal, 1 local) and none of the patients who did not receive radiation died over a median follow-up of 54 months. Of 15 patients with complete surgical staging who had adjuvant HDR brachytherapy (5 received concomitant chemotherapy), none experienced local, regional, or distant failure over 48 months of follow-up (6). In another small series of completely surgically staged patients, only 1 of 11 (9%) patients with stage I UPSC received adjuvant brachytherapy and that patient developed a pelvic sidewall recurrence. In that series, WPRT was given to 5 of 7 (71%) patients with surgical stage II disease and one developed a recurrence in the radiated field. Overall, the recurrence rate for stage I and II UPSC in this series was 16.7%, but two of the three patients who experienced recurrences died of their disease (12). Sood et al. examined multiple treatment modalities in all stages of UPSC. All patients were completely surgically staged. In this series, there were six stage I and eight stage II patients. Of the seven stage I and II patients who received adjuvant radiation (WPRT, vaginal brachytherapy, or both), two failed (29%) and both of these failures included an abdominal (distant) component. Both patients died of their disease (22). Huh and colleagues reviewed 60 patients with surgical stage I UPSC (omentectomy was not required) from multiple institutions. Forty patients did not receive adjuvant treatment and 7 of 40 (17.5%) had recurrences, four locally and three distally. Six of seven patients with recurrence died of their disease. Twelve patients in this study received adjuvant radiation (WPRT and brachytherapy in 42%, WART in 25%, and brachytherapy alone in 33%). Two of 12 patients in the radiotherapy group (16.7%) had recurrences (both distal), and both patients died of their disease (25). Mehta et al. examined a group of stage I and II UPSC patients who were not uniformly completely staged. Overall, they found that none of the ten early-stage patients who received whole pelvic and/or vaginal brachytherapy had a pelvic recurrence versus 5 of 13 patients without radiotherapy. A literature review suggested that there was little variation in the rate of abdominal failures in early-stage UPSC patients treated with or without WART, but there was a decrease in the overall number of pelvic recurrences when WPRT or vaginal brachytherapy was employed in the adjuvant setting (from 27% without radiation versus 11% with pelvic radiation) (23). The utility of pelvic radiotherapy in preventing local recurrence has recently been supported in a study of combined modality therapy. Of 43 patients who received vaginal brachytherapy, none had a local recurrence. In contrast, 6 of 31 (19%) patients treated without brachytherapy had local recurrences (20). The importance of adjuvant radiation in early-stage UPSC was further substantiated by Hamilton and colleagues. They retrospectively analyzed 68 stage I and II UPSC patients (omentectomy was not a routine part of staging) of whom 33 received no adjuvant treatment. Out of 26 patients treated with radiation (WPRT or WART) alone, 4 had recurrences (15.4%); half of them being intraabdominal (both in the WART group). There were 14 recurrences in the stage I and II UPSC patients who did not receive adjuvant treatment. Six of 14 (43%) were in the vagina and the rest were abdominal/distant. The authors argued that the 5-year OS was improved in patients receiving adjuvant radiation or chemotherapy versus expectant management (85% versus 54% respectively) (26). In completely staged patients (including omentectomy) with UPSC limited to the endometrium, one study did not demonstrate a benefit of any adjuvant therapeutic modality (27).

Pelvic recurrences appear to be well-controlled with the addition of adjuvant pelvic radiation (6, 20, 23, 25, 26), but distal recurrences are problematic as almost all patients who experience distant recurrences will die of their disease. Interestingly, overall, WART has not been able to control abdominal recurrences (23, 26) and, moreover, in one study (21), 2 of 58 patients receiving WART for UPSC died of toxicity potentially related to treatment.

Chemotherapy

There are a few retrospective series that have examined the role of chemotherapy as a single adjuvant treatment modality for stage I and II UPSC. Table 3 provides a summary of treatment failures in several retrospective adjuvant chemotherapy studies. Sood et al. reported on one patient who received chemotherapy in a population of patients who underwent complete surgical staging. The patient received single agent therapy (doxorubicin, paclitaxel, or cisplatin), recurred distally in the bone, and ultimately died of disease (22). Using platinum-based combination chemotherapy

Table 3. Stage I and II UPSC chemotherapy treatment failures

Reference	Modality	Recurrence rate (%)	Failures
Huh et al. (25)	Platinum combined	0	N/A
Dietrich et al. (28)	Carboplatin/paclitaxel	4.8	Local
Hamilton et al. (26)	Platinum combined	14	Local and distant

Platinum combined refers to cisplatin- or carboplatin-based chemotherapy combined with another cytotoxic agent with cyclophosphamide, doxorubicin, or paclitaxel, Huh et al. reported more encouraging results. Of seven patients who received platinum-based chemotherapy as adjuvant treatment, none experienced recurrence over a mean follow-up of 32 months (25). In a multi-institutional review of surgically staged patients with stage I UPSC, 21 patients received adjuvant combination chemotherapy with carboplatin (AUC 6) and paclitaxel (135–175 mg/m^2). In this group, there was one vaginal recurrence (salvaged) with a median follow-up of 41 months. Six patients were treated with single agent platinum, and in this group two recurred (33%) (28). This study highlights the potential value of adding a taxane to the treatment regimen. Paclitaxel at a dose of 200 mg/m^2 given every 3 weeks has demonstrated activity in advanced or recurrent UPSC with a reported objective response rate of 77%, but with significant hematologic toxicity (29). Another retrospective series showed the potential efficacy of platinum-based combination chemotherapy with paclitaxel. Of six stage I UPSC patients treated adjuvantly with a platinum/paclitaxel combination, there were no recurrences. One stage II UPSC patient treated with platinum/doxorubicin failed at multiple sites including vagina and abdomen (26).

Combined Modality Therapy

One of the first groups to study combined modality therapy for early-stage UPSC was Rosenberg and colleagues (2). They examined outcome in ten UPSC patients with clinical stage I disease treated with complete surgical staging without omentectomy. All patients received adjuvant WPRT and four cycles of combination chemotherapy consisting of cisplatinum and epirubicin. None of the patients treated with both surgery and radiation recurred with a median follow-up of 32 months. Table 4 summarizes combined modality therapy and treatment failures in UPSC. Sood et al. reviewed five patients who had combined modality therapy with WPRT and single agent chemotherapy with either doxorubicin, paclitaxel, or cisplatin. All these patients were surgically staged as stage I or II UPSC. There were three

Table 4. Stage I and II UPSC: Combined modality treatment failures

Reference	Modality	Recurrence rate (%)	Failures
Rosenberg et al. (2)	WPRT/platinum combination	0	N/A
Sood et al. (22)	WPRT/single agent	60	Distant
Low et al. (31)	WPRT/BT/platinum combination	7.7	Distant
Kelly et al.[a] (20)	WPRT/WART/BT/ platinum combination	4.5	Local
Fakiris et al. (32)	Intraperitoneal ^{32}P/BT	17.6	Local and distant

WPRT whole pelvic radiotherapy; BT brachytherapy; WART whole abdominal radiotherapy; *Platinum combination* platinum-based regimen with another cytotoxic agent; *Single agent* adriamycin (doxorubicin), paclitaxel, or cisplatin
[a]Excludes patients with IA disease who did not receive adjuvant treatment

recurrences (60%), all with a distant component, but only one patient died of disease (22). Bancher-Todesca et al. reviewed all types of adjuvant therapy in a heterogeneous group of 23 patients with all stages of UPSC (lymphadenectomy performed in 74%). All patients were offered chemotherapy and/or radiation therapy. Irradiation consisted of vault and WPRT. Chemotherapy was given as single agent carboplatin or as combination of cisplatin and cyclophosphamide. Eight patients had stage I or II tumors; six received some form of adjuvant therapy, and four received both chemotherapy and WPRT. None of the patients died of their disease. When all stages were considered, the benefit of combined modality therapy was more apparent. Three of ten (30%) patients who had single modality (chemo-therapy or radiation) and seven of eight (87%) patients with combined modality therapy were alive with a median follow-up of 39 months. This translated into a 80% 5-year OS for patients treated with both chemotherapy and radiation and a 30% 5-year OS for patients treated with single modality therapy (30). Low et al. reviewed 26 patients with surgically staged UPSC (including omentectomy) of which 13 (50%) had stage I or II tumors. All patients were treated similarly with four cycles of adjuvant platinum-based chemotherapy (either cisplatin/epirubicin or carboplatin/paclitaxel) followed by WPRT and HDR brachytherapy. A selected group of stage I patients with minimal myometrial invasion received HDR alone. Of the 13 stage I or II patients, 4 received HDR alone. Only one patient had a distant recurrence and died of disease while another patient died without evidence of disease. Stage-specific 5-year OS in this study was 72.9% for patients with stage I and 100% for patients with stage II tumors. Of note, no patient developed vaginal vault recurrences (31). In the largest study of surgically staged, early-stage UPSC to date, Kelly et al. found a statistically significant improvement in disease-free survival (DFS) and OS in patients who received platinum-based chemotherapy. Seventy four patients with surgical stage I UPSC reviewed adjuvant therapy with a variety of adjuvant chemo-therapy and radiation protocols. In a multivariate analysis controlled for substage, only chemotherapy with or without vaginal brachytherapy was associated with a significant decrease in recurrences ($P < 0.003$). When broken down by substage, patients with IA disease who did not have any residual tumor in the hysterectomy specimen ($N = 7$) and did not receive adjuvant therapy, none of them experienced recurrences. Among patients with stage IA tumor with residual disease in the uterus at the time of hysterectomy who did not receive adjuvant therapy, 6 of 14 (43%) had recurrences. The same trend was maintained for patients with stage IB and IC tumors. When combined, 1 out of 22 (4.5%) patients with stage IB and IC tumors who received adjuvant chemotherapy had recurrences while 14 of 18 (77%) had recur-rences in the no adjuvant chemotherapy group. Interestingly, 5 of 12 (42%) patients who received brachytherapy alone as treatment had recurrences, but no patient who received irradiation (brachytherapy or pelvic) with chemotherapy had vaginal recur-rences (20). In the only prospective phase II therapeutic trial in surgically staged UPSC and clear-cell carcinomas, Fakiris et al. found that out of 17 stage I and II UPSC patients treated with intraperitoneal 32P and brachytherapy, 3 (17.6%) had recurrences and 2 of them died of disease. The median follow-up in this study was 39.4 months, and the two-year OS for all stages was excellent (89.2%) (32).

Summary

Uterine papillary serous carcinoma is a rare histologic subtype of endometrial cancer, representing approximately 5% of all endometrial cancers. It is an aggressive tumor that has a unique spectrum of genetic alterations that contribute to its tumorigenesis (15). Multiple retrospective studies have demonstrated that there is a high frequency of extrapelvic disease even in clinical stage I tumors and that tumor spread tends to mimic that of serous ovarian cancer rather than endometrioid endometrial adenocarcinoma. If 10% or more of the preoperative biopsy specimen contains UPSC, an extended surgical staging laparotomy should be performed (14). Extended surgical staging includes TAH/BSO/pelvic and para-aortic lymph node dissection /infracolic omentectomy or omental biopsy/peritoneal cytology and should be performed in all patients with clinical stage I or II tumors. Serum CA-125 is a reliable marker to monitor therapy in the majority of patients (13).

Multiple adjuvant treatment modalities for early-stage UPSC have been employed (Tables 2, 3, 4). Taken together, radiation alone affords some degree of local control while still leaving patients at risk for distant failure. Chemotherapy as a single treatment modality is likely best given as a platinum agent combined with a taxane. Single agent chemotherapy alone is associated with a high rate of distant failures (22). Combined modality therapy with chemotherapy and radiation appears to offer the lowest recurrence rates with acceptable morbidity. Vaginal recurrences can be significantly reduced with brachytherapy alone (20, 32), likely with lower morbidity than WPRT or WART. In patients with residual disease in the hysterectomy specimen, it is currently our recommendation to treat all early-stage UPSC patients with chemoradiation (20). The optimal radiation techniques as well as optimal chemotherapeutic agents are yet to be determined. Multi-institutional phase II or III trials should be designed to answer these questions.

Carcinosarcoma

Epidemiology and Natural History

Uterine carcinosarcomas represent ≤ 5% of all endometrial cancers. Like UPSCs, they are biologically aggressive neoplasms with high rate of extrauterine disease, high recurrence rates (about 50% across multiple series), and poor disease-free and overall survival rates. Whether carcinosarcomas should be classified as epithelial or mesenchymal tumors has been debated. In most of the clinical literature to date, carcinosarcomas have been included with uterine sarcomas, likely because their prognosis is dismal. However, there is mounting molecular evidence that these tumors are clonal (33–37) and epithelial in origin. The malignant epithelial component has been shown to be capable of inducing a mesenchymal component when injected into nude mice whereas the mesenchymal component could not (35). Furthermore, patterns of metastases indicate the prominent role of the epithelial component as well. Silverberg et al. found a carcinoma component in 30/34 (88%) lymph node metastases (38). Autopsy data, however, have shown no difference in metastatic spread between uterine carcinosarcomas and leiomyosarcomas (39). Clinically, carcinosarcoma behaves like a combination of aggressive adenocarcinoma and sarcoma with a propensity for both lymphatic and hematogenous spread and uniformly poorer outcome when compared to other high-risk histologic subtypes of endometrial cancer. Amant et al. compared outcomes among three groups of high risk, early-stage endometrial cancer patients including grade 3 endometrioid adenocarcinomas, carcinosarcomas, UPSC, and clear-cell carcinomas. Although only 45% of the patients had lymphadenectomy at the time of staging laparotomy, carcinosarcomas were more likely to spread to pelvic and para-aortic lymph nodes. Long-term survival was 86% for grade 3 endometrioid adenocarcinomas and 44% for carcinosarcomas. After a median follow-up of 24 months, 58% of patients with carcinosarcoma had died of their disease compared to 43% with UPSC and clear cell and 28% with grade 3 endometrioid adenocarcinomas (40).

Uterine carcinosarcomas occur more commonly in older (postmenopausal) patients and a recent review of SEER data found a higher frequency of carcinosarcomas in African American versus Caucasian women (4.3 versus 1.7/100,000, $P <$ 0.001) (41). Like most histologic variants of endometrial cancer, carcinosarcomas commonly present with vaginal bleeding or pelvic pain (42). A summary of common clinical findings is presented in Table 5. Grossly, they often grow as fleshy, polypoid masses filling or prolapsing out of the endometrial cavity. There may be an association between long-term tamoxifen use and development of carcinosarcomas (43). Complete surgical staging is paramount in these patients. In one study, 32% of patients with clinical stage I disease (thought to be confined to the uterine corpus) were upstaged based on omental involvement (three of nine patients) or positive lymph nodes (42). The importance of evaluation of extrauterine disease is highlighted in a landmark clinicopathologic study of 203 early-stage (clinical stage I and II) carcinosarcomas (38). In this study, 40 patients were identified with metastatic disease. The majority of the tumors (25 out of 40) had >50% myometrial invasion, but 10% (4 patients) had no myometrial invasion. Notably, the recurrence rate at 31 months for carcinosarcomas without myometrial invasion was 25%.

Multiple attempts have been made to identify pathologic variables associated with outcome and the results have been controversial. Because prognosis is poor even in early-stage disease, it is difficult to identify pathologic variables that will be statistically

Table 5. Carcinosarcomas: clinical features

Median age at diagnosis = 66 years
More common in African American women
May be associated with long-term tamoxifen use
Postmenopausal bleeding most common
Grossly bulky polypoid masses

associated with outcome. In a study of 301 stage I and II (clinical) carcinosarcomas, adnexal spread, lymph node metastases, heterologous type of mesenchymal component, and grade of sarcomatous component were all associated with decreased progression-free survival (PFS) (44). The overall recurrence rate in this study was 53% and 21% of tumors recurred in the pelvis. In other longitudinal studies of carcinosarcoma, no significant associations have been found between carcinoma grade, sarcoma component, mitotic count, LVSI, sarcoma histologic subtype, or tumor size and overall survival (42, 45). It has been argued that prognosis is worse when the epithelial component is a serous carcinoma (46, 47), but this has not been definitively proven.

Treatment

As outlined above, uterine carcinosarcoma carries a particularly poor prognosis even when diagnosed at an early stage. Ideally, treatment should address the high rate of both local (pelvic) and distant recurrences. Because carcinosarcomas are rare, the majority of clinical studies are retrospective. The few prospective, randomized trials include other types of uterine sarcomas or include all stages of carcinosarcomas. Therapeutic trials directed specifically to early-stage carcinosarcoma are rare. Current clinical management of these tumors is therefore evolving and more randomized clinical trials are needed.

Initial evaluation of uterine carcinosarcomas is similar to that for other forms of endometrial cancer. A preoperative chest X-ray should be obtained to rule out pulmonary metastases. Abdomino-pelvic CT scan is warranted if surgical resection does not seem clinically/technically feasible to evaluate disease extent and determine protocol eligibility. Complete surgical resection and staging is advisable including TAH, BSO, peritoneal cytology, and pelvic/ para-aortic lymph node dissection. The value of routine omentectomy in carcinosarcomas has not been established, but in the presence of grossly positive lymph nodes, removal/ biopsy of the omentum may convey prognostic value. Adjuvant treatment with radiation, chemotherapy, or combination of both is advisable even in early-stage disease. As in UPSC, patients with carcinosarcoma are likely to benefit most from combined modality therapy, but this has not yet been proven in prospective trials.

Adjuvant Radiation

There is only one prospective, randomized controlled trial of adjuvant radiation on uterine carcinosarcomas (GOG 150). This trial randomized patients with all stages of optimally debulked uterine carcinosarcoma to adjuvant whole abdominal radiotherapy (WAR) or cisplatin 20 mg/m^2 plus ifosfamide 1.5 g/m^2 with mesna for three cycles. Preliminary results suggest improved results for patients receiving

Table 6. Uterine carcinosarcoma: single modality therapy

Reference	N	Modality	Recurrence
Gerszten et al. (49)	20	WPRT +/– brachytherapy	0%[a]
	24	Surgery	22% (local and distant)
Knocke et al. (51)	33	WPRT +/– brachytherapy	Local = 4.8% stage I, 25% stage II Distant = 18.3% stage I, 33.3% stage II
Chi et al. (52)	28	WPRT (10 neoadjuvant)	21% pelvic, 43% distant[b]
	10	Surgery	50% pelvic, 40% distant
Le (53)	12	WPRT	58%[b]
	16	Surgery	44%
Omura et al. (56)	93	Adriamycin	38%[b]
		Surgery	51%
Sutton et al. (59)	65	Cisplatin/ifosfamide	Overall = 35%; pelvic = 15.4%, distant/multiple site = 20%
Resnik et al. (60)	23	Cisplatin, doxorubicin, etoposide	22%
Odunsi et al. (65)	8	CYVADIC	38%

WPRT whole pelvic radiotherapy; CYVADIC cyclophosphamide, vincristine, doxorubicin (Adriamycin), dacarbazine
[a]Significant difference in overall survival favoring radiation therapy
[b]No difference observed in overall survival versus surgery

chemotherapy (48). There are multiple retrospective studies analyzing the role of adjuvant radiotherapy in early-stage carcinosarcoma. Although overall survival benefit was identified in a small number of studies, the majority did not require strict surgical staging. Despite these limitations, local control appears to be improved with the addition of WPRT +/– vaginal brachytherapy. Table 6 summarizes recurrence rates in early-stage carcinosarcomas treated with adjuvant radiation.

Gerszten et al. reviewed their experience with 44 early-stage (FIGO stage I and II) uterine carcinosarcomas. Twenty patients received WPRT with or without vaginal brachytherapy and 24 were managed with surgery alone. Over the whole cohort of all stages ($N = 60$), 73% had lymph nodes removed as part of the surgical staging. The investigators noted a decrease in local failures (22% in surgery group and 0% in RT group) as well as a decrease in combined local and distant failures (32% and 4%, respectively). Median survival in the surgically managed group was 12 months compared to 77 months in patients who received adjuvant RT ($P = 0.07$ for all stages). Survival was also improved in patients with stage I and II tumors ($P = 0.02$). In this study, local failure was predictive of distant recurrence and death even when adjusted for clinical stage (49). Molpus et al. retrospectively examined outcomes in 43 early-stage uterine carcinosarcoma and found a significant survival advantage in patients who were treated with surgery and adjuvant radiation compared to surgery alone. As it has proven typical for this aggressive disease, 29% of patients with clinical stage I were upstaged at the time of laparotomy and the 5-year OS was only 38% when the disease was confined to the uterus (50), suggesting that surgical staging was incomplete. Interestingly, a benefit was seen in patients who received RT suggesting that improved local control may decrease distant failure rate. Yamada et al. reviewed 62 patients with clinical stage I uterine carcinosarcoma. Ninety percent of the patients had pelvic lymphadenectomy and 42% para-aortic lymph node sampling. Of 28 patients who were considered stage I or II, only 11 received adjuvant WPRT. The authors identified an overall survival benefit in these patients, but were unable to show a decrease in pelvic recurrences across all stages. Of note, in this study, occult extrauterine disease was identified in 61% of 62 patients. The overall recurrence rate was 50% and 43% of patients had distal recurrences (47). Local and distant control was also achieved in a retrospective analysis by Knocke et al. There were 33 patients with early stage tumors (out of a total of 63 reviewed), but only 41% had some form of lymph node sampling. WPRT +/− vaginal brachytherapy was employed in all patients and local control rates were 95.2% for patients with stage I and 75% for patients with stage II tumors. Distant control rates were equally impressive at 81.7% for stage I and 66.7% for stage II tumors. Only 3.2% of patients receiving radiotherapy had grade 3 toxicity (51).

Although these studies demonstrated survival advantage and decreased local and (potentially) distal failures using adjuvant WPRT +/− vaginal brachytherapy, there are several studies that question the therapeutic benefit of adjuvant RT in early-stage uterine carcinosarcomas. Chi et al. reviewed 38 patients with stage I and II carcinosarcomas. Surgical staging was incomplete with only 45% of patients having some form of lymph node sampling. Out of ten patients managed by surgery alone, 50% had a pelvic recurrence, 40% had a distant recurrence, with a 60% 5-year OS. Out of 28 patients treated with WPRT (10 had RT as neo-adjuvant treatment), 21% had a pelvic recurrence, 43% a distant recurrence, with a 59% 5-year OS. Although the overall survival and rate of distant failures were unchanged, pelvic recurrences were reduced by 50% in the second group (52). In a review of 32 carcinosarcoma patients (19 stage I and II) with complete surgical staging, Le et al. found similar recurrence rates among those treated with surgery alone or surgery plus adjuvant irradiation; 44% (7 of 16) in the surgery only group and 58% (7 of 12) in the surgery plus adjuvant radiation group recurred. Overall survival was equally dismal in both groups with 27% of patients surviving among those treated with RT versus 33% of patients who had surgery alone (53). In another study that examined clinical stage I–III uterine carcinosarcomas, patients who were treated with adjuvant or neo-adjuvant (only 35 of 300 patients had surgery followed by RT), WPRT was associated with fewer pelvic recurrences than surgery alone (28% vs. 48%, $P < 0.0002$). Pelvic radiotherapy appeared to lengthen the time to distant relapse from 7 to 17 months, but the overall rate of distant failure was similar between surgery and surgery plus radiation groups (54% versus 57%, respectively) (54). Sartori et al. also found that adjuvant radiation conferred a decrease in the local failure rate but no improvement in overall recurrence rates. Of 66 clinical stage I and II uterine carcinosarcomas, the overall recurrence rates were 38.2% (stage I) and 63.6% (stage II). As a combined group, 40% of early-stage carcinosarcomas failed locally, 40% failed distally, and 20% failed at multiple sites. When all stages were included, WPRT reduced pelvic recurrence rates from 21% to 10.7% in patients who received adjuvant RT (55). Finally, in one of the only randomized trials conducted in early-stage uterine sarcomas, pelvic radiotherapy appeared to reduce the rate of vaginal recurrences, but was not found to improve distant failure rates even in the doxorubicin (Adriamycin) arm of this trial (56) (to be discussed further in the "Chemotherapy" section of this chapter).

Although the majority of these studies feature admixtures of different surgical stages with a wide variety of therapeutic RT (some neo-adjuvant, some adjuvant), it appears that pelvic radiotherapy offers a decrease in local relapse rates. The effect on overall survival varies among studies and will only be adequately addressed in prospective trials. Distant failures are common in patients treated with surgery or a combination of surgery plus irradiation, therefore chemotherapy should be included as part of the adjuvant regimen.

Chemotherapy

As mentioned above, the high-distant failure rate (from 19–50%) across multiple studies in early-stage uterine carcinosarcoma suggests that adding chemotherapy could improve survival. Interestingly, as understanding of the molecular basis of carcinosarcomas has improved, the chemotherapeutic regimens have changed. Initial therapeutic trials assumed that carcinosarcomas behaved clinically like sarcomas and were treated with the same agents. Over time, the epithelial component has been shown to drive tumorigenesis and clinical behavior of this malignancy and therapeutic strategies have shifted accordingly. Although the majority of chemotherapeutic trials include advanced stage patients with measurable disease, it can be extrapolated that agents with activity in advanced or recurrent uterine carcinosarcoma may have activity in early-stage disease as well. A summary of recurrence rates in patients treated with adjuvant chemotherapy is found in Table 6.

Omura et al. performed a phase III trial of adjuvant Adriamycin (60 mg/m^2) versus observation in patients with clinical stage I and II sarcomas. Lymphadenectomy was not required for surgical staging, but all patients were required to have no residual disease after primary surgery. Pelvic radiotherapy was allowed at the discretion of the treating physician. Of 156 evaluable patients, 93 had a diagnosis of carcinosarcoma. The recurrence rate was 38% in the adjuvant Adriamycin group and 51% in patients without further treatment (not statistically different). For clinical stage I tumors, the median survival was 67.2 months. The addition of adjuvant Adriamycin did not prolong OS or PFS, and no difference was seen when a subgroup analysis was performed in patients who received adjuvant pelvic radiotherapy as well. For patients with carcinosarcomas in the Adriamycin arm, 75% of the recurrences occurred in the pelvis and vagina compared to 33% in the no chemotherapy arm. Distant metastases (lung and abdomen) were reduced from 66% in the no treatment group to 25% in patients treated with Adriamycin. Although no overall statistical differences were seen between treatment and no treatment arms of this trial, there appears to be a trend to reduce distant failure in patients with carcinosarcoma with adjuvant treatment (56). Other agents have been evaluated as adjuvant therapy in the advanced/recurrent setting. Sutton et al. performed a phase II trial of ifosfamide and mesna in patients with advanced/recurrent uterine carcinosarcoma and found an objective response rate (OR) of 32.2% with a 18% complete response (CR) rate. There was one death attributed to therapy among 29 evaluable patients (57). Sutton et al. also then examined the role of combination chemotherapy with ifosfamide plus or minus cisplatin in a large phase III trial of patients with advanced or recurrent uterine carcinosarcomas. Treatment consisted of 1.5 gm/m^2/day ifosfamide for 5 days (a reduced dose was given to patients with a history of radiation therapy) with or without 20 mg/m^2 cisplatin × 5 days. The overall response rate in the combination arm was 54% compared to 36% in the ifosfamide alone arm (36%). There was no change in OS with the addition of cisplatin, but a slight prolongation of PFS was observed. The combination regimen was toxic with six treatment-related deaths seen with full (1.5 gm/m^2) doses of ifosfamide (58). Given the improved OR with combination cisplatin and ifosfamide, Sutton et al. examined the same combination regimen in a phase II trial of 65 evaluable patients with clinical stage I and II uterine carcinosarcomas. Lymphadenectomy was not required as part of the surgical staging, and all patients were scheduled to receive three cycles of adjuvant combination chemotherapy. The primary outcome measures were disease-free survival (DFS) and OS. The dosing was similar to the phase III trial (58). The majority of patients (89%) completed three cycles. Grade 3 or 4 thrombocytopenia was seen in 63% of evaluable patients, and 26% had grade 3 or 4 neutropenia. The two-year PFS was 69% while the 2-year and 5-year OS were 82% and 62%, respectively. Of the patients that had recurrences (35% of whole cohort), half of them were in the pelvis (59). Note that there was no adjuvant radiation allowed in this trial. Resnik et al. studied combination chemotherapy with cisplatin doxorubicin, and etoposide in 42 patients with uterine carcinosarcoma. In this phase II trial, 23 patients had stage I or II disease. Almost all (22 of 23) patients had complete surgical staging with lymph node sampling with or without omentectomy. Preoperative or postoperative radiotherapy was allowed. Out of the 23 patients with early-stage tumors, 5 had recurrences (22%). Of note, UPSC was identified as the carcinoma component in 3/5 (60%) of the patients with recurrences. In this study, patients with early stage disease had a 92% two-year survival rate and a 83% PFS. Only 22% of patients experienced grade 3 complications (60). Other phase II trials in advanced/recurrent carcinosarcoma have not been successful (61, 62). Recent phase III data suggest that adding paclitaxel to ifosfamide has improved OS and PFS when compared to ifosfamide alone. In this study, 179 patients with advanced/recurrent uterine carcinosarcoma were randomized to receive ifosfamide alone at a dose of 2g/m^2 or ifosfamide at 1.6g/m^2 plus paclitaxel at 135mg/m^2 every 21 days for a maximum of eight cycles. The combination arm had significantly better overall response and a 29% decrease in the adjusted hazard of death or progression ($P = 0.03$), although alopecia and neuropathy were more commonly seen (63). One retrospective study in patients with advanced/recurrent carcinosarcoma found four of five evaluable patients (80%) to have a complete response to combination therapy with carboplatin (AUC 6) and paclitaxel (175 mg/m^2) (64). Another group followed 24 stage I uterine sarcoma patients with complete surgical staging who received combination chemotherapy with vincristine, doxorubicin (Adriamycin), cyclophosphamide, and dacarbazine (CYVADIC). Eight of the 24 patients evaluable for response had uterine carcinosarcoma and 3 (38%) recurred on this regimen (65).

The optimal chemotherapeutic regimen for uterine carcinosarcoma (all stages) has not been identified. Given improved response rates with the addition of platinum (58, 59, 64), it is likely that future trials will incorporate a platinum arm. Recurrence remains a significant problem in patients with early-stage uterine carcinosarcoma treated with chemotherapy alone (or in combination with radiotherapy), and more effective multimodality treatments are required to reduce the rates of local and distant failures.

Multimodality Therapy

It is evident that recurrence rates are high in uterine carcinosarcomas treated with adjuvant single-modality therapy (either chemotherapy or radiation). This has prompted several investigators to explore combination therapy with radiation and chemotherapy to address local and distant recurrences. Currently, there are no prospective trials open for multimodality therapy in uterine carcinosarcomas, thus, treatment benefit must be extrapolated from small numbers of patients evaluated retrospectively. Table 7 summarizes DFS and OS in patients with uterine carcinosarcoma treated with multimodality therapy.

Kohorn et al. found that four of five (80%) patients treated with radiation, surgery, and adjuvant chemotherapy (with doxorubicin/cyclophosphamide or doxorubicin/cisplatin) were disease free after a follow-up of 36–60 months (66). Manolitsas et al. examined outcome in 38 clinical stage I or II (lymphadenctomy not required) patients with uterine carcinosarcoma that received primary surgery followed by pelvic radiation and combination chemotherapy with four to six cycles of cisplatin (75 mg/m^2) and epirubicin (75 mg/m^2). Nine of 38 patients (24%) were upstaged at the time of

Table 7. Uterine carcinosarcoma: multimodality therapy

Reference	N	Modalities	DFS (%)	OS (%)
Kohorn et al. (66)	5	Surgery/RT/ Chemotherapy[a]	80	
Manolitsas et al. (67)	21	Surgery/WPRT/cisplatin, epirubicin	90	95
Menczer et al. (68)	10	Surgery/cisplatin, Ifosfamide/WPRT	70	75[b]

RT radiation therapy, WPRT whole pelvic radiotherapy
[a]Chemotherapy consisted of doxorubicin/cyclophosphamide or doxorubicin/cisplatin
[b]OS for patients treated with WPRT alone = 50% and 22% for chemotherapy alone

surgery. Chemoradiation was administered in a sequential or "sandwich" fashion with two cycles of chemotherapy given prior to pelvic radiotherapy, followed by completion of the chemotherapy. Patients were treated with WPRT unless a complete lymphadenectomy was performed and lymph nodes were documented to be negative. Those patients received vaginal brachytherapy only. Eleven patients (29%) received no chemotherapy. Only one patient experienced a grade 3 toxicity. Impressively, survival for patients who completed multimodality therapy was 95% (20 of 21 patients) and DFS was 90% with a median follow-up of 55 months. In contrast, OS among patients who did not receive the recommended treatment protocol was 47%. There was one death (and one recurrence) among the 21 patients who received combination therapy. This patient experienced local and distant failure and was originally staged as IA (disease confined to a polyp) (67). A recent study has reviewed all stages of uterine carcinosarcoma treated with chemotherapy alone, WPRT alone, or combined modality (chemotherapy followed by radiation). Out of 49 patients, 25 had clinical stage I tumors. Radiation was delivered as WPRT with HDR brachytherapy. Patients were treated with cisplatin and ifosfamide combination therapy as a single modality and in combination with radiation. Patients who received sequential therapy were administered a higher dose of cisplatin (80 mg/m^2 vs. 60 mg/m^2) and a lower dose of ifosfamide (1.2 gm/m^2/day vs. 1.5 gm/m^2/day). Ten patients received combined modality therapy with a 75% 5-year OS compared to that of WPRT alone (50.5%) and chemotherapy alone (22.2%). Although sites of failure were not explicitly addressed in this study, multi-site failure (both pelvic and distant) appeared to be most common (68).

Summary

Uterine carcinosarcoma is a particularly aggressive neoplasm with high rates of treatment failure even when disease is confined to the uterus (38). Molecular evidence points toward a clonal epithelial origin of these malignancies (33–37) and some evidence suggests more aggressive behavior if the epithelial component consists of serous carcinoma (46, 60). However, both hematogenous and lymphatic spread have been described (38, 39). Results from single modality therapy remain disappointing. There is some promise in combining pelvic radiation therapy with chemotherapy, but the optimal chemotherapeutic regimen has yet to be determined. The most active chemotherapeutic regimen to date is cisplatin and ifosfamide (58, 59) and despite its high toxicity will likely serve as the standard of care arm in future therapeutic trials. The most active chemotherapeutic regimen to date is ifosfamide plus paclitaxel and despite its toxicity will serve as the control arm in future trials (63). Currently, there are six phase II GOG protocols evaluating various cytotoxic as well as biologic therapies in the adjuvant and recurrent setting for uterine carcinosarcoma. Radiation appears to offer local control (52, 53), but distant failure remains problematic. With results from GOG 150 (whole abdominal radiotherapy versus combination chemotherapy with cisplatin and ifosfamide), the contribution of adjuvant radiation to overall survival will be clearer. Protocols that include multimodality therapy in early-stage patients are necessary as combination modality therapy appears to offer the best chance to decrease local and distant failures.

Clear Cell Carcinoma and Tumors of Mixed Histology

Epidemiology and Natural History

Clear cell carcinoma represents <5% of all endometrial cancers in the United States. It was first described by Scully and Barlow who identified these tumors to originate from Mullerian epithelium (69). Microscopically, they show tubulocystic, papillary, and/or solid patterns (70). The clear histologic appearance of the tumor cells is due to their high glycogen content. Other histologic hallmarks are eosinophilic and hobnail cells. All tumors are graded as poorly differentiated (grade 3) by FIGO convention, and unlike clear cell carcinoma of the cervix, in the corpus it does not appear to be associated with maternal exposure to diethylstilbestrol. These cancers have a very similar clinical course to that seen in UPSC with regards to pattern of spread, lack of apparent precursor lesions, and poor prognosis when compared to endometrioid cancers. Thus, clinical outcomes in clear cell cancers have often been reported in combined series with UPSC.

Tumors of mixed histology are more common than pure serous or clear cell carcinomas. Craighead et al. reported that 11% of their patients had tumors of mixed histology including some combination of endometrioid, clear cell, and serous carcinoma (71). Most reports define mixed histology as the coexistence of two or more cell types each of which constitutes at least 10% of the tumor. Cirisano et al. found that tumors with mixed histology (at least 25% of serous or clear cell carcinoma) behave similarly to UPSC (72). The amount of unusual histology needed in a mixed carcinoma to confer a poor prognosis is unclear. Some investigators believe that any amount of poor-prognosis histology (serous or clear cell carcinoma) is sufficient, whereas others think that a small focus of high-risk histology does not affect prognosis. It has been demonstrated that if 10% of the tumor is composed of serous carcinoma, the prognosis is worse than that of poorly differentiated endometrioid adenocarcinoma (14).

Clear cell carcinoma is most commonly seen in thin, postmenopausal patients, is not likely related to estrogen exposure, and is more common in African American women. As with other high-risk types of endometrial cancer, there is a high risk of extrauterine spread. A complete staging laparotomy is therefore indicated. Cirisano et al. showed that nearly 40% of patients with clear cell carcinoma clinically confined to the uterus had extrauterine spread and a small number had extrauterine disease even in the absence of myometrial invasion (72). As with UPSC, survival is highly variable and depends on the extent of surgical staging with most series not requiring retroperitoneal nodal sampling or omentectomy. Abeler et al.

reported the Norwegian Radium Hospital experience with 97 patients diagnosed with clear cell carcinoma and unclear surgical staging. They found a 42% 5-year survival for all stages of clear cell carcinoma compared to 27% for UPSC. The 5-year OS rate was 90% for patients without myometrial invasion, 59% for patients with disease limited to the corpus, and 27% for patients with stage II disease. In this series, myometrial invasion and LVSI were poor prognostic factors (73). Carcangiu et al. reviewed 29 patients with surgical stage I and II clear cell carcinoma. Eleven of 29 patients had retroperitoneal nodal sampling. The 5-year survival for patients with stage I clear cell carcinoma was 73% and 59% for those with stage II tumors (74). Creasman et al. reviewed the FIGO annual data and reported a 5-year survival rate of 81% for surgical stage I clear cell carcinoma compared to 72% for UPSC and 76% for grade 3 endometrioid cancers (75). Large studies of clear cell carcinoma patients in which all have been "comprehensively" staged, including lymph nodes and omentectomy, have not been reported.

Treatment

Given the rarity of these tumors, there are no prospective trials involving only early-stage clear cell carcinoma or mixed tumors. Most trials completed by the National Cancer Institute sponsored Gynecologic Oncology Group (GOG) have only included patients at the point of relapse with measurable disease for salvage chemotherapy. GOG 99, a large prospective randomized trial of intermediate risk (stage I and II) endometrial cancer patients, specifically excluded high-risk histologic subtypes (24). Our recommendations for therapy must, therefore, be extrapolated from retrospective trials involving heterogeneous cohorts of patients (UPSC, grade 3 endometrioid, and mixed histology). The initial therapy is surgery with a comprehensive staging procedure including TAH, BSO, pelvic and para-aortic lymph node resection, omentectomy, and possibly multiple peritoneal biopsies and diaphragm cytology. Patients with no residual disease at the time of hysterectomy (high-risk tumor only on dilation curettage or endometrial biopsy) and possibly other stage IA patients can be observed. All other patients should be considered for adjuvant therapy.

As clear cell carcinoma appears to behave clinically like UPSC and other aggressive histologic variants of endometrial cancer, we recommend consideration of adjuvant cytotoxic chemotherapy for these patients based on available retrospective data for UPSC. Unfortunately, clear cell carcinomas are less responsive to conventional cytotoxic chemotherapy than other high-risk histologic subtypes of endometrial cancer. McMeekin et al. reported the GOG experience of 1,203 patients with measurable recurrent or advanced endometrial cancer treated with a variety of different regimens (doxorubicin, cisplatin, paclitaxel, or combinations). The overall response rate was 42% for the entire cohort, being 44% for endometrioid carcinoma, 44% for UPSC, and 32% for clear cell carcinoma (76). The decreased response for the clear cell carcinoma tumors was statistically significant.

Thus the most appropriate chemotherapeutic regimen is not known and toxicity should be taken into account when selecting adjuvant therapies. Therefore, there may be a role for novel biologic agents in treating this malignancy. Although there is limited data available for patients with clear-cell carcinomas and mixed histology, it is likely that they will benefit from some form of pelvic radiotherapy to decrease the risk of local recurrence. As with UPSC, chemoradiation is likely to have the lowest failure rates in early-stage clear-cell carcinomas and mixed-histology tumors. Our current recommendation is to use vaginal brachytherapy or intensity-modulated radiation therapy (IMRT) to the pelvis in combination with carboplatin and paclitaxel. This regimen is not based on evidence of superior efficacy to other regimens, but on the manageable toxicity of this regimen.

Conclusions

- Serous carcinoma, carcinosarcoma, clear cell carcinoma and mixed histology tumors although representing 3–5% of all endometrial cancers, are responsible for a significant percentage of endometrial cancer mortality.
- These tumors are understudied in randomized-controlled trials and available retrospective data are limited by non-standardized surgical staging and variable treatment regimens applied.
- As significant risk of disease spread outside the uterus exists, comprehensive surgical staging is of paramount importance.
- High local and distant failure rates in patients with early-stage disease have prompted testing of combined modality therapy with chemotherapy and localized radiation, utilizing both high-dose rate brachytherapy to the vaginal cuff or IMRT to the pelvis.

References

1. Jemal A, Siegel R, Ward E, Murray T, Xu J, Smigal C, et al. Cancer Statistics, 2008. CA Cancer J Clin 2008;58(2):271–296.
2. Rosenberg P, Blom R, Hogberg T, Simonsen E. Death rate and recurrence pattern among 841 clinical stage I endometrial cancer patients with special reference to uterine papillary serous carcinoma. Gynecol Oncol, 1993;51: 311–315.
3. Lauchlan SC. Tubal (serous) carcinoma of the endometrium. Arch Pathol Lab Med, 1981;105: 615–618.
4. Hendrickson M, Ross J, Eifel P, Martinez A, Kempson R. Uterine papillary serous carcinoma: a highly malignant form of endometrial adenocarcinoma. Am J Surg Pathol, 1982;6: 93–108.
5. Kato DT, Ferry JA, Goodman A, et al. Uterine papillary serous carcinoma (UPSC): a clinicopathologic study of 30 cases. Gynecol Oncol, 1995;59: 384–389.
6. Turner BC, Knisely JP, Kacinski BM, et al. Effective treatment of stage I uterine papillary serous carcinoma with high dose-rate vaginal apex radiation (192Ir) and chemotherapy. Int J Radiat Oncol Biol Phys, 1998;40: 77–84.

7. Cirisano FD, Jr, Robboy SJ, Dodge RK, et al. The outcome of stage I-II clinically and surgically staged papillary serous and clear cell endometrial cancers when compared with endometrioid carcinoma. Gynecol Oncol, 2000;77: 55–65.
8. Platz CE, Benda JA. Female genital tract cancer. Cancer, 1995;75: 270–294.
9. Grice J, Ek M, Greer B, et al. Uterine papillary serous carcinoma: evaluation of long-term survival in surgically staged patients. Gynecol Oncol, 1998;69: 69–73.
10. Goff BA, Kato D, Schmidt RA, et al. Uterine papillary serous carcinoma: patterns of metastatic spread. Gynecol Oncol, 1994;54: 264–268.
11. Tay EH, Ward BG. The treatment of uterine papillary serous carcinoma (UPSC): are we doing the right thing? Int J Gynecol Cancer, 1999;9: 463–469.
12. Bristow RE, Asrari F, Trimble EL, Montz FJ. Extended surgical staging for uterine papillary serous carcinoma: survival outcome of locoregional (Stage I-III) disease. Gynecol Oncol, 2001;81: 279–286.
13. Abramovich D, Markman M, Kennedy A, Webster K, Belinson J. Serum CA-125 as a marker of disease activity in uterine papillary serous carcinoma. J Cancer Res Clin Oncol, 1999;125: 697–698.
14. Boruta DM, 2nd, Gehrig PA, Groben PA, et al. Uterine serous and grade 3 endometrioid carcinomas: is there a survival difference? Cancer, 2004;101: 2214–2221.
15. Lax SF. Molecular genetic pathways in various types of endometrial carcinoma: from a phenotypical to a molecular-based classification. Virchows Arch, 2004;444: 213–223.
16. Slomovitz BM, Burke TW, Eifel PJ, et al. Uterine papillary serous carcinoma (UPSC): a single institution review of 129 cases. Gynecol Oncol, 2003;91: 463–469.
17. Chan JK, Loizzi V, Youssef M, et al. Significance of comprehensive surgical staging in non-invasive papillary serous carcinoma of the endometrium. Gynecol Oncol, 2003;90: 181–185.
18. Geisler JP, Geisler HE, Melton ME, Wiemann MC. What staging surgery should be performed on patients with uterine papillary serous carcinoma? Gynecol Oncol, 1999;74: 465–467.
19. Carcangiu ML, Chambers JT. Uterine papillary serous carcinoma: a study on 108 cases with emphasis on the prognostic significance of associated endometrioid carcinoma, absence of invasion, and concomitant ovarian carcinoma. Gynecol Oncol, 1992;47: 298–305.
20. Kelly MG, O'Malley DM, Hui P, et al. Improved survival in surgical stage I patients with uterine papillary serous carcinoma (UPSC) treated with adjuvant platinum-based chemotherapy. Gynecol Oncol, 2005;98: 353–359.
21. Lim P, Al Kushi A, Gilks B, Wong F, Aquino-Parsons C. Early stage uterine papillary serous carcinoma of the endometrium: effect of adjuvant whole abdominal radiotherapy and pathologic parameters on outcome. Cancer, 2001;91: 752–757.
22. Sood BM, Jones J, Gupta S, et al. Patterns of failure after the multimodality treatment of uterine papillary serous carcinoma. Int J Radiat Oncol Biol Phys, 2003;57: 208–216.
23. Mehta N, Yamada SD, Rotmensch J, Mundt AJ. Outcome and pattern of failure in pathologic stage I-II papillary serous carcinoma of the endometrium: implications for adjuvant radiation therapy. Int J Radiat Oncol Biol Phys, 2003;57: 1004–1009.
24. Keys HM, Roberts JA, Brunetto VL, et al. A phase III trial of surgery with or without adjunctive external pelvic radiation therapy in intermediate risk endometrial adenocarcinoma: a Gynecologic Oncology Group study. Gynecol Oncol, 2004;92: 744–751.
25. Huh WK, Powell M, Leath CA, 3rd, et al. Uterine papillary serous carcinoma: comparisons of outcomes in surgical Stage I patients with and without adjuvant therapy. Gynecol Oncol, 2003;91: 470–475.
26. Hamilton CA, Liou WS, Osann K, et al. Impact of adjuvant therapy on survival of patients with early-stage uterine papillary serous carcinoma. Int J Radiat Oncol Biol Phys, 2005;63: 839–844.
27. Elit L, Kwon J, Bentley J, Trim K, Ackerman I, Carey M. Optimal management for surgically Stage 1 serous cancer of the uterus. Gynecol Oncol, 2004;92: 240–246.
28. Dietrich CS, Modesitt SC, DePriest PD, et al. The efficacy of adjuvant platinum-based chemotherapy in Stage I uterine papillary serous carcinoma (UPSC). Gynecol Oncol, 2005;99: 557–563.

29. Ramondetta L, Burke TW, Levenback C, Bevers M, Bdurka-Bevers D, Gershenson DM. Treatment of uterine papillary serous carcinoma with paclitaxel. Gynecol Oncol, 2001;82: 156–161.
30. Bancher-Todesca D, Neunteufel W, Williams KE, et al. Influence of postoperative treatment on survival in patients with uterine papillary serous carcinoma. Gynecol Oncol, 1998;71: 344–347.
31. Low JS, Wong EH, Tan HS, et al. Adjuvant sequential chemotherapy and radiotherapy in uterine papillary serous carcinoma. Gynecol Oncol, 2005;97: 171–177.
32. Fakiris AJ, Moore DH, Reddy SR, et al. Intraperitoneal radioactive phosphorus (32P) and vaginal brachytherapy as adjuvant treatment for uterine papillary serous carcinoma and clear cell carcinoma: a phase II Hoosier Oncology Group (HOG 97-01) study. Gynecol Oncol, 2005;96: 818–823.
33. Bitterman P, Chun B, Kurman RJ. The significance of epithelial differentiation in mixed mesodermal tumors of the uterus. A clinicopathologic and immunohistochemical study. Am J Surg Pathol, 1990;14: 317–328.
34. Kounelis S, Jones MW, Papadaki H, Bakker A, Swalsky P, Finkelstein SD. Carcinosarcomas (malignant mixed mullerian tumors) of the female genital tract: comparative molecular analysis of epithelial and mesenchymal components. Hum Pathol, 1998;29: 82–87.
35. Emoto M, Iwasaki H, Kikuchi M, Shirakawa K. Characteristics of cloned cells of mixed mullerian tumor of the human uterus. Carcinoma cells showing myogenic differentiation in vitro. Cancer, 1993;71: 3065–3075.
36. Wada H, Enomoto T, Fujita M, et al. Molecular evidence that most but not all carcinosarcomas of the uterus are combination tumors. Cancer Res, 1997;57: 5379–5385.
37. Fujii H, Yoshida M, Gong ZX, et al. Frequent genetic heterogeneity in the clonal evolution of gynecological carcinosarcoma and its influence on phenotypic diversity. Cancer Res, 2000;60: 114–120.
38. Silverberg SG, Major FJ, Blessing JA, et al. Carcinosarcoma (malignant mixed mesodermal tumor) of the uterus. A Gynecologic Oncology Group pathologic study of 203 cases. Int J Gynecol Pathol, 1990;9: 1–19.
39. Fleming WP, Peters WA, Kumar NB, Morley GW. Autopsy findings in patients with uterine sarcoma. Gynecol Oncol, 1984;19: 168–172.
40. Amant F, Cadron I, Fuso L, et al. Endometrial carcinosarcomas have a different prognosis and pattern of spread compared to high-risk epithelial endometrial cancer. Gynecol Oncol, 2005;98: 274–280.
41. Brooks SE, Zhan M, Cote T, Baquet CR. Surveillance, epidemiology, and end results analysis of 2677 cases of uterine sarcoma 1989–1999. Gynecol Oncol, 2004;93: 204–208.
42. Inthasorn P, Carter J, Valmadre S, Beale P, Russell P, Dalrymple C. Analysis of clinicopathologic factors in malignant mixed Mullerian tumors of the uterine corpus. Int J Gynecol Cancer, 2002;12: 348–353.
43. McCluggage WG, Abdulkader M, Price JH, et al. Uterine carcinosarcomas in patients receiving tamoxifen. A report of 19 cases. Int J Gynecol Cancer, 2000;10: 280–284.
44. Major FJ, Blessing JA, Silverberg SG, et al. Prognostic factors in early-stage uterine sarcoma. A Gynecologic Oncology Group study. Cancer, 1993;71: 1702–1709.
45. Nielsen SN, Podratz KC, Scheithauer BW, O'Brien PC. Clinicopathologic analysis of uterine malignant mixed mullerian tumors. Gynecol Oncol, 1989;34: 372–378.
46. Ramondetta LM, Burke TW, Jhingran A, et al. A phase II trial of cisplatin, ifosfamide, and mesna in patients with advanced or recurrent uterine malignant mixed mullerian tumors with evaluation of potential molecular targets. Gynecol Oncol, 2003;90: 529–536.
47. Yamada SD, Burger RA, Brewster WR, Anton D, Kohler MF, Monk BJ. Pathologic variables and adjuvant therapy as predictors of recurrence and survival for patients with surgically evaluated carcinosarcoma of the uterus. Cancer, 2000;88: 2782–2786.
48. Wolfson AH, Brady MF, Rocereto T, et al. A gynecologic oncology group randomized phase III trial of whole abdominal irradiation (WAI) vs. cisplatin-ifosfamide and mesna (CIM) as post-surgical therapy in stage I–IV carcinosarcoma of the uterus. Gynecol Oncol 2007; 107(2): 177–85.

49. Gerszten K, Faul C, Kounelis S, Huang Q, Kelley J, Jones MW. The impact of adjuvant radiotherapy on carcinosarcoma of the uterus. Gynecol Oncol, 1998;68: 8–13.
50. Molpus KL, Redlin-Frazier S, Reed G, Burnett LS, Jones HW. Postoperative pelvic irradiation in early stage uterine mixed mullerian tumors. Eur J Gynaecol Oncol, 19: 541–546, 1998.
51. Knocke TH, Weitmann HD, Kucera H, Kolbl H, Pokrajac B, Potter R. Results of primary and adjuvant radiotherapy in the treatment of mixed Mullerian tumors of the corpus uteri. Gynecol Oncol, 1999;73: 389–395.
52. Chi DS, Mychalczak B, Saigo PE, Rescigno J, Brown CL. The role of whole-pelvic irradiation in the treatment of early-stage uterine carcinosarcoma. Gynecol Oncol, 1997;65: 493–498.
53. Le T. Adjuvant pelvic radiotherapy for uterine carcinosarcoma in a high risk population. Eur J Surg Oncol, 27: 282–285, 2001.
54. Callister M, Ramondetta LM, Jhingran A, Burke TW, Eifel PJ. Malignant mixed Mullerian tumors of the uterus: analysis of patterns of failure, prognostic factors, and treatment outcome. Int J Radiat Oncol Biol Phys, 2004;58: 786–796.
55. Sartori E, Bazzurini L, Gadducci A, et al. Carcinosarcoma of the uterus: a clinicopathological multicenter CTF study. Gynecol Oncol, 1997;67: 70–75.
56. Omura GA, Blessing JA, Major F, et al. A randomized clinical trial of adjuvant adriamycin in uterine sarcomas: a Gynecologic Oncology Group study. J Clin Oncol, 1985;3: 1240–1245.
57. Sutton GP, Blessing JA, Rosenshein N, Photopulos G, DiSaia PJ. Phase II trial of ifosfamide and mesna in mixed mesodermal tumors of the uterus (a Gynecologic Oncology Group study). Am J Obstet Gynecol, 1989;161: 309–312.
58. Sutton G, Brunetto VL, Kilgore L, et al. A phase III trial of ifosfamide with or without cisplatin in carcinosarcoma of the uterus: a Gynecologic Oncology Group study. Gynecol Oncol, 79: 147–153, 2000.
59. Sutton G, Kauderer J, Carson LF, et al. Adjuvant ifosfamide and cisplatin in patients with completely resected stage I or II carcinosarcomas (mixed mesodermal tumors) of the uterus: a Gynecologic Oncology Group study. Gynecol Oncol, 2005;96: 630–634.
60. Resnik E, Chambers SK, Carcangiu ML, Kohorn EI, Schwartz PE, Chambers JT. A phase II study of etoposide, cisplatin, and doxorubicin chemotherapy in mixed mullerian tumors (MMT) of the uterus. Gynecol Oncol, 1995;56: 370–375.
61. Curtin JP, Blessing JA, Soper JT, DeGeest K. Paclitaxel in the treatment of carcinosarcoma of the uterus: a Gynecologic Oncology Group study. Gynecol Oncol, 2001;83: 268–270.
62. Miller DS, Blessing JA, Schilder J, Munkarah A, Lee YC. Phase II evaluation of topotecan in carcinosarcoma of the uterus: a Gynecologic Oncology Group study. Gynecol Oncol, 2005;98: 217–221.
63. Homesley HD, Filiaci V, Markman M, et al. Phase III trial of ifosfamide with or without paclitaxel in advanced uterine carcinosarcoma: a Gynecologic Oncology Group study. J Clin Oncol 2007;25(5):526–31.
64. Toyoshima M, Akahira J, Matsunaga G, et al. Clinical experience with combination paclitaxel and carboplatin therapy for advanced or recurrent carcinosarcoma of the uterus. Gynecol Oncol, 2004;94: 774–778.
65. Odunsi K, Moneke V, Tammela J, et al. Efficacy of adjuvant CYVADIC chemotherapy in early-stage uterine sarcomas: results of long-term follow-up. Int J Gynecol Cancer, 2004;14: 659–664.
66. Kohorn EI, Schwartz PE, Chambers JT, Peschel RE, Kapp DS, Merino M. Adjuvant therapy in mixed mullerian tumors of the uterus. Gynecol Oncol, 1986;23: 212–221.
67. Manolitsas TP, Wain GV, Williams KE, Freidlander M, Hacker NF. Multimodality therapy for patients with clinical Stage I and II malignant mixed Mullerian tumors of the uterus. Cancer, 2001;91: 1437–1443.
68. Menczer J, Levy T, Piura B, et al. A comparison between different postoperative treatment modalities of uterine carcinosarcoma. Gynecol Oncol, 2005;97: 166–170.
69. Scully RE, Barlow JF. "Mesonephroma" of ovary. Tumor of Mullerian nature related to the endometrioid carcinoma. Cancer, 1967;20: 1405–1417.

70. Kanbour-Shakir A, Tobon H. Primary clear cell carcinoma of the endometrium: a clinicopathologic study of 20 cases. Int J Gynecol Pathol, 1991;10: 67–78.
71. Craighead PS, Sait K, Stuart GC, et al. Management of aggressive histologic variants of endometrial carcinoma at the Tom Baker Cancer Centre between 1984 and 1994. Gynecol Oncol, 2000;77: 248–253.
72. Cirisano FD Jr, Robboy SJ, Dodge RK, et al. Epidemiologic and surgicopathologic findings of papillary serous and clear cell endometrial cancers when compared to endometrioid carcinoma. Gynecol Oncol, 1999;74: 385–394.
73. Abeler VM, Kjorstad KE. Clear cell carcinoma of the endometrium: a histopathological and clinical study of 97 cases. Gynecol Oncol, 1991;40: 207–217.
74. Carcangiu ML, Chambers JT. Early pathologic stage clear cell carcinoma and uterine papillary serous carcinoma of the endometrium: comparison of clinicopathologic features and survival. Int J Gynecol Pathol, 1995;14: 30–38.
75. Creasman WT, Kohler MF, Odicino F, Maisonneuve P, Boyle P. Prognosis of papillary serous, clear cell, and grade 3 stage I carcinoma of the endometrium. Gynecol Oncol, 2004;95: 593–596.
76. McMeekin DS, Filiaci VL, Thigpen JT, Gallion HH, Fleming GF, Rodgers WH. The relationship between histology and outcome in advanced and recurrent endometrial cancer patients participating in first-line chemo therapy trials: a Gynecologic Oncology Group study. Gynecol Oncol, 2007;106:16–22.

Treatment of Advanced and Recurrent Carcinoma: Hormonal Therapy

Franco Muggia and Stephanie V. Blank

Abstract Progestins were the first drugs to be used in systemic therapy of endometrial cancer. After four decades of clinical trials, their role has been narrowed to a relatively small percentage of tumors that have metastasized but are well differentiated and rich in hormonal receptors. Nevertheless, with better selection of patients likely to benefit from hormonal therapy and the exploration of potential role after chemotherapy, one may look forward to new directions of interest.

Keywords Endometrial cancer • Progestins • Hormone receptors

Introduction

Endocrine therapy is applicable to a relatively small percentage of patients with endometrial adenocarcinoma that present at advanced stage or eventually recur with disseminated disease. Its importance, thus far, is primarily historical. Progestins occupied the center stage in the treatment of metastatic endometrial cancer since the 1961 landmark report of Kelley and Baker on their activity (1, 2). We provide an overview of the clinical experience with these agents, focussing on current recommendations and future directions.

Clinical Experience (1961–2000)

After the initial report, a number of trials evaluated parenteral and oral progestational agents, mostly in patients with recurrent disease. These agents were appealing in this role because they offered potential for response with minimal toxicity. The following conclusions have been reached after four decades of clinical trials:

F. Muggia (✉) and S.V. Blank
Division of Medical Oncology, NYU Cancer Institute, NYU Medical Center, New York, NY
e-mail: Franco.Muggia@nyumc.org

F. Muggia and E. Oliva (eds.), *Uterine Cancer*, Current Clinical Oncology,
DOI: 10.1007/978-1-60327-044-1_11,
© Humana Press, a Part of Springer Science+Business Media, LLC 2009

Table 1. Features of endometrial cancer that predict response to hormonal versus cytotoxic therapy[a]

Feature	Response to hormonal therapy	Response to cytotoxic therapy
ER and PR+	Predictive of response with well-differentiated tumors (more likely to be ER and PR+)	Not predictive; better if negative?
Tumor grade	Well to moderately differentiated	Better if poorly differentiated?
Interval from diagnosis	Longer, more likely to respond	Not predictive
Disease sites	Lung and bones: more response	Not predictive

ER estrogen receptor, PR progesterone receptor
[a]Modified from reference (3)

1. Progestin therapy is applicable to a small percentage of patients who develop metastases from endometrial cancer. The characteristics of patients who respond to a wide variety of progestational agents differ substantially from those who show benefit from cytotoxic therapy (Table 1).
2. Escalating the progestin dose beyond megestrol acetate 200 mg daily does not yield improved results (4).
3. Tamoxifen has shown some activity, with a regimen alternating tamoxifen and a progestin having received the widest testing (4, 5), while other hormonal therapies such as aromatase inhibitors and GnRH agonists have not gone on to further development.
4. There is no evidence that adding progestins to chemotherapy results in additional benefit.

Current Status of Hormonal Therapy

Representative results from one large institutional study and three Gynecologic Oncology Group (GOG) studies of hormonal agents in disseminated endometrial cancer are shown in Table 2. The best outcome reported is the original one from the Mayo Clinic that undoubtedly reflects favorable patient selection and may be indicative of what could be obtained by narrowing the criteria for treatment of recurrent endometrial cancer with hormones.

The alternating regimen, representing the last large GOG study of hormonal therapy for recurrent and advanced endometrial cancer, running between July 1994 and November 1995, has become widely used because of the activity that was documented, and survival results that compare favorably to preceding studies. This trial was also notable for achieving an unexpectedly high response rate of 22% among patients with poorly differentiated tumors. The alternating treatment rationale is also soundly based on up-regulation of PR when exposed to estrogen – in this case

Table 2. Achievements of hormones in recurrent endometrial cancer: Selected series

First author (reference)	Drug(s)	Patients	Response rates (%)	Outcome
Reifenstein (4)	Hydroxyprogesterone caproate	314	30	Median S: 20 m
Thigpen (5) (GOG 81)	MPA 200 mg versus 1,000 mg	145, 144	25, 15	Median PFS: 3.2 m, S: 11.1 m versus PFS: 2.5 m, S: 7.0 m
Thigpen (6) (GOG 81F)	Tamoxifen 20 mg bid	68	10	Median PFS: 3.2 m, S: 8.8 m
Whitney (7) (GOG 119)	1 w MPA 200 mg, alt 1 w tamoxifen 40 mg	60	33	Median PFS: 4.0 m, S: 12.0 m
Fiorica (8) (GOG 153)	3 w megestrol acetate 80 mg bid, alt 3 w tamoxifen 20 mg bid	56	27	Median PFS: 2.7 m, S: 14 m

MPA medroxyprogesterone acetate (Provera), PFS progression-free survival, S survival, bid twice daily, m months, w weeks

substituted by the weak agonist tamoxifen. Moreover, tamoxifen has single agent activity, albeit modest. Finally, weight gain, the most common problem encountered with progestin therapy (although this is not well documented in these trials), is less likely to be as steep on an intermittent regimen (reported as grade 1 in 7 and grade 2 in 5 of 56 patients in GOG 153).

An aspect lacking validation in large trials of hormonal agents is the relationship of hormone receptors to response, partly because the trials were mostly run when such receptors were determined by the more laborious biochemical assays. GOG 81 pooled receptor data in 132 patients from the standard and high-dose arms of megestrol acetate and observed a noteworthy correlation between response and receptor status. Only 7 of 86 patients with tumors being negative for PR and 17 of 46 with positive receptors showed responses ($p < .001$). Not unexpectedly, a marked association between receptor status and tumor grade was recorded in this trial. Thus, it is likely that the results of hormonal therapy are highly dependent on patient selection, and could certainly be improved by hormone receptor determinations and knowledge of tumor grade. The GOG studies included a varying proportion of well differentiated tumors that may account for the variability in results (Table 3).

The best survival outcome was obtained in GOG 153, the trial in which patients had the highest percentage of grade 1 tumors. These findings reinforce the validity of patient selection based on differentiation and receptor status. The standard treatment is progestin-based, and treatment course is indefinite, as hormonal therapy is continued until progression is evident. There is no established role for secondary hormonal treatment following failure of initial hormonal therapy.

Table 3. GOG studies: Patient entry by grade

Study	Tumor grade and number of patients per arm	Grade I/total (%)	Grade 1 and 2/total (%)
GOG 81 MPA 200 mg	I: 32 II: 57 III: 56	22	61
GOG 81 MPA 1,000 mg	I: 27 II: 56 III: 71	17	53
GOG 119 MPA/Tam	I: 15 II: 17 III: 27	25	53
GOG 153 MA/Tam	I: 16 II: 17 III: 22	29	59

MPA/Tam = medroxyprogesterone acetate alternating with tamoxifen every week,
MA/Tam = megestrol acetate alternating with tamoxifen every 3 weeks

Future Directions

In Chapter 7, Duska described ongoing studies of progesterone action on endometrial neoplasias prior to surgery (GOG 211), an approach utilized with increasing frequency for select endometrial cancer patients desiring fertility preservation. It also discusses the issues in progestin treatment of early endometrial cancer and provides an informative background on future directions that may, to some extent, be applicable to more advanced presentations. Chapter 13 reviews further combined hormonal approaches.

As reviewed above, the data on hormonal therapy for advanced and recurrent endometrial cancer are outdated but do yield key information for future studies; the focus should be on well-differentiated cancers that have metastasized and on progestin-based therapy. There is little or no point in studying other hormonal approaches before refining our knowledge on how to optimize selection for progestin-based therapy. In this regard, hormonal therapy bears resemblance to more modern targeted therapies for which proper patient selection maximizes response. Additionally, as with biologic therapies, the definition of successful treatment with hormonal agents might include stable disease and not necessarily be limited to partial and complete responses.

The last large study by GOG concerning hormonal therapy for recurrent disease attempted to compare the alternating MA/Tam every 3 weeks to cisplatin, doxorubicin, and paclitaxel chemotherapy (GOG 189). The study was activated in May 2001 but closed early in August 2002 after accruing only 21 patients per arm. Early progression and relative rarity of well-differentiated tumors rendered hormonal treatment an inadequate choice for most endometrial cancers to be able to test in such a sequential strategy. Nevertheless, introduction of hormonal therapy as maintenance after chemotherapy remains an untested strategy that is potentially attractive.

Emphasis on continued treatment also emerges from studies of hormonal therapy. As long as an objective response or stability is achieved, the treatment should be continued indefinitely, a point that was made by Taylor several years ago (3).

The last chapter of this book discusses targeted therapies based on emerging biological characteristics of this disease. This chapter emphasizes the historical development of the first of such targets: the progesterone receptor. Future studies of this hormonal approach including translational components should probably be directed to both endometrial and ovarian tumors that share the importance of such signaling and also to atypical endometrial hyperplasia. For most endometrial carcinomas that are prone to metastasize, the future lies in chemotherapy and in other non-hormonal targeted therapies.

Conclusions

- Patients with endometrial cancers that are well-differentiated but have metastasized, may benefit from progestin-based therapy; other patient selection factors have not been well studied in spite of the many years this treatment has been available.
- Patients benefitting from hormonal approaches have tumors that are biologically different than most that are the target of chemotherapy treatments.
- Alternating tamoxifen with progestin megestrol acetate has gained favor as a hormonal approach because it has potentially better tolerance than continuous progestin.
- A number of other hormonal approaches have been introduced but data are quite preliminary and are not likely to be superior to progestins.
- Chemotherapy should be also be considered in these patients if hormonal therapy fails (see Chapter 12).

References

1. Kelley RM, Baker WH. Progestational agents in the treatment of carcinoma of the endometrium. N Eng J Med 1961; 264:216–8.
2. Kelley RM, Baker WH. The role of progesterone in human endometrial cancer. Cancer Res 1965; 25:1190–2.
3. Taylor RW. In Endometrial Cancer–International Symposium Marburg 1986 – K-D Schulz, RJB King, K Pollow, and RW Taylor, Editors. Treatment of disseminated, recurrent endometrial cancer with progestational agents. W Zuckscherdt Verlag, Munchen, 1987. pp. 155–6.
4. Reifenstein EC. The treatment of advanced endometrial cancer with hydroxyprogesterone caproate. Gynecol Oncol 1974; 2: 377–414.
5. Thigpen JT, Brady MF, Alvarez RD, et al. Oral medroxyprogesterone acetate in the treatment of advanced or recurrent endometrial carcinoma: a dose response study by the Gynecologic Oncology Group. J Clin Oncol 1999; 17: 1736–44.

6. Thigpen T, Brady MF, Homesley HD, Soper JT, Bell J. Tamoxifen in the treatment of advanced or recurrent endometrial carcinoma: a Gynecologic Oncology Group study. J Clin Oncol 2001; 19(2):364–7.
7. Whitney CW, Brunetto VL, Zaino RJ, et al. Phase II study of medroxyprogesterone acetate plus tamoxifen in advanced endometrial carcinoma: Gynecologic Oncology Group study. Gynecol Oncol 2004; 92 (1): 4–9.
8. Fiorica JV, Brunetto VL, Hanjani P, Lentz SS, Mannel R, Andersen W. Phase II trial of alternating courses of megestrol acetate and tamoxifen in advanced endometrial carcinoma: Gynecologic Oncology Group study. Gynecol Oncol 2004; 92 (1): 10–14.

Treatment of Advanced and Recurrent Carcinoma: Chemotherapy

Halla Nimeiri and Gini F. Fleming

Abstract The development of chemotherapy in endometrial cancer took place over two decades, but finally drug combinations have convincingly been shown to have a role in the treatment of advanced and recurrent endometrial cancer. Agents with antitumor activity include doxorubicin, cisplatin, and paclitaxel. A combination of paclitaxel with the cisplatin analog carboplatin and the combination of the three drugs are currently the most commonly used regimens.

Keywords Endometrial cancer • Chemotherapy • Doxorubicin • Cisplatin • Paclitaxel • Carboplatin

Introduction

Over the past two decades, major advances have been made in the exploration of systemic chemotherapy in the setting of metastatic or recurrent endometrial carcinoma. Recently, benefit to chemotherapy in the adjuvant setting has been demonstrated. Single agent anthracyclines, platinum compounds, and taxanes have produced response rates of over 20% in chemotherapy-naïve patients. Combination chemotherapy typically produces higher response rates and doxorubicin plus cisplatin is one of the best studied combinations. One study reported that the addition of paclitaxel to a platinum-based combination significantly improved response rate, PFS, and OS. However, the prognosis of recurrent or metastatic endometrial cancer remains poor, with median survival rates of only about a year in trials of patients with measurable disease (1, 2).

H. Nimeiri and G.F. Fleming (✉)
Section of Hematology/Oncology, Department of Medicine,
University of Chicago Medical Center, Chicago, IL
e-mail: gfleming@medicine.bsd.uchicago.edu

F. Muggia and E. Oliva (eds.), *Uterine Cancer*, Current Clinical Oncology,
DOI: 10.1007/978-1-60327-044-1_12,
© Humana Press, a Part of Springer Science+Business Media, LLC 2009

Data for the chemotherapeutic treatment of uterine carcinosarcomas are more limited, but similar agents appear to have activity in endometrial carcinomas and carcinosarcomas. Carcinosarcomas confer a dismal prognosis and median survivals on trials for women with measurable disease are only 7–9 months (3).

Single Agent Chemotherapy

A large number of cytotoxic agents have been tested in endometrial carcinoma since the early 1960s. Results of single-agent trials for drugs that are commercially available are presented in Table 1 (chemotherapy-naïve) and Table 2 (previously treated patients).

Anthracyclines were among the first agents proven to be effective. Doxorubicin has been studied in phase II and III clinical trials at doses of 50–60 mg/m^2, yielding overall response rates between 25% to 37% (4, 5). Epirubicin produced a similar

Table 1. Single-agent trials – No prior chemotherapy

	Dose	N	RR (%)
Doxorubicin (4)	50 mg/m^2 q 3 weeks	21	19
Doxorubicin (5)	60 mg/m^2 q 3 weeks	43	37
Epirubicin (48)	80 mg/m^2 q 3 weeks	27	26
Liposomal doxorubicin (49)	40 mg/m^2 q 4 weeks	52	11.5
Paclitaxel (50)	250 mg/m^2/24 h + G-CSF q 21 days	28	36
Paclitaxel (51)	210 mg/m^2 q 3 weeks	10	60
Docetaxel (13)	35 mg/m^2 q week	34	21
Docetaxel (14)	70 mg/m^2 q 3 weeks	19	37
Cisplatin (11)	50 mg/m^2 q 3 weeks	11	36
Cisplatin (9)	50–100 mg/m^2 q 4 weeks	26	42
Cisplatin (7)	60 mg/m^2 q 21 days	14	21
Cisplatin (10)	50 mg/m^2 q 21 days	49	20
Carboplatin (8)	400 mg/m^2 q 28 days	23	33
Carboplatin (6)	360 mg/m^2 q 28 days	27	32
Carboplatin (12)	400 mg/m^2 q 28 days	33	24
Cyclophosphamide (4)	666 mg/m^2 q 3 weeks	19	0
Hexamethylmelamine (52)	8 mg/kg/day	20	30
Hexamethylmelamine (53)	280 mg/m^2/day × 14 days q 28 days	34	9
Ifosfamide (54)	5 g/m^2/24 h q 21 days	16	12.5
Ifosfamide (55)	1.2 g/m^2/day × 5 days q 4 weeks	33	24
Ifosfamide (19)	5 g/m^2/24 h q 3 weeks	16	25
Cyclophosphamide (19)	1,200 mg/m^2/24 h q 3 weeks	14	14
Vinblastine (36)	1.5 mg/m^2/24 h × 5 days q 3 weeks	34	12
Vincristine (56)	1.4 mg/m^2 q week × 4 then q 2 weeks	33	18
Methotrexate (57)	40 mg/m^2/week	33	6
Etoposide PO (58)	50 mg/day × 21 days q 28 days	44	14
Topotecan (20)	0.8–1.5 mg/m^2 × 5 days q 21 days	40	20

RR response rate
G-CSF granulocyte colony stimulating factor

Table 2. Single-agent trials – prior chemotherapy

Agent	Dose	N	RR (%)
Doxorubicin (4)	50 mg/m^2	9	11
Mitoxantrone (59)	10–12 mg/m^2	15	0
Liposomal doxorubicin (60)	50 mg/m^2 q 4 weeks	42	9.5
Paclitaxel (16)	175 mg/m^2 q 3 weeks	19	37
Paclitaxel (61)	170 mg/m^2 q 3 weeks	7	43
Paclitaxel (15)	200 mg/m^2 q 3 weeks	44	27
Paclitaxel (51)	210 mg/m^2 q 3 weeks	13	7.7
Docetaxel (14)	70 mg/m^2 q 3 weeks	13	23
Cisplatin (62)	3 mg/kg q 3 weeks	13	31
Cisplatin (63)	50 mg/m^2 q 3 weeks	25	4
Carboplatin (12)	300 mg/m^2 q 4 weeks	17	0
Oxaliplatin (47)	130 mg/m^2 q 21 days	52	13.5
Ifosfamide (64)	1.2 g/m^2/day × 5 q 4 weeks	40	15
Ifosfamide (19)	5 g/m^2/24 h q 3 weeks	16	0
Cyclophosphamide (19)	1,200 mg/m^2/24 h q 3 weeks	15	0
Etoposide IV (65)	100 mg/m^2 days 1, 3, 5 q 28	29	3
Teniposide (66)	100 mg/m^2/week	22	9
Etoposide PO (67)	50 mg/m^2 × 21 q 28 days	22	0
Vincristine (68)	0.25–0.5 mg/m^2 CIV × 5 days	5	0
Fludarabine (69)	18 mg/m^2/day × 5 q 28 days	19	0
Dactinomycin (70)	2 mg/m^2 q 4 weeks	25	12
Topotecan (18)	0.5–1.5 mg/m^2 × 5 q 21 days	22	9

RR response rate

response rate of 26% in one small phase II study. Pegylated liposomal doxorubicin (Doxil®) proved disappointing in first-line treatment, producing a response rate of only 11.5%.

Platinum agents also have good activity. Cisplatin and its less neurotoxic analog, carboplatin, have produced response rates between 20% and 42% in a number of single-agent trials (6–12). A trial of oxaliplatin by the GOG in patients with prior platinum therapy reported a response rate of 13.5% (47). The taxanes, paclitaxel and docetaxel, are the only agents ever shown to have meaningful activity in previously treated patients and have, therefore, now been incorporated into most front-line regimens (13–16).

There are few other drugs with known activity. In the 1970s, six trials investigated the efficacy of 5-fluorouracil as a single agent and reported response rates up to 20% (17). This might be lower if modern standards for efficacy reporting were applied. Finally, topotecan and cyclophosphamide have marginal activity (18–20) and gemcitabine is a promising cytotoxic agent for which no data are yet available in endometrial cancer.

Combination Chemotherapy

Six randomized trials of first-line chemotherapy for recurrent or metastatic endometrial cancer have been published in the past 15 years (Table 3), but only two have shown a survival benefit to one of the two arms being tested. GOG 107 compared single agent doxorubicin to the combination of cisplatin and doxorubicin. Patients receiving the combination arm demonstrated a significant improvement in overall response rate (42% versus 25%) and progression-free interval (6.2 months versus 3.9 months), but OS was similar (median 9 months) (21). However, a similar trial conducted by the European Organization of Research and Treatment of Cancer (EORTC 55872), which likewise compared single agent doxorubicin to the combination of cisplatin and doxorubicin, found not only a higher response rate (43% versus 17%), but also a longer OS (median 9 months versus 7 months) for the combination regimen (22).

Table 3. Randomized chemotherapy trials (first-line)

	Regimen	N	RR (%)	Median OS (mo)
Aapro	Dox 60 mg/m^2 q 4 weeks	87	17	7
EORTC-55872 (2003) (57)	Dox 60 mg/m^2 + Cis 50 mg/m^2 q 4 weeks	90	43	9 ($p = 0.06$)
Thigpen	Dox 60 mg/m^2 q 3 weeks	150	25	9.2
GOG-107 (2004) (21)	Dox 60 mg/m^2 + Cis 50 mg/m^2 q 3 weeks	131	42	9.0 (NS)
Thigpen	Dox 60 mg/m^2 q 3 weeks	132	22	6.7
GOG-48 (1994) (71)	Dox 60 mg/m^2 + Ctx 500 mg/m^2 q 3 weeks	144	30	7.3 (NS)
Gallion	Dox 60 mg/m^2 + Cis 60 mg/m^2 q 3 weeks	169	46	11.2
GOG-139 (2003) (72)	Dox 60 mg/m^2 (6 am) + Cis 60 mg/m^2 (6 pm) q 3 weeks	173	49	13.2 (NS)
Fleming	Dox 60 mg/m^2 + Cis 50 mg/m^2 q 3 weeks	157	40	12.6
GOG-163 (2004) (2)	Dox 50 mg/m^2 + Tax 150 mg/m^2/24 h + G-CSF	160	43	13.6 (NS)
Fleming	Dox 60 mg/m^2 + Cis 50 mg/m^2 q 3 weeks	129	34	12.3
GOG-177 (2004) (1)	Dox 45 mg/m^2 + Cis 50 mg/m^2 + Tax 160 mg/m^2 + G-CSF	134	57	15.3 ($p = 0.037$) 2-sided
GOG-209 ongoing	Tax 175 mg/m^2 + Carbo AUC 6 vs Dox 45 mg/m^2 + Tax 160 mg/m^2 + G-CSF	–	–	–

Dox doxorubicin, CTX cyclophosphamide, Cis cisplatin, Tax paclitaxel (TAXOL), Carbo Carboplatin, G-CSF granulocyte colony stimulating factor, 24h 24 hour infusion

Table 4. Advanced or recurrent endometrial carcinoma[a]: Phase II trials of combination chemotherapy

Author	Regimen	N	RR (%)	PFS median (months)	Overall median (months)
Dimopoulos (2000) (73)	Paclitaxel 175 mg/m^2 + Cisplatin 75 mg/m^2 q 3 weeks	24	67	8.4	17.6
Hoskins (2001) (23)	Carbo AUC5-7 + Paclitaxel 175 mg/m^2 q 4 weeks	46	61	N/A	N/A
Gebbia (2001) (74)	Cisplatin 80 mg/m^2 + Vinorelbine 25 mg/m^2 on D1/8	35	57	6	8.5
Scudder (2005) (26)	Carbo AUC6 + Paclitaxel 175 mg/m^2 + Amifostine 740 mg/m^2 q 4 weeks	47	40	7	14

[a]Selected prospective trials of platinum doublets in chemotherapy-naïve patients

The first randomized trial (GOG 163) using paclitaxel compared the combination of doxorubicin and cisplatin (AP) to doxorubicin plus 24-h infusional paclitaxel given every 3 weeks using G-CSF support. There was no difference between the two arms in terms of response rate, PFS or OS (2). However, when paclitaxel was added to doxorubicin plus cisplatin with filgrastim support (TAP), the three drug combination was superior to doxorubicin plus cisplatin in terms of response rate (57% versus 34%), PFS (median 8.3 months versus 5.3 months), and OS (median 15.3 months versus 12.3 months) (1). Neurologic toxicity was worse for those receiving TAP, with 12% grade 3 and 27% grade 2 peripheral neuropathy compared to 1% and 4%, respectively, in those receiving AP. Whether sequential therapy (AP followed by paclitaxel) could have produced similar survival to the three drug combination was not addressed by GOG 177.

As chemotherapy in the setting of metastatic/recurrent disease is generally palliative, quality of life issues are of major importance. Multiple nonrandomized phase II trials have suggested efficacy and tolerable toxicity for the regimen of carboplatin plus paclitaxel in recurrent or metastatic endometrial cancer with reported response rates of 27–63% (23–27) (Table 4). The GOG is currently conducting a large phase III trial (GOG-209) in women with stage III, IV, or recurrent endometrial cancer comparing carboplatin plus paclitaxel to the three drug TAP regimen.

Adjuvant Chemotherapy

Evaluating the benefit of adjuvant treatment in high-risk patients with endometrial cancer is difficult because of the relative rarity of poor-prognosis early-stage disease. Known risk factors for relapse include deep myometrial invasion, high grade, serous, or clear cell histology, and involvement of pelvic or paraaortic lymph nodes.

Until recently, no systemic therapy had been shown to reduce the risk of recurrence for any stage of endometrial carcinoma. However, there is now one published study, GOG 122, demonstrating a benefit to adjuvant AP chemotherapy when compared to whole abdominal irradiation (28). Women with stage III and low-volume (<2 cm residual disease after debulking surgery) stage IV endometrial carcinoma were randomized to receive WAI with a pelvic boost or to AP chemotherapy with no radiotherapy. The hazard ratio for progression was 0.71 favoring AP (95% CI, 0.55–0.91; $p < .01$). Women with both stage III and stage IV disease appeared to benefit from treatment. However, an Italian trial in women with somewhat lower risk disease failed to demonstrate a benefit to adjuvant cisplatin plus doxorubicin plus cyclophosphamide (CAP) regimen compared to standard pelvic irradiation. Eligible women had stage III or stage IC G3 or II G3 carcinomas with >50% myometrial invasion; clear cell and serous cancers were excluded. There was no overall survival benefit [hazard ratio for death 0.95 (95% CI, 0.66–1.36; $p = 0.77$)] or disease-free survival benefit [hazard ratio for event 0.88 (95% CI, 0.63–1.23; $p = 0.45$)] (29) using chemotherapy. A Japanese GOG (JGOG) randomized trial which predominantly included women with stage I deeply invasive disease also failed to show an overall benefit for CAP chemotherapy compared to pelvic irradiation, although a subgroup of high to intermediate risk patients did better with chemotherapy (75).

Recurrence in the pelvis was common in both arms of GOG 122. Twenty-five percent of recurrences in patients treated with WAI and 35% of recurrences in those treated with chemotherapy were initially limited to the pelvis. Therefore, a combination of chemotherapy and radiotherapy in the adjuvant setting seems reasonable. A subsequent GOG trial 184 treated women with stage III endometrial carcinoma with "involved field" radiotherapy (i.e., pelvic with or without para aortic fields) followed by randomization to either TAP or AP chemotherapy. Granulocyte-colony stimulating factor was administered in both arms. Preliminary results do not suggest a benefit to the addition to paclitexel in this setting. The Radiation Therapy Oncology Group published a phase II trial testing the addition of chemotherapy to adjuvant radiation therapy in women with grade 2 or 3 tumors with >50% myometrial invasion, cervical stromal invasion, or pelvic-confined extrauterine disease (30). Assessment of lymph node status was not required. Women received pelvic radiation therapy with cisplatin 50 mg/m^2 on days 1 and 28 followed by vaginal brachytherapy and then 4 cycles of cisplatin 50 mg/m^2 and paclitaxel 175 mg/m^2. A total of 46 patients were accrued between 1997 and 1999 with a median follow up of 4.3 years. Pelvic, regional, and distant recurrence rates were 2%, 2%, and 19%, respectively, while OS and disease-free survival were 85% and 81%, respectively. Unfortunately, a randomized successor trial was closed because of poor accrual. Other randomized trials of radiotherapy versus chemotherapy plus radiotherapy are ongoing, and their results will better clarify which patients will benefit from adjuvant chemotherapy or combinations of chemotherapy plus radiotherapy.

Despite the absence of randomized data, many centers administer adjuvant chemotherapy to women with early-stage serous carcinomas. There is a very high likelihood that a woman with apparent stage I serous carcinoma has distant spread of disease at the time of diagnosis. Since patients without meticulous staging frequently have stage III or IV disease, chemotherapy can be presumed to have benefit in this setting. Whether well-staged earlier-stage high-risk disease, such as a stage I serous or grade 3 tumors, will benefit from chemotherapy is not known.

Carcinosarcomas

Uterine carcinosarcomas (also known as malignant mixed müllerian tumors) have been traditionally classified as a subtype of uterine sarcoma and studied in trials with sarcomas. Adjuvant and systemic treatments have been similar to those used for uterine sarcomas. However, in recent years, clinical, histopathologic, and molecular evidence have suggested that carcinosarcomas are closely related to carcinomas. Regardless, carcinosarcomas are aggressive malignancies with a 35% overall 5-year survival (31, 32).

Response rates for single agent chemotherapy in carcinosarcomas range from 0–10% for doxorubicin (33, 34), 18–42% for cisplatin (35, 36), 32% for ifosfamide, and 18% for paclitaxel (37, 38). As with endometrial carcinomas, combination chemotherapy regimens have been shown to improve response rates at the expense of added toxicity. GOG 194 randomized women with advanced, recurrent, or persistent carcinosarcoma to treatment with ifosfamide alone or ifosfamide plus cisplatin (3). The combination regimen produced better response rates (54% versus 36%), but there was no significant difference in OS (7.6 months versus 9.4 months, $p = .071$). A subsequent study randomized chemotherapy-naïve women with stage III or IV disease to ifosfamide alone or ifosfamide plus paclitaxel (39). The combination arm produced a significant improvement in response rate, PFS, and OS (hazard of death 0.69; 95% CI, 0.49–0.97; $p = 0.03$).

One randomized trial of adjuvant chemotherapy for women with carcinosarcoma has been published. The GOG compared cisplatin plus ifosfamide plus mesna (CIM) to WAI in optimally debulked stages I–IV carcinosarcomas. Results, adjusted for stage and age, showed a 21% lower recurrence rate for CIM relative to WAI (hazard ratio 0.79, 95%CI; 0.530–1.176, $p = 0.245$ and 29%) and lower estimated death rate for CIM relative to WAI (hazard ratio 0.712, 95%CI; 0.484–1.048, $p = 0.085$) (40). Whether the less toxic regimens used in carcinomas (such as paclitaxel/carboplatin) will produce as much benefit as the ifosfamide-containing regimens that were developed based on sarcoma treatment remains to be seen.

New Directions

A greater understanding of cancer biology and major advances in biotechnology in the last decade have led to the development of agents targeted against specific abnormalities in cancers, especially to aberrant growth signal transduction and microenvironment factors. While trials of new agents in endometrial cancer generally lag behind studies in the more common tumors, a number of these novel therapeutic agents are currently being investigated in advanced endometrial cancer.

Erlotinib, a small-molecule inhibitor of the EGFR tyrosine kinase, has been tested in a phase II trial for chemotherapy-naïve recurrent and advanced endometrial cancer patients. There were 2 out of 27 patients with partial responses (7%) and 14 patients with stable disease (57%) for a median of 3.7 months (41). Whether molecular factors, such as specific mutations in EGFR, will predict response of women with endometrial carcinoma to this category of agents is unknown.

The human Her-2/*neu* gene product, also known as p185[HER2] or c-*erb*B2, is a member of the epidermal growth factor receptor transmembrane receptor tyrosine kinase family. Overexpression of Her-2/*neu* has been found to play a role in cellular transformation, tumorigenesis, and metastasis. Twenty-five percent to 30% of breast cancers overexpress Her-2/*neu*, which is associated with a shorter disease-free interval and worse OS in that setting. This poor prognosis is markedly improved by trastuzumab (anti-HER-2/neu monoclonal antibody). Several series have reported that Her-2/*neu* overexpression and amplification may also be present in endometrial cancers (42). It appears to be more common in serous tumors and in carcinosarcomas (43). One complete response to single agent trastuzumab in a patient with a serous carcinoma of the endometrium has been reported, and an ongoing phase II GOG trial is testing single agent trastuzumab (44) in women whose tumors demonstrate HER-2/*neu* amplification.

Temsirolimus (CCI-779), a rapamycin analog that inhibits the mammalian target of rapamycin (mTOR), appears to have promise in the treatment of endometrial cancer. mTOR is downstream of the phosphoinositide 3-kinase/Akt pathway that is negatively regulated by the PTEN tumor suppressor gene. PTEN deficiency can lead to activation of mTOR, which ultimately directs the translation of specific mRNA subpopulations important for cell proliferation and survival. In cell lines, PTEN deficient tumors are particularly sensitive to mTOR inhibitors. As loss of PTEN is very common in endometrioid endometrial carcinomas, these tumors were logical candidates for therapy with mTOR inhibitors (45). Results of the first stage of a phase II trial testing CCI-779 in chemotherapy-naïve women with advanced or recurrent endometrial carcinoma have been reported (abstract form), and showed a response rate of 31% (46).

Bevacizumab, a monoclonal antibody targeting vascular endothelial growth factor (VEGF), is of great interest because of its high levels of activity against ovarian cancer. A single agent phase II trial of this agent has been completed by the GOG.

It is hoped that judicious application of adjuvant therapy and incorporation of newer agents into treatment will improve the outlook for women with poor-prognosis endometrial cancers in the future.

Conclusions

• Patients with advanced or recurrent endometrial carcinoma have a median survival of about a year.

- Platinum/taxane-based chemotherapy produces response rates between 40% to 60% in the setting of metastatic endometrial carcinoma.
- A survival benefit has recently been demonstrated for the use of adjuvant chemotherapy in stage III endometrial carcinoma.
- Uterine carcinosarcomas are aggressive cancers with a 35% overall 5-year survival. Preliminary data suggest a benefit to adjuvant chemotherapy.

References

1. Fleming GF, Brunetto VL, Cella D, et al. Phase III trial of doxorubicin plus cisplatin with or without paclitaxel plus filgrastim in advanced endometrial carcinoma: a Gynecologic Oncology Group study. J Clin Oncol 2004;22:2159–2166.
2. Fleming GF, Filiaci VL, Bentley RC, et al. Phase III randomized trial of doxorubicin + cisplatin versus doxorubicin + 24-h paclitaxel + filgrastim in endometrial carcinoma: a Gynecologic Oncology Group study. Ann Oncol 2004;15:1173–1178.
3. Sutton G, Brunetto VL, Kilgore L, et al. A phase III trial of ifosfamide with or without cisplatin in carcinosarcoma of the uterus: a Gynecologic Oncology Group study. Gynecol Oncol 2000;79: 147–153.
4. Horton J, Begg CB, Arseneault J, Bruckner H, Creech R, Hahn RG. Comparison of adriamycin with cyclophosphamide in patients with advanced endometrial cancer. Cancer Treat Rep 1978;62:159–161.
5. Thigpen JT, Buchsbaum HJ, Mangan C, Blessing JA. Phase II trial of adriamycin in the treatment of advanced or recurrent endometrial carcinoma: a Gynecologic Oncology Group study. Cancer Treat Rep 1979;63:21–27.
6. Burke TW, Munkarah A, Kavanagh JJ, et al. Treatment of advanced or recurrent endometrial carcinoma with single-agent carboplatin. Gynecol Oncol 1993;51:397–400.
7. Edmonson JH, Krook JE, Hilton JF, et al. Randomized phase II studies of cisplatin and a combination of cyclophosphamide-doxorubicin-cisplatin (CAP) in patients with progestin-refractory advanced endometrial carcinoma. Gynecol Oncol 1987;28:20–24.
8. Green JB, 3rd, Green S, Alberts DS, O'Toole R, Surwit EA, Noltimier JW. Carboplatin therapy in advanced endometrial cancer. Obstet Gynecol 1990;75:696–700.
9. Seski JC, Edwards CL, Herson J, Rutledge FN. Cisplatin chemotherapy for disseminated endometrial cancer. Obstet Gynecol 1982;59:225–228.
10. Thigpen JT, Blessing JA, Homesley H, Creasman WT, Sutton G. Phase II trial of cisplatin as first-line chemotherapy in patients with advanced or recurrent endometrial carcinoma: a Gynecologic Oncology Group study. Gynecol Oncol 1989;33:68–70.
11. Trope C, Grundsell H, Johnsson JE, Cavallin-Stahl E. A phase II study of Cis-platinum for recurrent corpus cancer. Eur J Cancer 1980;16:1025–1026.
12. van Wijk FH, Lhomme C, Bolis G, et al. Phase II study of carboplatin in patients with advanced or recurrent endometrial carcinoma. A trial of the EORTC Gynaecological Cancer Group. Eur J Cancer 2003;39:78–85.
13. Gunthert AR, Ackerman S, Beckmann MW et al. Phase II study of weekly docetaxel in patients with recurrent or metastatic endometrial cancer: AGO Uterus-4. Gynecol Oncol 2007;104:86–90.
14. Katsumata N, Noda K, Nozawa S, et al. Phase II trial of docetaxel in advanced or metastatic endometrial cancer: a Japanese Cooperative Study. Br J Cancer 2005;93:999–1004.
15. Lincoln S, Blessing JA, Lee RB, Rocereto TF. Activity of paclitaxel as second-line chemotherapy in endometrial carcinoma: a Gynecologic Oncology Group study. Gynecol Oncol 2003;88:277–281.

16. Lissoni A, Zanetta G, Losa G, Gabriele A, Parma G, Mangioni C. Phase II study of paclitaxel as salvage treatment in advanced endometrial cancer. Ann Oncol 1996;7:861–863.
17. Carbone PP, Carter SK. Endometrial cancer: approach to development of effective chemotherapy. Gynecol Oncol 1974;2:348–353.
18. Miller DS, Blessing JA, Lentz SS, Waggoner SE. A phase II trial of topotecan in patients with advanced, persistent, or recurrent endometrial carcinoma: a Gynecologic Oncology Group study. Gynecol Oncol 2002;87:247–251.
19. Pawinski A, Tumolo S, Hoesel G, et al. Cyclophosphamide or ifosfamide in patients with advanced and/or recurrent endometrial carcinoma: a randomized phase II study of the EORTC Gynecological Cancer Cooperative Group. Eur J Obstet Gynecol Reprod Biol 1999;86: 179–183.
20. Wadler S, Levy DE, Lincoln ST, Soori GS, Schink JC, Goldberg G. Topotecan is an active agent in the first-line treatment of metastatic or recurrent endometrial carcinoma: Eastern Cooperative Oncology Group Study E3E93. J Clin Oncol 2003;21:2110–2114.
21. Thigpen JT, Brady MF, Homesley HD, et al. Phase III trial of doxorubicin with or without cisplatin in advanced endometrial carcinoma: a Gynecologic Oncology Group study. J Clin Oncol 2004;22:3902–3908.
22. Aapro MS, van Wijk FH, Bolis G, et al. Doxorubicin versus doxorubicin and cisplatin in endometrial carcinoma: definitive results of a randomised study (55872) by the EORTC Gynaecological Cancer Group. Ann Oncol 2003;14:441–448.
23. Hoskins PJ, Swenerton KD, Pike JA, et al. Paclitaxel and carboplatin, alone or with irradiation, in advanced or recurrent endometrial cancer: a phase II study. J Clin Oncol 2001;19: 4048–4053.
24. Nakamura T, Onishi Y, Yamamoto F, Kouno S, Maeda Y, Hatae M. Evaluation of paclitaxel and carboplatin in patients with endometrial cancer. Gan To Kagaku Ryoho 2000;27: 257–262.
25. Price FV, Edwards RP, Kelley JL, Kunschner AJ, Hart LA. A trial of outpatient paclitaxel and carboplatin for advanced, recurrent, and histologic high-risk endometrial carcinoma: preliminary report. Semin Oncol 1997;24:S15–78–S15–82.
26. Scudder SA, Liu PY, Wilczynski SP, et al. Paclitaxel and carboplatin with amifostine in advanced, recurrent, or refractory endometrial adenocarcinoma: a phase II study of the Southwest Oncology Group. Gynecol Oncol 2005;96:610–615.
27. Weber B, Mayer F, Bougnoux P, et al. What is the best chemotherapy regimen in recurrent or advanced endometrial carcinoma? Preliminary results. Paper presented at: Proc Am Soc Clin Oncol, 2003.
28. Randall ME, Brunetto G, Muss H, et al. Whole abdominal radiotherapy versus combination doxorubicin-cisplatin chemotherapy in advanced endometrial carcinoma: a randomized phase III trial of the Gynecologic Oncology Group. Paper presented at: Proc Am Soc Clin Oncol, 2003.
29. Maggi R, Lissoni A, Spina F, et al. Adjuvant chemotherapy vs radiotherapy in high-risk endometrial carcinoma: results of a randomised trial. Br J Cancer 2006;95:266–271.
30. Greven K, Winter K, Underhill K, Fontenesci J, Cooper J, Burke T. Preliminary analysis of RTOG 9708: Adjuvant postoperative radiotherapy combined with cisplatin/paclitaxel chemotherapy after surgery for patients with high-risk endometrial cancer. Int J Radiat Oncol Biol Phys 2004;59:168–173.
31. Dinh TV, Slavin RE, Bhagavan BS, Hannigan EV, Tiamson EM, Yandell RB. Mixed mullerian tumors of the uterus: a clinicopathologic study. Obstet Gynecol 1989;74:388–392.
32. George M, Pejovic MH, Kramar A. Uterine sarcomas: prognostic factors and treatment modalities--study on 209 patients. Gynecol Oncol 1986;24:58–67.
33. Gershenson DM, Kavanagh JJ, Copeland LJ, Edwards CL, Freedman RS, Wharton JT. High-dose doxorubicin infusion therapy for disseminated mixed mesodermal sarcoma of the uterus. Cancer 1987;59:1264–1267.
34. Omura GA, Major FJ, Blessing JA, et al. A randomized study of adriamycin with and without dimethyl triazenoimidazole carboxamide in advanced uterine sarcomas. Cancer 1983;52: 626–632.

35. Thigpen JT, Blessing JA, Orr JW, Jr, DiSaia PJ. Phase II trial of cisplatin in the treatment of patients with advanced or recurrent mixed mesodermal sarcomas of the uterus: a Gynecologic Oncology Group study. Cancer Treat Rep 1986;70:271–274.

36. Thigpen JT, Kronmal R, Vogel S, et al. A phase II trial of vinblastine in patients with advanced or recurrent endometrial carcinoma. A Southwest Oncology Group Study. Am J Clin Oncol 1987;10:429–431.

37. Curtin JP, Blessing JA, Soper JT, DeGeest K. Paclitaxel in the treatment of carcinosarcoma of the uterus: a Gynecologic Oncology Group study. Gynecol Oncol 2001;83:268–270 .

38. Sutton GP, Blessing JA, Rosenshein N, Photopulos G, DiSaia PJ. Phase II trial of ifosfamide and mesna in mixed mesodermal tumors of the uterus (a Gynecologic Oncology Group study). Am J Obstet Gynecol 1989;161:309–312.

39. Homesley HD, Filiaci VL, Bitterman P, et al. Phase III trial of ifosfamide plus paclitaxel as first line of advanced or recurrent uterine carcinosarcoma (mixed mesodermal tumors). Gynecol Oncol 2006;101:S31.

40. Wolfsen AH, Brady MF, Rocereto T, et al. A gynecologic oncology group randomized phase III trial of whole abdominal irradiation (WAI) vs Cisplatin-Ifosfamide and mesna (CIM) as Post-surgical therapy in stage I-IV carcinosarcoma (CS) of the uterus. Gynecol Oncol 2007; 107(2):177–185 PMID 17822748.

41. Jasa KV, Fyles A, Elit L, et al. Phase II study of erlotinib (OSI 774) in women with recurrent or metastatic or metastatic endometrial cancer: NCIC CTG IND-148. Paper presented at ASCO, 2004.

42. Grushko TA, Ridderstrale K, Olopade OI, Mundt A, Fleming GF. Identification of HER-2/ NEU oncogene amplification by fluorescence in situ hybridization in endometrial carcinoma from patients included in Gynecologic Oncology Group trial. Proc Am Soc Clin Oncol 2003;22:468.

43. Villella JA, Cohen S, Tiersten A, Smith DH, Hibshoosh H, Hershman D. Her2/neu expression in uterine papillary serous cancers. Proc Am Soc Clin Oncol 2003;22:465.

44. Fleming GF, Sill MA, Thigpen JT, et al. Phase II evaluation of trastuzumab in patients with advanced or recurrent endometrial carcinoma: a report on GOG 181B. Proc Am Soc Clin Oncol 2003;22:453.

45. Slomovitz BM, Wu W, Broaddus RR, et al. mTOR inhibition is a rational target for the treatment of endometrial cancer. J Clin Oncol 2004:22.

46. Oza AM, Elit L, Biagi J, et al. A phase II study of Temisrolimus (CCI-779) in Patients patients with Metastatic metastatic and/or Locally locally Recurrent recurrent Endometrial endometrial Cancer cancer - NCIC CTG IND 160. Paper presented at: AACR-NCI-EORTC Molecular Targets and Cancer Therapeutics, 2005.

47. Fracasso PM, Blessing JA, Molpus KL, Adler LM, Sorosky J, Rose PG. Phase II study of oxiliplatin as second-line chemotherapy in endometrial adenocarcinoma: a Gynecologic Oncology Group study. Gynecol Oncol 2006;103:523–26.

48. Calero F, Asins-Codoner E, Jimeno J, et al. Epirubicin in advanced endometrial adenocarcinoma: a phase II study of the Grupo Ginecologico Espanol para el Tratamiento Oncologico (GGETO). Eur J Cancer 1991;27:864–866.

49. Homesley HD, Blessing JA, Sorosky J, Reid G, Look KY. Phase II trial of liposomal doxorubicin at 40 mg/m(2) every 4 weeks in endometrial carcinoma: a Gynecologic Oncology Group study. Gynecol Oncol 2005;98:294–298.

50. Ball HG, Blessing JA, Lentz SS, Mutch DG. A phase II trial of paclitaxel in patients with advanced or recurrent adenocarcinoma of the endometrium: a Gynecologic Oncology Group study. Gynecol Oncol 1996;62:278–281.

51. Hirai Y, Hasumi K, Onose R, et al. Phase II trial of 3-h infusion of paclitaxel in patients with adenocarcinoma of endometrium: Japanese Multicenter Study Group. Gynecol Oncol 2004;94:471–476.

52. Seski JC, Edwards CL, Copeland LJ, Gershenson DM. Hexamethylmelamine chemotherapy for disseminated endometrial cancer. Obstet Gynecol 1981;58:361–363.

53. Thigpen JT, Blessing JA, Ball H, Hanjani P, Manetta A, Homesley H. Hexamethylmelamine as first-line chemotherapy in the treatment of advanced or recurrent carcinoma of the endometrium: a phase II trial of the Gynecologic Oncology Group. Gynecol Oncol 1988;31: 435–438.
54. Barton C, Buxton EJ, Blackledge G, Mould JJ, Meanwell CA. A phase II study of ifosfamide in endometrial cancer. Cancer Chemother Pharmacol 1990;26(Suppl):S4–S6.
55. Sutton GP, Blessing JA, DeMars LR, et al. A phase II Gynecologic Oncology Group trial of ifosfamide and mesna in advanced or recurrent adenocarcinoma of the endometrium. Gynecol Oncol 1996;63:25–27.
56. Broun GO, Blessing JA, Eddy GL, Adelson MD. A phase II trial of vincristine in advanced or recurrent endometrial carcinoma. A Gynecologic Oncology Group study. Am J Clin Oncol 1993;16:18–21.
57. Muss HB, Blessing JA, Hatch KD, Soper JT, Webster KD, Kemp GM. Methotrexate in advanced endometrial carcinoma. A phase II trial of the Gynecologic Oncology Group. Am J Clin Oncol 1990;13:61–63.
58. Poplin EA, Liu PY, Delmore JE, et al. Phase II trial of oral etoposide in recurrent or refractory endometrial adenocarcinoma: a Southwest Oncology Group Study. Gynecol Oncol 1999;74: 432–435.
59. Hilgers RD, Von Hoff DD, Stephens RL, Boutselis JG, Rivkin SE. Mitoxantrone in adenocarcinoma of the endometrium: a Southwest Oncology Group Study. Cancer Treat Rep 1985;69: 1329–1330.
60. Muggia FM, Blessing JA, Sorosky J, Reid GC. Phase II trial of the pegylated liposomal doxorubicin in previously treated metastatic endometrial cancer: a Gynecologic Oncology Group study. J Clin Oncol 2002;20:2360–2364.
61. Woo HL, Swenerton KD, Hoskins PJ. Taxol is active in platinum-resistant endometrial adenocarcinoma. Am J Clin Oncol 1996;19:290–291.
62. Deppe G, Cohen CJ, Bruckner HW. Treatment of advanced endometrial adenocarcinoma with cis-dichlorodiammine platinum (II) after intensive prior therapy. Gynecol Oncol 1980;10: 51–54.
63. Thigpen JT, Blessing JA, Lagasse LD, DiSaia PJ, Homesley HD. Phase II trial of cisplatin as second-line chemotherapy in patients with advanced or recurrent endometrial carcinoma. A Gynecologic Oncology Group study. Am J Clin Oncol 1984;7:253–256.
64. Sutton GP, Blessing JA, Homesley HD, McGuire WP, Adcock L. Phase II study of ifosfamide and mesna in refractory adenocarcinoma of the endometrium. A Gynecologic Oncology Group study. Cancer 1994;73:1453–1455.
65. Slayton RE, Blessing JA, Delgado G. Phase II trial of etoposide in the management of advanced or recurrent endometrial carcinoma: a Gynecologic Oncology Group study. Cancer Treat Rep 1982;66:1669–1671.
66. Muss HB, Bundy BN, Adcock L. Teniposide (VM-26) in patients with advanced endometrial carcinoma. A phase II trial of the Gynecologic Oncology Group. Am J Clin Oncol 1991;14: 36–37.
67. Rose PG, Blessing JA, Lewandowski GS, Creasman WT, Webster KD. A phase II trial of prolonged oral etoposide (VP-16) as second-line therapy for advanced and recurrent endometrial carcinoma: a Gynecologic Oncology Group study. Gynecol Oncol 1996;63:101–104.
68. Jackson DV Jr., Jobson VW, Homesley HD, et al. Vincristine infusion in refractory gynecologic malignancies. Gynecol Oncol 1986;25:212–216.
69. Von Hoff DD, Green S, Alberts DS, et al. Phase II study of fludarabine phosphate (NSC-312887) in patients with advanced endometrial cancer. A Southwest Oncology Group Study. Am J Clin Oncol 1991;14:193–194.
70. Moore DH, Blessing JA, Dunton C, Buller RE, Reid GC. Dactinomycin in the treatment of recurrent or persistent endometrial carcinoma: a Phase II study of the Gynecologic Oncology Group. Gynecol Oncol 1999;75:473–475.
71. Thigpen JT, Blessing JA, DiSaia PJ, Yordan E, Carson LF, Evers C. A randomized comparison of doxorubicin alone versus doxorubicin plus cyclophosphamide in the management of

advanced or recurrent endometrial carcinoma: a Gynecologic Oncology Group study. J Clin Oncol 1994;12:1408–1414.

72. Gallion HH, Brunetto VL, Cibull M, et al. Randomized phase III trial of standard timed doxorubicin plus cisplatin versus circadian timed doxorubicin plus cisplatin in stage III and IV or recurrent endometrial carcinoma: a Gynecologic Oncology Group study. J Clin Oncol 2003;21:3808–3813.

73. Dimopoulos MA, Papadimitriou CA, Georgoulias V, et al. Paclitaxel and cisplatin in advanced or recurrent carcinoma of the endometrium: long-term results of a phase II multicenter study. Gynecol Oncol 2000;78:52–57.

74. Gebbia V, Testa A, Borsellino N, Ferrera P, Tirrito M, Palmeri S. Cisplatin and vinorelbine in advanced and/or metastatic adenocarcinoma of the endometrium: a new highly active chemotherapeutic regimen. Ann Oncol 2001;12:767–772.

75. Susumu N, Sagae S, Udagawa Y, Niwak, Kuramoto H, Satch S, Kudo R. Randomized phase III trial of pelvic radiotherapy versus asplatin-based combined chemotherapy in patients with intermediatic - and high - risk endometrial cancer: A Japanese Gynecologic Oncology Group study. Gynecol Oncel 2008;108:226–233.

Treatment for Advanced and Recurrent Carcinoma: Combined Modalities

Marcela G. del Carmen and Neil S. Horowitz

Abstract The contribution of chemotherapy has provided new opportunities for exploring the combination of local and systemic modalities in both early and advanced stages of endometrial carcinoma. The following circumstances are discussed: (1) radiation therapy for locally recurrent endometrial cancer; (2) surgery for stage IV and recurrent endometrial cancer; and (3) advanced stage endometrial cancer consolidating with postoperative and post-chemotherapy radiation therapy. Integration of hormones is also discussed.

Keywords Endometrial cancer • Radiation • Surgery in stage IV and recurrences • Chemotherapy • Hormones

Introduction

Endometrial cancer is generally associated with a good prognosis. This is largely because approximately 75% and 13% of patients present with stage I and stage II disease, respectively (1). For these women, surgery alone or in combination with local therapy is generally curative. For patients with stage III or IV disease, or for those with recurrent endometrial cancer, prognosis remains poor and the optimal adjuvant therapy is yet to be established (Table 1). A subset of these patients may benefit from hormonal manipulation, systemic chemotherapy, or combination treatment with volume-directed radiotherapy and systemic chemotherapy. The choice of therapy depends on extent of residual disease after initial surgery, site and nature of the recurrence, prior therapy used, and the intent of treatment, be it curative or palliative. As the use of hormonal therapy and chemotherapy for treatment of advanced or recurrent

M.G. del Carmen (✉) and N.S. Horowitz
Division of Gynecologic Oncology, Vincent Obstetrics and Gynecology Service,
Massachusetts General Hospital, Boston, MA
e-mail: mdelcarmen@partners.org

F. Muggia and E. Oliva (eds.), *Uterine Cancer*, Current Clinical Oncology,
DOI: 10.1007/978-1-60327-044-1_13,
© Humana Press, a Part of Springer Science+Business Media, LLC 2009

Table 1. [a]Five-year survival for patients with endometrial cancer by [b]FIGO staging

FIGO staging	Five-year survival (%)
IA	88.9
IB	90.0
IC	80.7
IIA	79.9
IIB	72.3
IIIA	63.4
IIIB	38.8
IIIC	51.1
IVA	19.9
IVB	17.2

[a]Adapted from Tarone and Chu (1, p. 221)

[b]FIGO: International Federation of Gynecology and Obstetrics

carcinoma is addressed elsewhere, the aim of this chapter is to focus on combined treatment modalities for this group of women.

Radiation Therapy for Locally Recurrent Endometrial Cancer

Site of recurrence, previous treatment with radiation therapy, relapse-free interval, and histology are important prognostic factors affecting survival in patients with recurrent endometrial cancer. A longer relapse-free interval, low-grade histology, isolated vaginal recurrence, and endometrioid adenocarcinomas are factors associated with improved survival in recurrent endometrial cancer (2, 3). In general, women with non-endometrioid histologies have a worse prognosis than those with endometrioid histologies. For women with a recurrent endometrial cancer following primary treatment with surgery alone, radical radiation therapy may be appropriate. For a select group of patients not previously radiated and with small vaginal recurrences, radiation therapy may be curative. The use of radiation therapy, as part of primary treatment, influences sites of recurrence and survival after relapse. As documented by the PORTEC trial, survival was longer for women with recurrent disease who had not been treated with adjuvant radiation following primary surgery (4, 5). This trial included women with stage I disease, not all of whom had complete surgical staging, and randomized them to surgery alone or adjuvant pelvic radiation therapy (4, 5). At 3 years, the actuarial survival after any relapse in the non-radiation therapy group was 51% compared to 19% for women in the adjuvant radiation therapy group (4, 5). After an isolated vaginal cuff recurrence, five-year survival for the non-radiated group was 65% compared to 43% for women randomized to the adjuvant radiation therapy arm of the study (4, 5). Overall, for women treated with radiation therapy in the recurrent setting, long-term survival is reported to range from 18–71% (6–9) and five-year survival is documented to range from 25 to 50% (9–11).

Successful local control depends on anatomic site of recurrence and tumor size at relapse. Local control is possible in 40–75% of women treated with salvage radiation therapy (3, 7, 9, 11). In a series of 91 patients with isolated vaginal recurrences, local control was seen in 75% of those treated with salvage radiation therapy (9). Tumor size at the time of recurrence also influences local control. In a series of 58 women with recurrent endometrial cancer, five-year local control was 80% for those with tumors ≤2 cm compared to 54% for those with larger tumors ($p = 0.02$) (11). Women with non-central recurrences have a worse prognosis than those with isolated vaginal relapse. Although only limited experience exists, salvage radiation therapy may be appropriate in the setting of a non-central recurrence (12). For women with a pelvic recurrence, three-year survival is reported to be 8%, compared to 73% for those with an isolated vaginal recurrence (4, 5). This survival is comparable to the three-year survival in patients with distant metastases (4, 5).

Patients with vaginal recurrences are usually treated with a combination of pelvic radiation and brachytherapy. For women with a previous history of pelvic radiation therapy, brachytherapy alone is utilized (13). In the presence of bulky disease, interstitial brachytherapy has been reported to result in excellent pelvic control rates (13, 14). It is important to underscore that in the recurrent setting, higher doses of radiation therapy are required than the ones used in the adjuvant setting. As a result, 3–12% of patients suffer from severe treatment-related side effects, especially in the gastrointestinal tract (3, 6, 9, 14). Patients with a previous history of radiation therapy are especially susceptible to severe toxicity at the time of radiation therapy in the recurrent setting (6, 14).

Surgery for Stage IV and Recurrent Endometrial Cancer

Cytoreductive surgery may play a role in the management of stage IV endometrial cancer. There are several retrospective reviews that suggest a survival advantage in those patients who have their tumor optimally cytoreduced (Table 2) (15–17). In all three series, successful cytoreduction was a statistically significant prognostic variable

Table 2. Surgical cytoreduction for stage IV endometrial cancer

Author	Reference number	Number of patients	Residual tumor diameter (cm)	Median survival (months)
Goff et al. 1994	(17)	47	Resected	18
			Unresected	8
Chi et al. 1997	(16)	55	≤2 cm	31
			>2 cm	12
			Unresected	3
Bristow et al. 2000	(15)	65	Microscopic	40
			≤1 cm	15
			>1 cm	11

by multivariant analysis. In the study by Bristow et al., young age (<58 years old) and a good performance status were also predictive of survival. Chi and his colleagues saw no difference in survival for those women who presented with optimal stage IV disease and those who were surgically cytoreduced to an optimal extent of disease, suggesting that aggressive surgery, in addition to the biology of the tumor, plays a role in survival (16).

Recurrent disease isolated to the central pelvis following radiation therapy is seen rarely. Selected patients with such a recurrence may be candidates for pelvic exenteration (18, 19). Pelvic exenteration has been associated with significant operative morbidity and poor overall survival in the setting of recurrent endometrial cancer (18, 19). In a series of 44 patients, nine long-term survivors were recorded (19). This highly morbid procedure may be the only potentially curative alternative for selected patients with a central recurrence following initial surgery and radiation therapy. However, radical pelvic resection extended pelvic resection in conjunction with intra-operative radiation have also been described as an option (20).

Other than pelvic exenteration for central recurrences, surgery does not have a definitive role in the treatment of patients with recurrent endometrial cancer. Two recent retrospective analyses have explored the role of surgery in this setting. Scarabelli and his colleagues operated on 20 women at the time of their first pelvic or abdominal recurrence (21). Patients were classified as having no residual tumor or having tumor at the end of surgery (21). Postoperative therapy was at the discretion of the treating surgeon but included both radiation and chemotherapy. Sixty-five percent of patients were left with no residual disease and had a median PFS and OS of 9.1 and 11.8 months, respectively. There were two perioperative deaths but otherwise morbidity was acceptable. These results were statistically significantly better than those for patients who were left with disease. The PFS for this group was 1.5 months and none was alive 9 months after surgery (21). The other review by Campagnutta et al. is an updated analysis from the same group (22). In this series of 75 patients, 56 (75%) were left with no residual disease but with a 30% rate of major surgical complications and 8% rate of postoperative mortality (22). Patients who did achieve optimal tumor cytoreduction had an improvement in their cumulative 5-year survival (36%) when compared to those with residual disease (0%) (22). Given the modest improvements in survival in both of these reviews and the morbidity and mortality of surgery, appropriate patient selection is critical prior to embarking on this management of recurrent disease.

Advanced Stage Endometrial Cancer

Approximately 5–10% of patients with endometrial cancer present with clinical stage III disease (23). Unfortunately, stage III disease includes women with quite varying risks, as the ultimate outcome for women with positive cytology as their only risk factor is obviously quite different from those with multiple positive pelvic or para-aortic lymph nodes. Radiotherapy alone as primary treatment for these patients is associated with a 15–40% five-year survival rate and a high rate of distant failures. As a consequence, surgery is often the mainstay of therapy (23). The role of adjuvant therapy and more importantly the type of adjuvant treatment for women with stage III disease remains controversial.

The management of patients with positive peritoneal cytology remains a challenge. These patients have been treated via numerous modalities including hormonal treatment, whole abdominal radiation therapy, and intraperitoneal chromic phosphate. In a series of 22 patients with stage IIIA endometrial cancer, defined as either positive peritoneal cytology and/or adnexal metastases, the reported 5-year disease-free survival was 90% with the use of whole abdominal radiation therapy (23).

Historically, intraperitoneal chromic phosphate has been used in the treatment of stage III endometrial cancer. In a study of 65 patients with clinical stage I–III, the reported two-year disease-free survival, following the administration of intraperitoneal chromic phosphate, for patients with stage I disease and positive peritoneal cytology, was documented to be 94% (24). Of note, in this study, the administration of intraperitoneal chromic phosphate with WPRT lead to important gastrointestinal tract toxicity, requiring surgical intervention in 29% of the patients (24). Although intraperitoneal chromic phosphate resulted in adequate disease-free survival, its concomitant use with radiation therapy is not appropriate, given the toxicity profile noted above. In a study by Creasman et al. among 23 patients with positive peritoneal cytology treated with intraperitoneal chromic phosphate, the recurrence rate was documented to be 13%, with a 9% mortality rate of (25). The highly controversial issue of positive peritoneal cytology as an isolated risk factor is evident in this study. Forty-six percent of patients with positive peritoneal cytology as an isolated factor were noted to be at risk of recurrence and death (25).

The use of hormonal therapy is an appropriate treatment approach to patients with malignant peritoneal cytology. In a series of 45 patients with malignant ascites as their only risk factor for adjuvant treatment, all treated with progesterone therapy, 80% were noted to have ER+ tumors and 90% were documented to have PR+ (26). Thirty-six of them underwent a second-look laparoscopic procedure with 94.5% having no evidence of disease (26). The remaining two patients were treated with progesterone therapy for an additional 2 years and had a negative third-look laparoscopy (26). Importantly, there were no documented recurrences or disease-related deaths (26).

The role of postoperative radiation therapy in conferring a survival advantage in patients with stage III endometrial cancer may be related to the impact of gross residual lymph nodal disease prior to initiating radiation therapy. In the GOG 33, the documented five-year survival for patients with para-aortic radiation therapy was noted to be 36% (27). In this series, 16 patients had pathologically confirmed para-aortic and pelvic nodal disease prior to initiation of radiation therapy (27). The radiation dose administered ranged from 4,500 to 5,075 cGy, delivered through 8 cm wide by 18 cm long portals, starting from the pelvic brim (27).

The documented five-year survival for patients with both para-aortic and pelvic nodal disease was 43% compared to 47% for those with para-aortic nodal disease only (27). In a series of 18 patients with para-aortic nodal disease treated with radiation therapy, the five-year OS for patients with microscopic nodal disease was noted to be 67% compared to 17% for patients with gross para-aortic nodal disease prior to commencing radiation therapy (28).

Trying to improve the results of radiation, many authors have attempted to combine cytotoxic chemotherapy with radiation. The safety and efficacy of combined postoperative chemo-radiation have been demonstrated in both ovarian and cervical carcinomas (29–31). The use of multimodality therapy in endometrial cancer addresses the fact that most relapses after adjuvant radiation occur outside the radiated field, and, there is a need for both local and systemic control in advanced staged endometrial cancer. Multiple chemotherapy agents have been combined with both volume directed and whole abdominal radiation with acceptable toxicity and response rates (Table 3) (32–36). Unfortunately, all of these studies are limited by their small size.

The GOG has recently published the results of a Phase III randomized trial for women with stage III and with low-volume stage IV disease (<2 cm of residual disease following surgical resection) (37). In this trial, patients were randomized to either WART versus combination chemotherapy (cisplatin plus doxorubicin). The study documented a significant PFS and OS benefiting patients treated with combination chemotherapy when compared to patients treated with WART (hazard for death, 0.68; 95% CI, 0.52–0.89; $p < 0.01$) (37). It is important to note that this trial commenced accrual in 1992. Since then, radiation techniques, chemothera-

Table 3. Phase I and II trials evaluating combination chemotherapy and radiation therapy in the management of stage III/IV and high-risk (papillary serous, clear cell) endometrial carcinoma

Author	Patients	Regimen	Comments
Duska 2005	20	Paclitaxel 160 mg/m^2, doxorubicin 45 mg/m^2, Carboplatin Auc 6 45 Gy WPRT	13 NED (median follow-up 16 months); SBO
Soper 2005	10	30 Gy WART + cisplatin 15mg/m^2 Doxorubicin 50 mg/m^2, Cisplatin 50 mg/m^2	7/10 chemo 10/10 Grade 4 neutropenia; five episodes FN Median survival 14 mo
Bruzzone 2004	45	Cisplatin 50 mg/m^2, epirubicin 60 mg/m^2, Cyclophosphamide 600 mg/m^2 50 Gy WPRT	8% Grade 4 neutropenia 9-year PFS: 30% OS: 53%
Frigerio 2000	13	Paclitaxel 60 mg/m^2 + 50 Gy WPRT	Minimal toxicity No survival data
Greven 2004	46	45 Gy WPRT + cisplatin 50 mg/m^2 dl + 28 Cisplatin 50 mg/m^2 + paclitaxel 175 mg/m^2	2% Grade 4 heme tox w/RT; 62% Grade 4 heme tox w/CT; 2-year DFS: 83%, OS: 90%

WPRT whole pelvic radiotherapy, WART whole abdominal radiotherapy, PFS progression-free survival, OS overall survival, FN febrile neutropenia

Table 4. Gynecologic Oncology Group trials for patients with stage III/IV endometrial cancer

Study number	Eligibility	Regimen
184	Stage III, <2 cm	WPRT +/– PA or VB → CDDP and doxorubicin +/– paclitaxel
210	Stage III/IV, measurable disease	CDDP 50 mg/m^2 + doxorubicin 45 mg/m^2 + paclitaxel 160 mg/m^2 v/s carboplatin AUC 6 + Paclitaxel 175 mg/m^2
9907	Stage III/IV, <2 cm	WART with weekly CDDP 25 mg/m^2 + paclitaxel 20 mg/m^2
9908	Stage III/IV, <2 cm	Doxorubicin + CDDP → WART

WPRT whole pelvic radiotherapy, WART whole abdominal radiotherapy, CDDP cisplatin, PA Para-aortic, VB vault brachytherapy, f/b

peutic regimens, and supportive care measures have improved and patients have more available options than in the early 1990s (38). As noted by Fleming, GOG 122 raised the question of the appropriateness of combining radiation therapy and chemotherapy for these patients (38). In GOG 184 patients were administered radiation therapy to the involved fields (either pelvis or pelvis and para-aortic lymph nodes) with subsequent delivery of six cycles of chemotherapy (Table 4). The randomization in GOG 184 was to different chemotherapeutic regimens, doxorubicin plus cisplatin versus doxorubicin, cisplatin, and paclitaxel. Accrual to GOG 184 has been completed and results will be available for publication in the near future.

However, is still controversial the timing of the chemotherapy and the most appropriate agents to use. It is unclear whether systemic treatment should be delivered prior to, after radiation, or delivered as a "sandwich" technique with some chemotherapy delivered before and after radiation. The GOG continues to investigate multimodality therapy and until the results of these studies are available, the answers to many of these questions will not be answered.

Combination Hormonal Therapy

The knowledge that development of endometrial cancer is associated with excess estrogen production has resulted in the use of a variety of progestational agents in the treatment of endometrial cancer (39, 40). A number of such agents have been used in the setting of recurrent and metastatic endometrial cancer. These agents include medroxyprogesterone acetate (MPA), hydroxyprogesterone caproate, and megestrol acetate. Reported response rates include 14–53% for MPA, 9–34% for hydroxyprogesterone caproate, and 11–56% for megestrol acetate (40–47). Overall, response rates of 30–35% have been reported (40–47), but recent data suggest that response rate to progestational therapy may be lower (15–20%) (46, 48). Responses to progestational agents are usually of short duration (median time of 4 months) (49). The use of these individual agents as hormonal therapy in advanced or recurrent endometrial cancer is discussed in detail in a different section.

The effectiveness of progestational agents has been theorized to be increased with the use of estrogenic compounds, such as tamoxifen (50, 51). Estrogenic substances have been documented to increase PRs in human endometrial cancer (50, 51). Progestins may downregulate PRs concentration so that the reduced effectiveness of progestational agents and their short duration may be the result of PRs' depletion in tumors treated with these agents (50). It has also been postulated that agents increasing PRs concentration, such as tamoxifen, may potentiate the effectiveness of progestin-based therapy (50). Tamoxifen has been associated with a 10–22% response rate in the treatment of endometrial cancer (52, 53).

Several studies have investigated the combination of progestational agents with tamoxifen in recurrent and advanced endometrial cancer. In the Eastern Cooperative Oncology Group (ECOG) study, there was no difference in the response rate between megestrol acetate as a single agent versus the combination of tamoxifen and megestrol acetate (54). In the GOG study, alternating tamoxifen and megestrol in the treatment of advanced or recurrent endometrial cancer, an overall response rate of 26% was noted (55). In this trial, megestrol (80 mg twice daily) was given for 3 weeks, followed by tamoxifen (20 mg twice daily) for 3 weeks (55). In another recent GOG study, patients with advanced endometrial cancer were treated with tamoxifen (20 mg twice daily) plus alternating weekly cycles of medroxyprogesterone (100 mg twice daily) (56). The response rate was 33%, with a median PFS of 3 months and median OS of 13 months. The results of this trial demonstrate the promising activity of combination daily tamoxifen and intermittent weekly medroxyprogesterone acetate in the treatment of advanced or recurrent endometrial cancer (56). The PFS and median survival in this trial are similar to those reported for progestin therapy alone (42, 44, 48). The adverse effects were also comparable to those reported in series of patients treated with progestin therapy alone. However, the reported 33% response rate is one of the highest seen among the GOG trials investigating the use of hormonal therapy in patients with advanced or recurrent endometrial cancer. Combination hormonal therapy for advanced or recurrent endometrial cancer is an attractive treatment alternative for selected patients, especially those with hormone receptor positive tumors. The potential response rate and the low toxicity profile associated with these agents make them a suitable therapeutic first choice for many such patients.

Combination Chemohormonal Therapy

Combination regimens utilizing chemotherapy and hormonal therapy have also been investigated in the treatment of advanced and recurrent endometrial cancer. The use of chemotherapy alone for recurrent or advanced endometrial cancer is discussed in detail in a different section. It is important to highlight the fact that only a few studies have evaluated the use of chemotherapy concurrently with hormonal therapy. These investigations have several and serious methodologic errors, are underpowered, and have not included the most active chemotherapeutic agents in endometrial cancer. Only a few of the Phase II clinical trials have accrued an excess of 20 patients. These trials documented response rates ranging from 40–50%, similar to the response rates seen with combination chemotherapeutic regimens without hormonal therapy (57, 58). A limited number of randomized trials have compared two different chemotherapeutic regimens containing progestins (57, 59). In the study by Ayoub et al., cyclophosphamide, doxorubicin, and 5-fluorouracil with sequential medroxyprogesterone acetate alternating with tamoxifen is compared to the same chemotherapeutic regimen without hormonal treatment (60). In this study of 43 patients, the response rate in the hormone-containing regimen was 43% compared to 15% in the chemotherapy-only arm. The documented median survival in the combination chemotherapy–hormone therapy arm was noted to be 14 months compared to 11 months for the chemotherapy-only arm. However, this difference in median survival was not statistically significant (60).

In the study by Cornelison et al., 50 consecutive patients were treated with melphalan, 5-fluorouracil, and medroxyprogesterone acetate as first-line therapy. Fifty additional patients were treated prospectively and at a later time with cisplatin, doxorubicin, etoposide, and megestrol acetate (61). The response rate for the two regimens was similar. A significant advantage at 2-year (45% versus 14%), 5-year (30% versus 5%), and median survival (22 versus 9 months) was seen with the second regimen (cisplatin, doxorubicin, etoposide, and megestrol acetate) when compared to the first regimen (melphalan, 5-fluorouracil, and medroxyprogesterone acetate) (61).

In a recent study, 23 patients were treated with carboplatin, methotrexate, and 5-fluorouracil, in combination with medroxyprogesterone acetate (62). Seventy-four percent of patients had an objective response, with a long-lasting response seen in two patients (9%). The documented median response duration was >10 months (3–45+), with a median survival >16 months (2–45+) (62). Even though, earlier trials have failed to show that simultaneous chemotherapy and hormonal therapy is superior to the more traditional treatment strategy of utilizing hormonal therapy followed by chemotherapy at the time of disease progression, the most recent trials are promising. However, the question of whether these regimens are better than paclitaxel-containing combination chemotherapy is not known yet and will require further investigation through randomized trials.

Conclusions

- Locally advanced or recurrent endometrial cancer can be treated by surgery, radiation therapy, hormonal therapy, or chemotherapy. The treatment modality of choice largely depends on localization of disease, patient's performance status, previous treatment history, and the tumor's hormonal receptor status.

- Isolated vaginal recurrences in patients with no previous history of radiation therapy are amenable to primary treatment with radiation therapy.
- Patients with recurrent low-grade tumors that express ER and PR may be treated with progestin therapy for prolonged periods of time, with adequate response rates and low toxicity.
- In the setting of hormone-receptor negative tumors or for tumors that have progressed after hormonal therapy, chemotherapy offers another treatment alternative with modest response rates.
- Combination chemotherapy, (especially regimens containing paclitaxel) or combinations of chemotherapy and hormonal therapy may achieve higher response rates.
- The best regimen is still unknown and the treatment of choice should be based on extent of disease recurrence, prior treatment history, patient preference, and performance status.

References

1. Tarone RE, Chu KC. Age-period-cohort analyses of breast, ovarian, endometrial and cervical cancer mortality rates for Caucasian women in the USA. J Epidemiol Biostat 2000;5:221–231.
2. Morgan JD, Reddy S, Sarin P, et al. Isolated vaginal recurrences of endometrial carcinoma. Radiology 1993;189:609–613.
3. Hoekstra CJ, Koper PC, van Putten WL. Recurrent endometrial adenocarcinoma after surgery alone: prognostic factors and treatment. Radiother Oncol 1998;27:164–166.
4. Creutzberg CL, van Putten WL, Koper PC, et al. Surgery and postoperative radiotherapy versus surgery alone for patients with stage 1 endometrial carcinoma: multicenter randomised trial. PORTEC study group. Post Operative Radiation Therapy in Endometrial Carcinoma. Lancet 2000;355:1404–1411.
5. Creutzberg CL, van Putten WL, Koper PC, et al. Survival after relapse in patients with endometrial cancer: results from a randomized trial small star, filled. Gynecol Oncol 2003;89:201–209.
6. Kuten A, Grigsby PW, Perez CA, et al. Results of radiotherapy in recurrent endometrial carcinoma: a retrospective analysis of 51 patients. Int J Radiat Oncol Biol Phys 1989;17:29–34.
7. Curran WJ, Whittington R, Peters AJ, Fanning J. Vaginal recurrences of endometrial carcinoma: the prognostic value of staging by a primary vaginal carcinoma system. Int J Radiat Oncol Biol Phys 1988;15:803–808.
8. Pai HH, Souhami L, Clark BG, Roman T. Isolated vaginal recurrences in endometrial carcinoma: treatment results using high-dose-rate intracavitary brachytherapy and external beam radiotherapy. Gynecol Oncol 1997;66:300–307.
9. Jhingran A, Burke TW, Eifel PJ. Definitive radiotherapy for patients with isolated vaginal recurrence of endometrial carcinoma after hysterectomy. Int J Radiat Oncol Biol Phys 2003;56:1366–1372.
10. Jereczek-Fossa B, Badzio A, Jassem J. Recurrent endometrial cancer after surgery alone: results of salvage radiotherapy. Int J Radiat Oncol Biol Phys 2000;48:405–413.
11. Wylie J, Irwin C, Pintilie M, et al. Results of radical radiotherapy for recurrent endometrial cancer. Gynecol Oncol 2000;77:66–72.
12. Monk BJ, Tewari KS, Puthawala AA, et al. Treatment of recurrent gynecologic malignancies with iodine-125 permanent interstitial irradiation. Int J Radiat Biol Phys 2002;52:806–815.

13. NagS, Yacoub S, Copeland LS, Fowler JM. Interstitial brachytherapy for salvage treatment of vaginal recurrences in previously unirradiated endometrial cancer patients. Int J Radiat Oncol Biol Phys 2002;54:1153–1159.

14. Tewari K, Cappuccini F, Brewster WR, et al. Interstitial brachytherapy for vaginal recurrences of endometrial carcinoma. Gynecol Oncol 1999;74:416–422.

15. Bristow RE, Zerbe MJ, Rosenshein NB, et al. Stage IVB endometrial carcinoma: the role of cytoreductive surgery and determinants of survival. Gynecol Oncol 2000;2:85–91.

16. Chi DS, Welshinger M, Venkatraman ES, et al. The role of surgical cytoreduction in Stage IV endometrial cancer. Gynecol Oncol 1997;1:56–60.

17. Goff BA, Goodman A, Muntz HG, Fuller AF, Nikrui N, and Rice L. Surgical stage IV endometrial carcinoma: a study of 47 cases. Gynecol Oncol 1994;52:237–240.

18. Morley GW, Hopkins MP, Lindenauer SM, et al. Pelvic exenteration, University of Michigan: 100 patients at 5 years. Obstet Gynecol 1989;74:934–943.

19. Barakat RR, Goldman NA, Patel DA, et al. Pelvic exenteration for recurrent endometrial cancer. Gynecol Oncol 1999;75:99–102.

20. Dowdy SC, Mariani A, Cliby WA, et al. Radical pelvic resection and intraoperative radiation therapy for recurrent endometrial cancer: technique and analysis of outcomes. Gynecol Oncol 2006;101:280–286.

21. Scarabelli C, Campagnutta E, Giorda G, et al. Maximal cytoreductive surgery as a reasonable therapeutic alternative for recurrent endometrial carcinoma. Gynecol Oncol 1998;70:90–93.

22. Campagnutta E, Giorda G, Depiero G, et al. Surgical treatment of recurrent endometrial carcinoma. Cancer 2004;100(1):89–96.

23. Potish RA, Twiggs LB, Adcock LL, Prem KA. Role of whole abdominal radiation therapy in the management of endometrial cancer: prognostic importance of factors indicating peritoneal metastases. Gynecol Oncol 1985;21:80–86.

24. Soper JT, Creasman WT, Clarke-Pearson DL, et al. Intraperitoneal chromic phosphate P 32 suspension therapy of malignant peritoneal cytology in endometrial carcinoma. Am J Obstet Gynecol 1985;153:191–196.

25. Creasman WT, Disaia PJ, Blessing J, et al. Prognostic significance of peritoneal cytology in patients with endometrial cancer and preliminary data concerning therapy with intreperitoneal radiopharmaceuticals. Am J Obstet Gynecol 1981;141:921–929.

26. Yazigi R, Piver MS, Blumenson L. Malignant peritoneal cytology as prognostic indicator in stage I endometrial cancer. Gynecol Oncol 1983;62:359–362.

27. Potish RA, Twigs LB, Adcock LL, et al. Paraaortic lymph node radiotherapy in cancer of the uterine corpus. Obstet Gynecol 1985;65:251–256.

28. Feuer GA, Calanog A. Endometrial carcinoma: treatment of positive paraaortic nodes. Gynecol Oncol 1987;27:104–109.

29. Rose PG, Bundy BN, Watkins EB, Thigpen JT, et al. Concurrent cisplatin-based radiotherapy and chemotherapy for locally advanced cervical cancer. N Engl J Med 1999;340(15):1144–1153.

30. Peters WA, Liu PY, Barrett RJ, et al. Concurrent chemotherapy and pelvic radiation therapy compared to pelvic radiation therapy alone as adjuvant therapy after radical surgery in high risk early stage cancer of the cervix. J Clin Oncol 2000;18(8):1606–1613.

31. Pickel H, Lahousen M, Petru E, et al. Consolidation radiotherapy after carboplatin-based chemotherapy in radically operated advanced ovarian cancer. Gynecol Oncol 1999; 72(2):215–219.

32. Duska LR, Berkowitz R, Matulonis U, et al. A pilot trial of TAC (paclitaxel, doxorubicin, and carboplatin) chemotherapy with filgastrim (r-met HuG-CSF) support followed by radiotherapy in patients with "high risk" endometrial cancer. Gynecol Oncol 2005;96:198–203.

33. Soper JT, Reisinger SA, Ashbury R, Jones E, Clarke-Pearson DL. Feasibility study of concurrent weekly cisplatin and whole abdominopelvic irradiation followed by doxorubicin/cisplatin chemotherapy for advanced stage endometrial carcinoma: a Gynecologic Oncology Group trial. Gynecol Oncol 2004;95:95–100.

34. Bruzzone M, Miglietta L, Frazone P, Gadducci A, Boccardo F. Combined treatment with chemotherapy and radiotherapy in high-risk FIGO stage III-IV endometrial cancer patients. Gynecol Oncol 2004;93(2):345–352.

35. Frigerio L, Mangili G, Aletti M, et al. Concomitant radiotherapy and paclitaxel for high-risk endometrial cancer: first feasibility study. Gynecol Oncol 2001;81:53–57.

36. Greven K, Winter K, Underhill K, Fontenesci J, Cooper J, Burke T. Preliminary analysis of RTOG 9708: Adjuvant postoperative radiotherapy combined with cisplatin/paclitaxel chemotherapy after surgery for patients with high-risk endometrial cancer. Int J Radiat Oncol Biol Phys 2004;59(1):168–173.

37. Randall ME, Filiaci VL, Muss H, et al. Randomized phase III trial of whole-abdominal irradiation versus doxorubicin and cisplatin chemotherapy in advanced endometrial carcinoma: a Gynecologic Oncology Group study. J Clin Oncol 2006;24:34–44.

38. Fleming GF. Major progress for a less common cancer. J Clin Oncol 2006;24:6–8.

39. Kohorn E. Gestagens and endometrial carcinoma. Gynecol Oncol 1976;4:398–411.

40. Kauppila A. Progestin therapy of endometrial, breast, and ovarian carcinoma. A review of clinical observations. Acta Gynecol 1989;63:441–450.

41. Kelley RM, Baker WH. Progestational agents in the treatment of carcinoma of the endometrium. N Engl J Med 1961;264:216–222.

42. Piver MS, Barlow JJ, Luain JR, et al. Medroxyprogesterone acetate versus hydroxyprogesterone caproate in women with metastatic endometrial adenocarcinoma. Am J Clin Oncol 1980;45:268–272.

43. Bonte J. Medroxyprogesterone in the management of primary and recurrent endometrial adenocarcinoma. Acta Obstet Gynecol Scand Suppl 1972;19:21–24.

44. Reifenstein EC. The treatment of advanced endometrial cancer with hydroxyprogesterone caproate. Gynecol Oncol 1974;2:337–414.

45. Geisler HE. The use of megestrol acetate in the treatment of advanced malignant lesions of the endometrium. Gynecol Oncol 1979;1:340–346.

46. Thigpen JT, Brady MF, Alvarez RD, et al. Oral medroxyprogesterone acetate in the treatment of advanced or recurrent endometrial carcinoma: a dose-response study by the Gynecologic Oncology Group. J Clin Oncol 1999;17:1736–1744.

47. Quinn MA, Cauchi M, Fortune D. Endometrial carcinoma: steroid receptors and response to medroxyprogesterone acetate. Gynecol Oncol 1985;21:314–319.

48. Thigpen JT, Blessing J, Disaia P. Oral medroxyprogesterone acetate in advanced or recurrent endometrial carcinoma: results of therapy and correlation with estrogen and progesterone receptor levels. In: Iacobelli S, editor. Endocrinology and Malignancy: Basic and Clinical Issues, The Proceedings of the First International Congress on Cancer and Hormones. CRC Press, Parthenon Publishers; Rome; 1986:446–447.

49. Barakat RR, Grigsby PW, Sabbatini P, et al. Corpus epithelial tumors. In: Hoskins WJ, Perez CA, Young RC, editors. Principles and Practices of Gynecologic Oncology. Second ed. Philadelphia, PA: Lippincott-Raven;1997:880–884.

50. Mortel R, Levy C, Wolff JP, et al. Female sex steroid receptors in postmenopausal endometrial carcinoma and biochemical response to an antiestrogen. Cancer Res 1981; 41:1140–1147.

51. Carlson JA, Allegra JC, Day TG, et al. Tamoxifen and endometrial carcinoma: alterations in estrogen and progesterone receptors in untreated patients and combination hormonal therapy in advanced neoplasia. Am J Obstet Gynecol 1984;149:149–153.

52. Thigpen JT, Brady MF, Homesley HD. Tamoxifen in the treatment of advanced or recurrent endometrial carcinoma. A Gynecologic Oncology Group study. J Clin Oncol 2001;19:364–367.

53. Moore TD, Phillips PH, Nerenstone SR, et al. Systemic treatment of advanced and recurrent endometrial carcinoma: current status and future directions. J Clin Oncol 1991; 9:1071–1077.

54. Pandya KJ, Yeap BY, Davis TE. Phase II study of megestrol and mestrol and tamoxifen in advanced endometrial carcinoma: an Eastern Cooperative Oncology Group (ECOG) study. Am J Clin Oncol 2001;24:43–46.

55. Fiorca JV, Brunetto VL, Hanjani P, et al. A phase II study of recurrent and advanced endometrial carcinoma treated with alternating courses of megestrol acetate (Megace) and tamoxifen citrate (Nolvadex). Proc ASCO (Abst # 1499); 2000;[abstract].
56. Whitney CW, Brunetto VL, Zaine RJ, et al. Phase II study of medroxyprogesterone acetate plus tamoxifen in advanced endometrial carcinoma: a Gynecologic Oncology study. Gynecol Oncol 2004;92:4–9.
57. Horton J, Elson P, Gordon P, et al. Combination chemotherapy for advanced endometrial cancer. An evaluation of three regimens. Cancer 1982;49:2441–2445.
58. Piver MS, Lele SB, Patsner B, et al. Melphalan, 5-fluoroiracil, and medroxyprogesterone acetate in metastatic endometrial carcinoma. Obstet Gynecol 1986;67:261–267.
59. Cohen CJ, Bruckner HW, Deppe G, et al. Multidrug treatment of advanced and recurrent endometrial carcinoma: a Gynecologic Oncology Group study. Obstet Gynecol 1984;63:719–726.
60. Ayoub J, Audet-Lapointe P, Methot Y, et al. Efficacy of sequential cyclical hormonal therapy in endometrial cancer and its correlation with steroid hormone receptor status. Gynecol Oncol 1988;31:327–337.
61. Cornelison TL, Baker TR, Piver MS, et al. Cisplatin, adriamycin, etoposide, megestrol acetate versus melphalan, 5-flurouracil, medroxyprogesterone acetate in the treatment of endometrial carcinoma. Gynecol Oncol 1995;59:243–248.
62. Bafaloukos D, Aravantinos G, Samonis G, et al. Carboplatin, methotrexate and 5-flurouracil in combination with medroxyprogesterone acetate (JMF-M) in the treatment of advanced or recurrent endometrial carcinoma: a Hellenic cooperative oncology group study. Oncology 1999;56:198–201.
63. Gallion HH, Brunetto VL, Cibull M, et al. Randomized phase III trial of standard timed doxorubicin plus cisplatin versus circadian timed doxorubicin plus cisplatin in stage III and IV or recurrent endometrial carcinoma: a Gynecologic Oncology Group study. J Clin Oncol 2003;21:3808–3813.

Management of Uterine Sarcomas

Carolyn Krasner and Martee L. Hensley

Abstract Leiomyosarcomas, endometrial stromal sarcomas, and carcinosarcomas differ widely in tumor biology and their treatment is being addressed in separate trials. Unfortunately, therapeutic progress is slow because of the relatively rarity of these tumors. Recent trials using well defined patient populations are helping to define the effect hormonal and chemotherapeutic strategies.

Keywords Uterine sarcomas • Carcinosarcoma • Leiomyosarcoma • Endometrial stromal sarcoma • Gemcitabine Docetaxel • Hormones

Introduction

Mesenchymal tumors of the uterus comprise only 3–5% of uterine neoplasms (about 2,000 cases per year in the United States) (1), yet account for a disproportionate percentage of deaths from uterine cancers, as high as 29% in one series (2). The rarity of these cancers makes randomized trials difficult to complete, even for cooperative groups, and thus, many of the larger studies conducted in uterine sarcomas have included various histologic subtypes, making application of the results to individual tumor types difficult. Careful histologic review is critical since sarcoma histologic subtypes vary in prognosis and management. Leiomyosarcoma and carcinosarcoma are the two most common histologic types of uterine sarcoma, accounting for approximately 80% of all uterine sarcomas. The remainder are endometrial stromal sarcomas (15%), high-grade undifferentiated uterine sarcomas, and müllerian adenosarcomas (5%).

C. Krasner (✉) and M.L. Hensley
Department of Medical Oncology, Gillette Center for Women's Cancers,
Massachusetts General Hospital, Boston, MA
e-mail: ckrasner@partners.org

F. Muggia and E. Oliva (eds.), *Uterine Cancer*, Current Clinical Oncology,
DOI: 10.1007/978-1-60327-044-1_14,
© Humana Press, a Part of Springer Science+Business Media, LLC 2009

Initial Surgical Management of Early-Stage Uterine Sarcomas

Surgery is the mainstay of treatment for all uterine sarcomas. Women typically present with abnormal bleeding, pelvic pain, or a pelvic mass; however, often, the diagnosis of malignancy, and of sarcoma specifically, is not known preoperatively. There are no radiographic procedures that are diagnostic of sarcoma preoperatively. Ultrasound, computed tomography, and MRI are all unreliable in distinguishing sarcomas from leiomyomata (3). Preoperative sampling such as Pap smear or endometrial curettage are unreliable as screening or diagnostic tests, since the tumor often does not involve the cervix or the endometrial cavity.

There is no staging system specifically for uterine sarcomas. Most often the FIGO (International Federation of Gynecologists and Obstetricians) staging system for endometrial cancer is used. Lymph node status is important for prognosis, but it is not therapeutic as shown when similarly staged patients did not consistently undergo lymphadnectomy (4). When lymph nodes are sampled, tumor is rarely upstaged in LMS (5), because normal-appearing lymph nodes are highly unlikely to be involved. In contrast, occult involvement of lymph nodes and other extrauterine tissues is much more common in carcinosarcoma (6–9). Most authors recommend lymph node dissection for a diagnosis of carcinosarcoma, but only if there is clinical suspicion of involvement for leiomyosarcoma (10, 11).

For women who underwent myomectomy for what was presumed to be leiomyomata, completion hysterectomy is indicated in the case of high-grade leiomyosarcoma, with strong consideration of bilateral salpingo-oophorectomy. In one report, two-thirds of patients had residual disease at completion hysterectomy (12). With low-grade leiomyosarcoma, limited data suggest that myomectomy may be adequate surgical treatment, but there remains a risk for late recurrences (13).

Low-grade endometrial stromal sarcoma is often cured by surgery alone. Extended surgical staging is not generally recommended (14). Surgical management should include removal of the adnexae, since these tumors are often hormonally responsive. One retrospective study found a significantly lower recurrence rate (43%) in patients who underwent oophorectomy in contrast to patients that did not (100%) (15), though other studies have not shown such difference (16).

Recent data regarding adjuvant treatment for women who have optimally debulked stage I, II, III, and IV carcinosarcoma suggest that even patients with advanced disease who can be debulked may have relatively favorable outcomes (17); thus, attempted resection for advanced carcinosarcoma is reasonable. Radiotherapy as a substitute of surgical debulking has been shown to result in worse outcomes (18). Patients with widely metastatic disease, regardless of histology (multi-site bone, lung, liver involvement for example) are generally not considered good candidates for extensive debulking surgery and an initial systemic approach is generally preferable.

Role of Adjuvant Therapies

Uterine sarcomas have varying biologic behaviors, with differing risks and patterns of recurrence and differences in responses to chemotherapeutic agents and radiation. Stage I and II carcinosarcoma have an approximately 50% risk of recurrence, with at least 20% of these involving the lungs (19–21). Stage I and II leiomyosarcomas have a 50–70% risk of recurrence, with >50% of such recurrences being limited to the lungs (22, 23). Low-grade endometrial stromal sarcomas have a much lower risk for recurrence, but both local and distant metastases may occur (24). Local (radiation) and systemic (chemotherapeutic and hormonal) adjuvant treatments have been tried to prevent or delay disease recurrence. Few data are prospective, and even fewer come from randomized-controlled trials, and many studies have not distinguished among histologic subtypes, making interpretation and application of results difficult.

Adjuvant Pelvic Radiation

Although the risk for local recurrence is high with high-risk histology uterine sarcomas (carcinosarcoma, leiomyosarcoma, and undifferentiated endometrial sarcoma), the risk of distant metastases with each of these cancer limits the role of adjuvant pelvic RT. In one retrospective review, 67% of patients had pelvic recurrences but only 14% had pelvis-only recurrence (25). Even if the hypothesis that improved local control leads to improved systemic control is correct, this benefit would only be seen in the small proportion of women destined to have a pelvic-only relapse. This hypothesis has seen various results among three studies (25–27). Even with the selection bias of retrospective studies, RT has not been shown to improve survival (4).

In GOG 20, a randomized trial of adjuvant doxorubicin versus observation for patients with uterine leiomyosarcoma, carcinosarcoma, or other histology sarcoma, pelvic radiation was permitted at the discretion of the treating physician (28). The incidence of first recurrence in the pelvis was 54% in the non-irradiated group compared to 23% in the radiated group ($p = .28$), with no difference in PFS or OS. This study reported a 77% pelvic control rate, which is comparable to that seen in other studies (26, 29). The EORTC has completed a trial in which 222 patients with stage I or II uterine sarcoma were randomized to receive external beam pelvic RT versus observation (study # 55874). A preliminary report suggested a lower incidence of local recurrence but no change in overall survival when pelvic RT was administered. A European study of 103 patients, treated with radiotherapy at the choice of their physician, demonstrated similar improvement in pelvic control, 76% as compared to 37% for patients who did not receive radiation. This study also showed an improvement in OS (73% versus 37%) (30), however, it is important to note that retrospective series are subject to considerable selection bias. A single small series addressing the effect of radiation in women with endometrial stromal sarcoma showed a 46% 5-year survival with surgery alone, increased to 62% with the addition of radiotherapy (31). Overall, there is no convincing data that survival is impacted by the addition of adjuvant radiotherapy.

Guidelines from the National Comprehensive Cancer Network (NCCN) suggest that adjuvant radiation therapy be considered for women with resected stage I–III leiomyosarcomas and carcinosarcomas and stage III endometrial stromal sarcomas (32). Prospective, stage- and histology-specific trials are needed in order to better define the role of adjuvant RT in uterine sarcomas.

Adjuvant Chemotherapy

Adjuvant chemotherapy is undertaken with the hope that it may improve outcome in the many patients that will develop distant disease failures by acting on micrometastases. Unfortunately, conclusive support for this approach is again hampered by the rarity of these diseases and the difficulty in conducting large randomized controlled trials powered to detect relatively small effect sizes.

There are two small trials comparing adjuvant doxorubicin to no further treatment. In GOG 20, 225 women with FIGO stage I or II uterine sarcoma were randomly assigned to eight cycles of doxorubicin versus no systemic treatment. Only 156 women were evaluable (95 women with carcinosarcoma, 48 with leiomyosarcoma, and 15 with sarcomas of other histologies). Patients were permitted to receive adjuvant pelvic radiotherapy at the discretion of the treating physician, either before or after chemotherapy. This trial did not show a statistically significant difference in OS or PFS between the two groups. The recurrence rate was 53% among patients assigned to observation versus 41% among those that received to doxorubicin (28). In unplanned subgroup analyses, when patients were examined by stage, histology, and adjuvant radiation, no group seemed to show a benefit in any of these parameters. Limitations of this study are many, including the high dropout rate and multiple protocol violations. No imaging was required prior to enrollment so that patients were not confirmed to lack evidence of metastatic disease prior to adjuvant treatment, and periodic imaging for evidence of recurrence was not required, as a result time to progression may have been artificially long. Radiation was given to more patients in the observation arm than in the doxorubicin arm, and doxorubicin has subsequently been shown to have limited activity in carcinosarcoma. The trial took 9 years to accrue and was powered to show what is likely an unobtainable benefit for the chemotherapy arm. In contrast, another randomized but small trial using doxorubicin for stage I sarcomas, showed an improvement in OS, 63% versus 36% at 5 years, as well as an improvement recurrence-free survival (33). These differing results are likely explained by the variety of histologies included on these trials.

There are multiple small, single-arm trials utilizing a number of adjuvant chemotherapeutic agents. Treatments employed have included both single agents as well as combinations: ifosfamide (34), cisplatin and epirubicin (3%), cisplatin plus adriamycin (36), vincristine, dacarbazine, and cyclophosphamide(37), cyclophosphamide, vincristine, adriamycin, dacarbazine (CyVADIC) (38), cyclophosphamide, actinomycin D and vincristine (39), ifosfamide and cisplatin (40), ifosfamide, cisplatin, and doxorubicin (41). These studies show that adjuvant chemotherapy is feasible, but none conclusively showed a benefit to this approach. These studies often showed surprisingly good survival rates which failed to correlate with the marginal benefit seen when these same drugs and combinations were utilized in the metastatic setting. This likely reflects patient selection bias inherent in single-institution phase II trials.

Recognizing the critical shortcomings of GOG 20, the GOG designed its subsequent adjuvant sarcoma study with two important differences: eligibility limited to women with carcinosarcoma, and chemotherapy tested had shown objective responses in patients with advanced, measurable disease. Thus, GOG 150 was a randomized trial for women with stage I, II, III, or IV completely resected carcinosarcomas. Patients had to have < 1 cm of visible residual disease, and enrolled within 8 weeks of surgery. The 207 evaluable women were assigned to receive WAR or three cycles of ifosfamide plus cisplatin. About 40% of the patients had stage I or II disease. This study suggested a role of adjuvant systemic therapy for completely resected sarcoma even though the authors did not find a statistically significant advantage in recurrent rate or survival for adjuvant chemotherapy (42).

For leiomyosarcoma, adjuvant chemotherapy after resection of disease is still considered experimental. The identification of dose-rate-based gemcitabine plus docetaxel as an active regimen for advanced disease (43) has led to a multi-institution trial of gemcitabine-docetaxel followed by doxorubicin as adjuvant therapy for resected stage I and II leiomyosarcoma, which is being conducted through the Sarcoma Alliance for Research through Collaboration (SARC).

Adjuvant Hormonal Therapy

Although ER and PR are present in most low-grade endometrial stromal sarcomas (44), and in up to 40% of high-grade leiomyosarcomas (45), there are no prospective studies assessing the effect of adjuvant hormonal therapy. Oophorectomy and avoidance of hormone replacement therapy are reasonable strategies for completely resected low-grade endometrial stromal sarcomas.

Treatment of Recurrent Disease

The management of recurrent uterine sarcoma is generally considered to be palliative, with a few exceptions. The treatments generally are similar to those utilized in the management of soft tissue sarcomas, with surgical resection considered for isolated recurrences, radiation therapy offered for palliation of symptoms from locoregional disease, and chemotherapy (or hormonal therapy in the case of low grade endometrial stromal sarcoma) for patients with more widespread disease or in whom the above modalities are not feasible.

Role of Surgical Resection

The limited efficacy of chemotherapy and radiotherapy underscores the importance of surgical resection in the treatment of recurrent uterine sarcomas. Care must be put into these decisions, but significant long-term survival is occasionally seen in patients undergoing patients with resection it metastases. This is most extensively studied in soft tissue sarcomas (46), but it has also been studied in uterine sarcomas. One series of patients with resection of pulmonary metastases showed a 5-year survival rate of 43% (47). Prognostic factors that influenced outcome included longer time from diagnosis to recurrence, fewer number and sites of metastases, and excellent performance status of the patient. The favorable outcomes reported represent highly selected patient populations and come from studies that lack a matched, non-surgical control group.

Other surgical maneuvers may also be considered. This approach may be curative, especially when performed for low-grade tumors. This appears to be especially warranted in the case of low-grade endometrial stromal sarcomas, if the surgical resection can be accomplished with limited morbidity (48).

Role of Radiotherapy

Radiotherapy may be effective in providing palliation of symptomatic, unresectable disease. It has a role in relieving pain, bleeding, and obstruction of ureters and bowels. The RTOG has a palliative schedule for these aims, which has been vetted in a phase II trial as producing a quality-of-life benefit (49). The regimen consisted of a split-course treatment, allowing patients to drop out if not receiving benefit or experiencing too great a degree of toxicity. The schedule for bulky pelvic disease consisted of 3.7 Gy twice daily for 2 days, separated by 2–4-week rest periods and repeated as many as three times.

Role of Systemic Therapies

The aim of systemic treatment for advanced disease is control of symptoms and prolongation of time to progression. To date, there are no data that demonstrate an improvement in overall survival with chemotherapy, although there are no randomized

Table 1. Gynecologic sarcomas: Randomized trials

Regimen	Patient # in treatment arm	Response rate (%)	Progression-free survival	Overall survival	Reference
Adriamycin (doxorubicin)	120	16		6.3 Months	(50)
Adriamycin, Dacarbazine	106	24		5.8 Months	
Adriamycin	50	19	5.1 Months	11.6 Months	(51)
Adriamycin Cyclophosphamide	54	20	4.9 Months	10.9 Months	
Ifosfamide	102	36	4 Months	7.6 Months	(52)
Ifosfamide, Cisplatin	92	54	6 Months[a]	9.4 Months	

[a]$p < .05$

trials in uterine sarcoma comparing chemotherapy to best supportive care for advanced, unresectable disease.

Many drugs have been evaluated in the treatment of sarcomas, both gynecologic and other soft tissue sites. In studies that included chemotherapy naïve and pre-treated patients, those who have not had chemotherapy before tend to have higher response rates. There does not seem to be improved response with higher doses of alkylating agents, such as ifosfamide and platinums, or anthracyclines. In gynecologic sarcomas, the most studied agents include doxorubicin, ifosfamide, cisplatin, and paclitaxel, with results shown in Table 1.

Combination chemotherapy, with two-, three-, or four-drug regimens, has also been tried. Table 2 summarizes results of combination regimens in phase II or III trials in gynecologic sarcomas. There are three sizable randomized phase III trials of combination regimens in gynecologic sarcomas. The first two trials included patients with either leiomyosarcoma or carcinosarcoma, while the last one enrolled only patients with carcinosarcoma. The first trial randomized 226 women to doxorubicin or the combination of doxorubicin and dacarbazine, with an OS of 6.3 months in the single agent arm and 5.8 months in the combination arm (50). The second trial randomly assigned 104 patients with either leiomyosarcoma or carcinosarcoma to treatment with doxorubicin or doxorubicin plus cyclophosphamide (51). This trial showed no difference in PFS or OS between the two groups of patients. The third randomized trial which included 200 patients with only carcinosarcoma, compared ifosfamide to the combination of ifosfamide plus cisplatin, and showed that the combination regimen did not result in improvement of OS and only in a small benefit in PFS (4 months versus 6 months) (52). This small benefit came at the expense of significantly increased toxicity with the combination of cisplatin plus ifosfamide, leading the authors to conclude that single-agent ifosfamide should remain the standard treatment for carcinosarcoma. When results of the phase II study of paclitaxel for second line treatment of advanced carcinosarcoma were known (58), GOG designed the next phase III study: ifosfamide versus ifosfamide plus paclitaxel and suggested improvement in response rates and survival outcomes for the combination regimen (59).

Table 2. Combination trials in gynecologic sarcomas

Combination	Doses	MMMT	LMS	ESS	NS	Reference
Ifosfamide	5 g/m² over 24 h	30% (30)	30.30%			(53)
Adriamycin	50 mg/m²					
Ifosfamide	5 g/m² over 24 h	30% (34)				(54)
Adriamycin	50 mg/m²					
Dacarbazine	250 mg/ m²/d × 5	23% (31)				(50)
Adriamycin	60 mg/m²					
Cyclophosphamide	500mg/m²				19% (26)	(51)
Adriamycin	60 mg/m²					
Ifosfamide	1.5 g/ m²/d × 5	54% (90)				(52)
Cisplatin	20 mg/ m²/d × 5					
Hydrea	500 mg q 6 h × 4		18% (38)			(54)
Dacarbazine	700 mg/m²					
Etoposide	100 mg/ m²/d × 3					
Vincristine	1.5 mg/ m²/d × 5	26% (27)	29% (14)	50% (2)		(56)
Actinomycin D	0.5 mg/ m²/d × 5					
Cyclophosphamide	300 mg/ m²/d × 5					
Gemcitabine	900 mg/m²		53% (34)			(57)
Docetaxel	d 1,8					

MMMT Malignant mixed müllerian tumor, LMS leiomyosarcoma, ESS endometrial stromal sarcoma, NS not specified

Histology-Specific Results

With older studies highlighting the differences in response profiles between carcinosarcomas and leiomyosarcomas, more recent studies have been designed as histology-specific phase II trials.

Carcinosarcoma

Carcinosarcoma (MMMT), thought to be the most common uterine sarcoma, may be the most chemotherapy-responsive tumor of the group. Recent evidence indicates that MMMT is the result of a de-differentiated epithelial malignancy rather than a true sarcoma (60). Earlier literature used to divide these tumors into homologous and heterologous types, depending on whether or not the mesenchymal components included tissue types normally found within the uterus. Additionally, metastatic implants may contain either epithelial elements (most common), mesenchymal elements, or remain a mixed population (61).

Single agents demonstrating activity in phase II trials for advanced, measurable carcinosarcoma include ifosfamide (response rate [RR] 32%) (62) and cisplatin (RR 19%) (63). Paclitaxel achieved an 18% RR as second-line therapy (58). Doxorubicin (RR 10%) (50), and topotecan (RR 10%) (64), have limited activity, and trimetrexate and diazoquone are inactive with response rates <5% (65, 66). Paclitaxel with carboplatin is currently under Phase II investigation in the GOG, based upon the similarity in clinical behavior of this tumor to epithelial ovarian cancer, trials that show activity in MMMTs of the ovary (53, 67) as well as responses in small series (68). Many clinicians have already adopted this combination into their practice for carcinosarcoma treatment. Gemcitabine and docetaxel are currently being tested prospectively within the GOG in carcinosarcoma as well as in leiomyosarcoma (69).

Leiomyosarcoma

Leiomyosarcoma is the second most common gynecologic sarcoma, and the least chemoresponsive, with frequent hematogenous dissemination. Agents tested in leiomyosarcoma that have minimal activity include cisplatin (response between 3–5%) (70), mitoxantrone (RR 0%) (71), amonifide, oral etoposide, topotecan, paclitaxel, thalidomide, and trimetrexate. Agents with modest response rates include doxorubicin (RR 25%) (72), Doxil (RR 16.1%) (73), ifosfamide (RR 17%) (74), gemcitabine (RR 20%) (75), and ecteinascidin (ET-743, Yondelis) (RR 8% as second line and 17% as first line treatment) (76, 77).

The combination of dose-rate-based gemcitabine plus docetaxel achieved a 53% objective response rate among 34 patients with leiomyosarcoma in a single institution trial. Among the patients with prior doxorubicin-based therapy, 50% responded (78). This regimen is being further tested in the cooperative group, multi-institution setting as second-line (GOG 131G) and first-line (GOG 87L) therapy. Both studies have shown a sufficient number of responses to proceed to their second stages of accrual.

Endometrial Stromal Sarcoma

From a clinical perspective, treatment of endometrial stromal sarcomas is based on dividing these tumors into low-grade and high-grade histology. Low-grade tumors (or endolymphatic stromal myosis) are indolent, their natural history often extends over decades, and they are often managed with repeat surgical interventions. These tumors rarely respond to chemotherapy, perhaps because of their low mitotic rates. However, many of these tumors express ER and PR and hormonal manipulations may be effective (see below).

Chemotherapy

High-grade stromal sarcoma is quite different from low-grade endometrial stromal sarcoma, with rapid recurrences and rare responses to chemotherapy. A single phase II GOG study showed a 33% response rate to ifosfamide (79). There have been also reports of responses, up to 50% with doxorubicin (80, 81) as well as a single patient with prolonged response to etoposide (82).

Hormonal Therapy

As these stromal neoplasms derive from endometrial stromal cells, there are multiple analyses documenting the presence of steroid receptors (ER and PR) in these neoplasms (57, 80, 83). The fact that hysterectomy with BSO seems to be associated with longer remissions than if the ovaries are preserved, supports the hormonal sensitivity of these tumors. One study showed rates of ER expression of 48.3% and PR expression of 30% (80). Analogous to the treatment of hormone-sensitive breast cancer, there have been attempts to treat low-grade endometrial stromal sarcomas with progestational agents such as megestrol acetate (85), anti-estrogens such as letrozole (86, 87), and GnRH agonists (88). Given the favorable toxicity profile of such agents, it is reasonable to consider using them in the adjuvant setting.

New Directions

Advances in the management of uterine sarcomas, as with all malignancies, are likely to come with better understanding of the molecular biology of these diseases, which may lead to the identification of appropriate therapeutic targets. The role of cell-cycle inhibitors, tyrosine kinase inhibitors, monoclonal antibodies, vascular growth factor inhibitor, and other targeted therapies is yet to be defined. New chemotherapeutic agents, such as Yondelis (ET-743), hold promise for improved outcomes. Cooperative efforts among institutions that include correlative science investigations in conjunction with treatment trials are necessary to elucidate appropriate targets and interventions, which should ultimately improve outcomes for women with these high-risk tumors.

Conclusions

- Management of uterine sarcomas of all stages requires careful histologic review and clinical expertise, but a role for adjuvant therapy in early-stage disease has not been established.
- In advanced and recurrent disease, management will depend on histology, time to recurrence, and site or sites of disease. Modalities to consider include surgical resection, radiation, and systemic therapies.
- Recent studies have led to the identification of active systemic regimens for leiomyosarcoma and carcinosarcoma.
- However, whenever possible, patients with uterine sarcomas should be encouraged to participate in clinical trials. The recent trend to design stage and histologic specific trials should improve management of these malignancies.

References

1. Brooks SE, Zhan M, Cote T, Baquet CR. Surveillance, epidemiology, and end results: analysis of 2677 cases of uterine sarcoma 1989–1999. Gynecol Oncol 2004;93:204.
2. Nordal RR, Thoresen SO. Uterine sarcomas in Norway 1956–1992: incidence, survival and mortality. Eur J Cancer 1997;33 (6):907–911.
3. Rha SE, Byun JY, Jung SE, et al. CT and MRI of uterine sarcomas and their mimickers. AJR Am J Roentgenol 2003;181:1369–1374.
4. Giuntoli RL 2nd, Metzinger DS, DiMarco CS, et al. Retrospective review of 208 patients with leiomyosarcoma of the uterus: prognostic indicators, surgical management, and adjuvant therapy. Gynecol Oncol 2003;89:460–469.
5. Yamada SD, Burger RA, Brewster WR, Anton D, Kohler MF, Monk BJ. Pathologic variables and adjuvant therapy as predictors of recurrence and survival for patients with surgically evaluated carcinosarcoma of the uterus. Cancer 2000;88:2782–2786.
6. Major FJ, Blessing JA, Silverberg SG, et al. Prognostic factors in early-stage uterine sarcoma. A Gynecologic Oncology Group study. Cancer 1993;71:1702–1709.
7. Ferrer F, Sabater S, Farrus, B, et al. Impact of radiotherapy on local control and survival in uterine sarcomas: a retrospective study from the Grup Oncologic Catala-Occita. Int J Radiat Oncol Biol Phys 1999;44:47–52.
8. Dinh TV, Slavin RE, Bhagavan BS, Hannigan EV, Tiamson EM, Yandell RB. Mixed mullerian tumors of the uterus: a clinicopathologic study. Obstet Gynecol 1989;74:388–392.
9. Silverberg SG, Major FJ, Blessing JA, et al. Carcinosarcoma (malignant mixed mesodermal tumor) of the uterus: a Gynecologic Oncology Group pathologic study of 203 cases. Int J Gynecol Pathol 1990;9:1–19.
10. Kahanpaa KV, Wahlstrom T, Grohn P, Heinonen E, Nieminen U, Widholm O. Sarcomas of the uterus: a clinicopathologic study of 119 patients. Obstet Gynecol 1986;67(3):417–424.
11. Parker WH, Fu YS, Berek JS. Uterine sarcoma in patients operated on for presumed leiomyoma and rapidly growing leiomyoma. Obstet Gynecol 1994;83(3):414–418.
12. Berchuck A, Rubin SC, Hoskins WJ, Saigo PE, Pierce VK, Lewis JLJR . Treatment of uterine leiomyosarcoma. Obstet Gynecol 1988;71:845–850.
13. O'Connor DM, Norris HJ. Mitotically active leiomyomas of the uterus. Hum Pathol 1990;21(2):223–227.
14. Goff BA, Rice LW, Fleischhacker D, et al. Uterine leiomyosarcoma and endometrial stromal sarcoma: lymph node metastases and sites of recurrence. Gynecol Oncol 1993;50:105–109.

15. Berchuck A, Rubin SC, Hoskins WJ, Soisson PA, Bast RC JR , Boyer CM. Treatment of endometrial stromal tumors. Gynecol Oncol 1990;36:60–65.
16. Norris HJ, Taylor HB. Mesenchymal tumors of the uterus. I. A clinical and pathologic study of 53 endometrial stromal tumors. Cancer 1966;19(6):755–766.
17. Wolfson AH, Brady MF, Rocereto TF, et al. A Gynecologic Oncology Group randomized trial of whole abdominal irradiation (WAI) vs cisplatin-ifosfamide+mesna (CIM) in optimally debulked stage I-IV carcinosarcoma (CS) of the uterus. Proc Amer Soc Clin Oncol 2006;24:5001, Abstract #185.
18. Hornback NB, Omura G, Major FJ. Observations on the use of adjuvant radiation therapy in patients with stage I and II uterine sarcoma. Int J Radiat Oncol Biol Phys 1986;12:2127–2130.
19. Podczaski ES, Woomert CA, Stevens CW, Jr, et al. Management of malignant, mixed meso-dermal tumors of the uterus. Gynecol Oncol 1989;32:240–244.
20. Callister M, Ramondetta LM, Jhingran A, Burke TW, Eifel PJ. Malignant mixed mullerian tumors of the uterus: Analysis of patterns of failure, prognostic factors, and treatment out-come. Int J Radiat Oncol Biol Phys 2004;58:786–796.
21. Spanos WJ Jr , Peters LJ, Oswald MJ. Patterns of recurrence in malignant mixed mullerian tumor of the uterus. Cancer 1986;57:155–159.
22. Major FJ, Blessing JA, Silverberg SG, et al. Prognostic factors in early-stage uterine sarcoma. A Gynecologic Oncology Group study. Cancer 1993;71:1702–1709.
23. Gadducci A, Landoni F, Sartori, E, et al. Uterine leiomyosarcoma: analysis of treatment fail-ures and survival. Gynecol Oncol 1996;62:25–32.
24. Gadducci A, Sartori E, Landoni F, et al. Endometrial stromal sarcoma: analysis of treatment failures and survival. Gynecol Oncol 1996;63:247–253.
25. Salazar OM, Bonfiglio TA, Patten SE, et al. Uterine sarcomas: analysis of failures with special emphasis on the use of adjuvant radiation therapy. Cancer 1978;42:1161–1170.
26. Knocke TH, Kucera H, Dorfler D, Pokrajac B, Potter R. Results of postoperative radiotherapy in the treatment of sarcoma of the corpus uteri. Cancer 1998;83(9):1972–1979.
27. Sorbe B. Radiotherapy and/or chemotherapy as adjuvant therapy of uterine sarcomas. Gyncol Oncol 1985;20:281–289.
28. Omura GA, Blessing JA, Major F, et al. A randomized clinical trial of adjuvantadriamycin in uterine sarcomas: a Gynecologic Oncology Group study. J Clin Oncol 1985;3:1240–1245.
29. Hornback NB, Omura G, Major FJ. Observations on the use of adjuvant radiation therapy in patients with stage I and II uterine sarcoma. Int J Radiat Oncol Biol Phys 1986;12:2127–2130.
30. Ferrer F, Sabater S, Farrus B, et al. Impact of radiotherapy on local control and survival in uterine sarcomas: a retrospective study from the Grup Oncologic Catala-Occita. Int J Radiat Oncol Biol Phys 1999;44:47–52.
31. Weitmann HD, Knocke TH, Kucera H, Potter R. Radiation therapy in the treatment of endometrial stromal sarcoma. Int J Radiat Oncol Biol Phys 2001;49(3):739–748.
32. National Comprehensive Cancer Network guidelines available online at www.nccn.org/pro-fessionals/physician_gls/default.asp.
33. Piver MS, Lele SB, Marchetti DL, Emrich LJ. Effect of adjuvant chemotherapy on time to recurrence and survival of stage I uterine sarcomas. J Surg Oncol 1988;38:233–239.
34. Kushner DM, Webster KD, Belinson JL, Rybicki LA, Kennedy AW, Markman M. Safety and efficacy of adjuvant single-agent ifosfamide in uterine sarcoma. Gynecol Oncol 2000;78:221–227.
35. Manolitsas TP, Wain GV, Williams KE, Freidlander M, Hacker NF. Multimodality therapy for patients with clinical Stage I and II malignant mixed Mullerian tumors of the uterus. Cancer 2001;91:1437–1443.
36. Peters WA 3rd, Rivkin SE, Smith MR, Tesh DE. Cisplatin and adriamycin combination chemo-therapy for uterine stromal sarcomas and mixed mesodermal tumors. Gynecol Oncol 1989;34:323–327.
37. van Nagell JR, Jr, Hanson MB, Donaldson ES, Gallion HH. Adjuvant vincristine, dactinomycin, and cyclophosphamide therapy in stage I uterine sarcomas. A pilot study. Cancer 1986;57:1451–1454.

38. Hannigan, EV, Freedman, RS, Elder, KW, Rutledge, FN. Treatment of advanced uterine sarcoma with adriamycin. Gynecol Oncol 1983;16:101–104.
39. Hannigan EV, Freedman RS, Elder KW, Rutledge FN. Treatment of advanced uterine sarcoma with vincristine, actinomycin D, and cyclophosphamide. Gynecol Oncol 1983;15:224–229.
40. Sutton G, Kauderer J, Carson LF, Lentz SS, Whitney CW, Gallion H. Gynecologic Oncology Group. Adjuvant ifosfamide and cisplatin in patients with completely resected stage I or II carcinosarcomas (mixed mesodermal tumors) of the uterus: a Gynecologic Oncology Group study. Gynecol Oncol 2005;9:630–634.
41. Pautier P, Rey A, Haie-Meder C, et al. Adjuvant chemotherapy with cisplatin, ifosfamide, and doxorubicin followed by radiotherapy in localized uterine sarcomas: results of a case-control study with radiotherapy alone. Int J Gynecol Cancer 2004;14:1112–1117.
42. Wolfson AH, Brady MF, Rocereto T, Mannel RS, Lee YC, Futoran RJ, Cohn DE, Ioffe OB. A gynecologic oncology group randomized phase III trial of whole abdominal irradiation (WAI) vs. cisplatin-ifosfamide and mensa (CIM) as post-surgical therapy in stage I–IV carcinosarcoma (CS) of the uterus. Gynecol Oncol 2007;107(2):177–85.
43. Hensley ML, Maki R, Venkatraman E, et al. Gemcitabine and docetaxel in patients with unresectable leiomyosarcoma: Results of a Phase II trial. J Clin Oncol 2002;20:2824–2831.
44. Reich O, Regauer S, Urdl W, Lahousen M, Winter R. Expression of oestrogen and progesterone receptors in low-grade endometrial stromal sarcomas. Br J Cancer 2000;82:1030–1034.
45. Leitao MM, Soslow RA, Nonaka D, et al. Tissue microarray immunohistochemical expression of estrogen, progesterone, and androgen receptors in uterine leiomyomata and leiomyosarcoma. Cancer 2004;101:1455–1462.
46. Mountain CF, McMurtrey MJ, Hermes RF. Surgery for pulmonary metastases: a 20-year experience. Ann Thorac Surg 1984;38:323–330.
47. Levenback C, Rubin SC, McCormack PM, Hoskins WJ, Atkinson EN, Lewis JL, Jr. Resection of pulmonary metastases from uterine sarcomas. Gynecol Oncol 1992;45:202–205.
48. Berchuck A, Rubin SC, Hoskins WJ, Saigo PE, Pierce VK, Lewis JL Jr . Treatment of endometrial stromal tumors. Gynecol Oncol 1990;36:60–65.
49. Spanos W, Guse C, Perez C, Grisby P, Doggett RL, Poulter C. Phase II study of multiple daily fractionations in the palliation of advanced pelvic malignancies: preliminary report of RTOG 8502. Int J Radiat Oncol Biol Phys 1989;17:659–661.
50. Omura GA, Major FJ, Blessing JA, et al. A randomized study of adriamycin with and without dimethyl triazenoimidazole carboxamide in advanced uterine sarcomas. Cancer 1983;52:626–632.
51. Muss HB, Bundy B, DiSaia PJ, et al. Treatment of recurrent or advanced uterine sarcoma. A randomized trial of doxorubicin versus doxorubicin and cyclophosphamide (a Phase III trial of the Gynecologic Oncology Group). Cancer 1985;55:1648–1653.
52. Sutton G, Brunetto VL, Kilgore L, et al. A phase III trial of ifosfamide with or without cisplatin in carcinosarcoma of the uterus: a Gynecologic Oncology Group study. Gynecol Oncol 2000;79:147–153.
53. Sit AS, Price FV, Kelley JL, et al. Chemotherapy for malignant mixed mullerian tumors of the ovary. Gynecol Oncol 2000;79:196–200.
54. Antman K, Crowley J, Balcerzak SP, et al. An intergroup phase III randomized study of doxorubicin and dacarbazine with or without ifosfamide and mesna in advanced soft tissue and bone sarcomas. J Clin Oncol 1993;11:1276–1285.
55. Currie J, Blessing JA, Muss HB, Fowler J, Berman M, Burke TW.Combination chemotherapy with hydroxyurea, dacarbazine (DTIC), and etoposide in the treatment of uterine leiomyosarcoma: a Gynecologic Oncology Group study. Gynecol Oncol 1996;61:27–30.
56. Piver MS, DeEulis TG, Lele SB, Barlow JJ. Cyclophosphamide, vincristine, adriamycin and dimethyl-triazeno imidazole carboxamide (CYVADIC) for sarcomas of the female genital track. Gynecol Oncol 1982;14:319–323.
57. Sabini G, Chumas JC, Mann WJ. Steroid hormone receptors in endometrial stromal sarcoma. A biochemical and immunohistochemical study. Am J Clin Pathol 1992;97(3):381–386.

58. Curtin JP, Blessing JA, Soper JT, DeGeest K. Paclitaxel in the treatment of carcinosarcoma of the uterus: a gynecologic oncology group study. Gynecol Oncol 2001;83:268–270.
59. Homesley HD, Filiaci V, Markan M, et al. Phase III trial of ifosfamide with or without paclitaxel in advanced uterine carcinosarcoma: A Gynecologic Oncology Group Study. J Clin Oncol 2007;25(5):526–31.
60. McCluggage WG. Malignant biphasic uterine tumours: carcinosarcomas or metaplastic carcinomas? J Clin Pathol 2002;55:321–325.
61. George E, Manivel JC, Denher LP, Wick MR. Malignant mixed mullerian tumors: an immunohistochemical study of 47 cases, with histogenetic considerations and clinical correlation. Hum Pathol 1991 Mar;22(3):215–223.
62. Sutton GP, Blessing JA, Rosenshein N, Photopulos G, DiSaia PJ. Phase II trial of ifosfamide and mesna in mixed mesodermal tumors of the uterus (a Gynecologic Oncology Group study). Am J Obstet Gynecol 1989;161:309–312.
63. Thigpen JT, Blessing JA, Beecham J, Homesley H, Yordan E. Phase II trial of cisplatin as first-line chemotherapy in patients with advanced or recurrent uterine sarcomas: a Gynecologic Oncology Group study. J Clin Oncol 1991;9:1962–1966.
64. Miller DS, Blessing JA, Schilder J, Munkarah A, Lee YC. Phase II evaluation of topotecan in carcinosarcoma of the uterus: a Gynecologic Oncology Group study. Gynecol Oncol 2005;98:217–221.
65. Fowler JM, Blessing JA, Burger RA, Malfetano JH. Phase II evaluation of oral trimetrexate in mixed mesodermal tumors of the uterus: a Gynecologic Oncology Group study. Gynecol Oncol 2002;85:311–314.
66. Slayton RE, Blessing JA, Clarke-Pearson D. A phase II trial of diaziquone (AZQ) in mixed mesodermal sarcomas of the uterus. A Gynecologic Oncology Group study. Invest New Drugs 1991;9:93–94.
67. Duska LR, Garrett A, Eltabbakh GH, Oliva E, Penson R, Fuller AF. Paclitaxel and platinum chemotherapy for malignant mixed mullerian tumors of the ovary. Gynecol Oncol 2002;85:459–463.
68. Toyoshima M, Akahira J, Matsunaga G, et al. Clinical experience with combination paclitaxel and carboplatin therapy for advanced or recurrent carcinosarcoma of the uterus. Gynecol Oncol 2004;94:774–778.
69. Hensley ML, Blessing JA, Mannel R, Rose PG. Fixed-dose rate gemcitabine plus docetaxel as first-line therapy for metastatic uterine leiomyosarcoma: a Gynecologic Oncology Group phase II trial. Gynecol Oncol 2008;109(3):329–34.
70. Thigpen T, Blessing JA, Beecham J, Homesley H, Yordan E. Phase II trial of cisplatin as first-line chemotherapy in patients with advanced or recurrent uterine sarcomas: a Gynecologic Oncology Group study. J Clin Oncol 1991;9:1962–1966.
71. Muss HB, Bundy BN, Adcock L, Beecham J. Mitoxantrone in the treatment of advanced uterine sarcoma. A phase II trial of the Gynecologic Oncology Group. Am J Clin Oncol 1990 Feb;13(1):32–34.
72. Omura GA, Major FJ, Blessing JA, et al. A randomized study of adriamycin with and without dimethyl triazenoimidazole carboxamide in advanced uterine sarcomas. Cancer 1983;52(4):626–632.
73. Sutton G, Blessing J, Hanjani P, Kramer P, Gynecologic Oncology Group. Phase II evaluation of liposomal doxorubicin (Doxil) in recurrent or advanced leiomyosarcoma of the uterus: a Gynecologic Oncology Group study. Gynecol Oncol 2005;96:749–752.
74. Sutton GP, Blessing JA, Barrett RJ, McGehee R. Phase II trial of ifosfamide and mesna in leiomyosarcoma of the uterus: a Gynecologic Oncology Group study. Am J Obstet Gynecol 1992;166:556–559.
75. Look KY, Sandler A, Blessing JA, et al. Phase II trial of gemcitabine as second-line chemotherapy of uterine leiomyosarcoma: a Gynecologic Oncology Group (GOG) study. Gynecol Oncol 2004;92:644–647.

76. Garcia-Carbonero R, Supko JG, Manola J, et al. Phase II and pharmacokinetic study of ecteinascidin 743 in patients with progressive sarcomas of soft tissues refractory to chemotherapy. J Clin Oncol 2004;22:1480–1490.
77. Delaloge S, Yovine A, Taamma A, et al. Ecteinascidin-743: a marine-derived compound in advanced, pretreated sarcoma patients--preliminary evidence of activity. J Clin Oncol. 2001;19:1248–1255.
78. Hensley ML, Maki R, Venkatraman E, et al. Gemcitabine and docetaxel in patients with unresectable leiomyosarcoma: Results of a Phase II Trial. J Clin Oncol 2002;20:2824–2831.
79. Sutton G, Blessing JA, Park R, DiSaia PJ, Rosenshein N. Ifosfamide treatment of recurrent or metastatic endometrial stromal sarcomas previously unexposed to chemotherapy: a study of the Gynecologic Oncology Group. Obstet Gynecol 1996;87:747–750.
80. Wade K, Quinn MA, Hammond I, Williams K, Cauchi M. Uterine sarcoma: steroid receptors and response to hormonal therapy. Gynecol Oncol 1990;39:364–367.
81. Berchuck A, Rubin, SC, Hoskins WJ, Saigo PE, Pierce VK, Lewis JL, Jr. Treatment of endometrial stromal tumors. Gynecol Oncol 1990;36:60–65.
82. Lin YC, Kudelka AP, Tresukosol D, et al. Prolonged stabilization of progressive endometrial stromal sarcoma with prolonged oral etoposide therapy. Gyencol Oncol 1995;58:262–265.
83. Baker VV, Walton LA, Fowler WC, Jr, Currie JL. Steroid receptors in endolymphatic stromal myosis. Obstet Gynecol 1984;63:72S–74S.
84. Chu MC, Mor G, Lim C, Zheng W, Parkash V, Schwartz PE. Low-grade endometrial stromal sarcoma: hormonal aspects. Gynecol Oncol 2003;90:170–176.
85. Spano JP, Soria JC, Kambouchner M, et al. Long-term survival of patients given hormonal therapy for metastatic endometrial stromal sarcoma. Med Oncol 2003;20:87–93.
86. Maluf FC, Sabbatini P, Schwartz L, Xia J, Aghajanian C. Endometrial stromal sarcoma: objective response to letrozole. Gynecol Oncol 2001;82:384–388.
87. Leunen, M, Breugelmans, M, De Sutter, P, et al.. Low-grade endometrial stromal sarcoma treated with the aromatase inhibitor letrozole. Gynecol Oncol 2004;95:769.
88. Mesia AF, Demopoulos RI. Effects of leuprolide acetate on low-grade endometrial stromal sarcoma. Am J Obstet Gynecol 2000;182:1140–1141.

Future Directions: New Targets

Franco Muggia, Leslie I. Gold, and John Curtin

Abstract The biology of endometrial cancer is providing new therapeutic targets. In this chapter we review (a) how the integration of chemotherapy has been taking place; (b) new targets worthy of consideration based on the biology of uterine cancers; (c) "targeted" therapies being tested in the treatment of these malignancies; and (d) future strategies.

Keywords Molecular targets • Immunotherapy • PTEN • mTOR • Hormone receptors

Introduction

The changes that are taking place in the treatment of uterine cancer are principally driven by clinical trials that during the past decade have firmly established a role for systemic chemotherapy in advanced stages of endometrial adenocarcinoma, and the advent of modern cancer therapeutics with drugs targeting hallmarks of malignancy beyond tumor cells. Nevertheless, the foundations for the successful application of these treatments to uterine cancer have come from careful surgical staging and study of pathologic prognostic factors. These concepts have been carefully delineated in the preceding chapters. Here we review (a) how the integration of chemotherapy has been taking place; (b) new targets worthy of consideration based on the biology of uterine cancers; (c) "targeted" therapies being tested in the treatment of these malignancies; and (d) future strategies.

F. Muggia (✉), L.I. Gold, and J. Curtin
Division of Medical Oncology, NYU Cancer Institute, NYU Medical Center, New York, NY
e-mail: Franco.Muggia@nyumc.org

F. Muggia and E. Oliva (eds.), *Uterine Cancer*, Current Clinical Oncology,
DOI: 10.1007/978-1-60327-044-1_15,
© Humana Press, a Part of Springer Science+Business Media, LLC 2009

Integration of Chemotherapy in Early Stages

The development of effective chemotherapeutic regimens against endometrial carcinoma dates to the 1970s with the introduction of doxorubicin (1) (use of progestins predated it and is covered in Chap. 12). A series of studies by the GOG made relatively slow progress in improving the outcome of patients with recurrences over what might be achieved with doxorubicin alone. Nevertheless, both the platinum compounds (cisplatin, carboplatin) and paclitaxel were convincingly shown to add to response rates and time to progression achievable with doxorubicin (2–4). Eventually, the three-drug combination, TAP (paclitaxel or Taxol, doxorubicin or Adriamycin, and cisplatin or Platinol) proved superior in survival in the latest fully published GOG study for recurrent endometrial carcinoma, over what could be achieved with AP (5). Because of toxicity considerations, however, some centers had built their treatment around carboplatin + paclitaxel and reported results that compared favorably with TAP (6). Accordingly, GOG-209 in this setting is a randomization between TAP and the above doublet. Noteworthy, aspects of these last studies are outcomes with median survivals that exceed 15 months for patients diagnosed with metastases beyond regional lymph nodes or who had disseminated recurrences after their initial treatments. These medians are in sharp contrast with studies by the same group over the past two decades with medians consistently under 1 year.

Another indication of improved outcomes resulting from chemotherapy is conveyed by the GOG-122 that compared whole abdominal radiation to AP chemotherapy for stages III and IV endometrial carcinoma with maximum size of residual disease limited to 2 cm. This study showed a 13% absolute difference in proportion of patients who were disease-free at 2 years in favor of chemotherapy (59% versus 46%) (7, 8). This study has stimulated the integration of chemotherapy in some of the early stages of patients with unusual histologies that are at high-risk for recurrence from the outset. Moreover, chemotherapy with limited field radiation has become the subject of study for stages III and IV with small volume or no residuum (e.g. GOG-184).

The treatment of carcinosarcoma of the uterus is similarly undergoing changes as various chemotherapeutic regimens show efficacy. Again, in a series of studies by the GOG, ifosfamide in combination with cisplatin (9), and subsequently in combination with paclitaxel (10) was proven superior to ifosfamide alone. In the last study, the superiority extended not only to response rates and time to progression, but also to survival. Finally, GOG-150 encompassing all stages of optimally resected uterine carcinosarcoma has shown that postoperative ifosfamide + cisplatin reduced recurrences, and prolonged survival in comparison with whole abdominal radiation (11). The demonstration of an impact on survival when given as an adjuvant to surgery, will stimulate further interest in chemotherapy of this aggressive malignancy. Already, experience indicates that the pattern of spread and the responsiveness of carcinosarcoma to chemotherapy are similar to the adenocarcinoma, and consistent with its presumed epithelial origin in spite of its tendency to spindling and association with rare mesenchymal differentiation. This tumor might be an example of the epithelial to mesenchymal transition (EMT), in vivo (12). A further stimulus in the systemic therapies of these uterine malignancies is the exploration of a role for combinations with targeted therapies (next two sections).

Identifying Potential Molecular Targets

Estrogen Receptors

Estrogen receptor has been a limited therapeutic target, perhaps because with tumor progression, receptors tend to be lost, and only a minority of patients with metastatic endometrial carcinoma show a response to treatments targeting ER and PR. One recent study, however, showed that 75% of endometrial carcinomas express PR and 25% ER (13). In addition, ER antagonists in the breast are agonists in the endometrium due to the differential recruitment of co-activators and co-repressors available in these respective tissues (14). Delineation of these co-activators and co-repressors in the endometrium may lead to identification of new targets. In uterine sarcomas ERs are often expressed but reports of endocrine interventions have remained largely anecdotal.

A great number of genes are likely regulated by the ER in the endometrium. The increase in lipogenesis associated with endometrial cancer stimulated interest in fatty acid synthase (FASN). Blocking FASN has the potential to decrease proliferation by decreasing ER activity (15). On the contrary, exposure to estrogen has sensitized endometrial cells to cisplatin (16).

Phosphatase and Tensin Homolog, p27kip1, Cables

Mutations in phosphatase and tensin homolog (PTEN; a dual lipid/protein phosphatase), which are widespread throughout the gene, controlling protein stability and localization, occur in more than half of type I endometrioid tumors whereas mutations in the K-Ras oncogene occur only in 10–30% of these tumors (17). Mutations in the tumor suppressor gene, p53, by contrast, are generally confined to grade 3 endometrioid carcinomas and type II UPSC (17–19). Specific genetic signatures of histologic subtypes of both endometrial and ovarian cancer have recently been described and, interestingly, show that there is both similarities within each organ and also, within serous and endometriod differentiation histiotypes between the organs (20). Further, ovarian and endometrial tumors with defects in β-catenin (Wnt pathway defective status) show a different pattern of gene expression than those with intact β-catenin status. Studies using both genomic and proteomic approaches to define new biomarker sets to categorize and individualize gynecologic cancers are emerging (21–27).

PTEN, p27kip1, and Cables are proteins that are lost or decreased in endometrial carcinogenesis (17, 28–30). As expected and importantly, these three proteins are upregulated by progesterone and downregulated by estrogen, although the mechanisms involved are likely quite disparate. An interesting clinical study revealed that an increase in p27 can be useful as a predictive marker for successful treatment of endometrial carcinoma by medroxyprogesterone acetate (MPA) (31). This study underscores the significance of p27 as a molecular target to control normal growth of the endometrium. As PTEN blocks Akt signaling, loss of PTEN activity leads to constitutive activation of the Akt pathway that affects cellular proliferation and survival. Loss of PTEN in the molecular pathogenesis of endometrial carcinoma is further corroborated by such findings in 20% of endometrial hyperplasias, a premalignant lesion of endometrioid-type I carcinomas; loss of expression is also seen in seemingly morphologically benign glands adjacent to tumors (17, 32). Mimicking human disease, heterozyogous mice lacking one PTEN allele (PTEN[+/−]) develop a number of tumors including endometrial complex atypical hyperplasia and carcinoma with high penetrance (33, 34) and further show accelerated disease following concomitant inactivation of p27[kip1] (35). p27 null mice are predisposed to endometrial carcinoma following gamma irradiation and urethane treatment (36, 37). The fact that loss of PTEN expression and p27 vary directly in both endometrioid and UPSC (38) suggests functional interaction between these two proteins in the pathogenesis of endometrial carcinoma. Interestingly, both are early events in this disease and both block cells late in G1 phase of the cell cycle. To support this idea, PTEN lipid phosphatase activity was shown to upregulate p27 levels in MCF-7 breast cancer cells (39) and, in addition, it appears that PTEN may act by preventing p27 degradation by lowering skp2 levels (40).

Expression of cables, another inhibitor of the cell cycle that acts by blocking cdk activity, is decreased in both type I and type II endometrial carcinomas (41). The cables-associated colon and endometrial cancer is related to lack of the cdk2 binding domain on cables due to alternative mRNA splicing (42). Mice genetically null for cables develop endometrial hyperplasia by 3–6 months of age (with no other tissue abnormalities) with ensuing well-differentiated adenocarcinomas following estrogen treatment (29). Taken together, knocking-out genes in mice that show proclivity for endometrial neoplasias have provided valuable information concerning proteins and their signaling pathways to pursue targeted therapy.

Activation of ERα was recently shown to involve increased phosphorylation of Ser[167] Akt as a consequence of loss of PTEN in mice both in vitro and in vivo studies (28). Similarly, PTEN increases p27 levels (31, 38) and TGF-β has been shown to increase PTEN and p27 (43). Primary cultures of endometrial epithelial cells show that inhibitors of MAPK block the ubiquitin-mediated degradation of p27 induced by estrogen (30) and, thus, have the potential to be useful anti-tumor agents. Since the pathogenesis of type I endometrial carcinoma is related to unopposed estrogen, MAPK inhibitors may be thought of in terms of blocking the apparent MAPK-driven estrogen-induced degradation of p27 (30). Further studies on PTEN, p27, TGF-β, and cables among other proteins implicated in endometrial carcinoma [e.g. Zeb1 (transcription factor), androgen receptor (AR)], may provide ideas for novel therapies for efficacy testing (44, 45).

Aberrant TGF-β Signaling

Primary cultures of endometrial cells derived from patient's tissues have been highly useful in providing mechanistic information and revealing potential molecular targets for therapy. As there are no "normal" cell lines, the use of primary cultures is the only manner in which one can compare normal and malignant cells for both behavior and specific responses. Exploiting this paradigm, Gold et al. showed that the signaling mechanism for transforming growth factor-β (TGF-β), a cytokine critical to growth suppression of epithelial cells, is disrupted early in endometrial carcinogenesis (46, 47). Thus, the serine kinase activity of TGF-β receptor I (TβRI) and the direct downstream transcription factors, Smads, that shuttle from the cytoplasm to the nucleus for gene regulation, are potential emerging targets for restoration of growth arrest in endometrial cancer cells. Genetic alterations of proteins in the TGF-β signaling pathway are present in many human cancers. These alterations subvert growth arrest and enable continuous cell cycling (48). However, the role of TGF-β in cancer has recently been shown to be complex. Although TGF-β is important in maintaining growth homeostasis early in cancer and is thus, antineoplastic, it plays an opposite role by mediating metastasis in malignant progression (49–52). The pro-oncogenic effects of TGF-β remain to be an enigma with respect to receptor signaling. Both monoclonal antibodies and small molecule inhibitors of TGF-β receptor I kinase are being tested clinically for advanced/aggressive cancers (53–56). Since TGF-β stimulates EMT, inhibitors of TGF-β signaling pathway might offer a therapeutic approach for carcinosarcomas, characterized by an EMT phenotype (12).

Effects of the Stroma

It has become increasingly clear, particularly in hormone-regulated organs, that the stromal cell compartment plays a critical role in promoting malignant progression, particularly, at earlier stages when stromal cells interact with epithelial cells (57–61). Hayward's group by using transplanted recombinant tissue technology combining stromal cells from malignant [termed cancer-associated fibroblasts (CAFs)] or normal prostate tissue with a non-tumorigenic human prostate epithelial cell line (BPH-1) and subsequently transplanted them to the renal capsule of nude mice, where the recombinant tissue transplant was well-perfused.

The recombinant tissues composed of stromal cells from malignant but not normal tissue, invaded the adjacent kidney tissue and the BPH-1 cells became irreversibly transformed as tumorigenic when adapted back to tissue culture. These cells had constitutively activated Akt and expressed high levels of TGF-β but lost their ability to respond to the growth inhibitory effect of this cytokine with a concomitant loss of p21 and Smad3 nuclear localization (62). In addition, the transformed BPH-1 cells had elevated levels of stromal-derived factor-1 (SDF-1/CXCL12), which is the receptor for CXCR4 chemokine, involved in mediating metastasis (63, 64). Importantly, these experiments provided potential targets involved in the switch in TGF-β function from tumor suppressor to pro-oncogenic factor during malignant progression. Other landmark studies by Bhowmick et al., blocking TGF-β signaling in mouse fibroblasts with a dominant negative TGF-β receptor (by homologous recombination), have promoted cancer of the forestomach and intraepithelial neoplasia of the prostate (65, 66).

Analogous transformation-associated effects of malignant stroma on endometrial epithelial cells have been observed by Gold et al. (unpublished data). In fact, the normal stromal cells and those adjacent to the tumor appear phenotypically quite different, implying that genetically altered premalignant or transformed epithelia influence the surrounding stroma. The incubation of normal endometrial epithelial cells in co-culture with stromal cells from malignant endometrium or their conditioned media stimulates epithelial cell growth while the normal stromal cells or their conditioned media do not have this effect. Similarly, conditioned media from stromal cells derived from malignant but not normal endometrium lowers p27 levels and increases cks1 levels in normal primary epithelial cells (67). These studies underscore the role of p27 as a major target for growth regulation of the endometrium and implicate the stroma in the regulation of p27 degradation in favor of malignant growth.

The ability of the neoplastic epithelia to hijack the stroma and the specific factors emanating from the stroma that aid in malignant progression are becoming important areas for study in understanding carcinogenesis. The use of co-cultures, tissue recombinant technology, and 3-dimensional (3-D) cultures are important tools in this endeavor (60, 62, 68–70). The inclusion of stromal cells in assays evaluating novel chemotherapies have already been undertaken as well as experimental protocols incorporating epithelial cells alone or in combination with stromal cells in 3-D cultures in which glands and stroma simulate their polar/normal morphology (60, 69–70). In addition, stromal cells are likely to become a target for therapy and the factors released from these cells may be considered for blocking by antibodies or inhibitors, as part of treatment protocols. Understanding cell/tissue dysfunction and therapeutic intervention on a molecular level using physiologically relevant model systems, such as co-cultures and 3-D cultures, provides an exciting new approach to determine which therapies or combinations thereof will yield the best response in vivo, for the treatment of endometrial cancer.

Exploration of Current "Targeted" Therapies

The term "targeted" therapies might best be applied to regimens selected based on the presence of known putative targets against a specific type of tumor tissue. Progestins, although empirically introduced, were the first "targeted therapies" against endometrial carcinoma (71, 72) with PR eventually validated as their target. Subsequently, studies have focused on other endocrine therapies such as tamoxifen by itself or alternating with progestins, LHRH agonists, aromatase inhibitors, and ER downregulators. Decades of clinical experience indicate that patients benefiting from such therapies are those who have certain tumor features: well-differentiated histology, positive hormone receptors, propensity to seed the lung, and >2 years between initial diagnosis and identification of metastases. Unfortunately, these represent the minority of patients with metastatic endometrial carcinoma and are discussed in Chap. 12. Non-hormonal targets are the focus of this section.

Angiogenesis Inhibitors

The monoclonal antibody, bevacizumab (Avastin) that binds the vascular endothelial growth factor (VEGF), thereby blocking angiogenesis, has been shown to have single agent activity against gynecologic cancer (73, 74). In a number of other malignancies, it potentiates the effects of chemotherapy improving response rates and progression-free survival, resulting in its approval for treatment of advanced colorectal cancer, recurrent breast cancer, and non-small cell lung cancer (75). Further, cytoskeletal-toxic chemotherapeutic agents, docetaxel and paclitaxel have anti-angiogenic activity by damaging endothelial cells (76). Finally, potentiation of the effects of radiation against rectal cancer has been attributed to its normalization of blood vessel function resulting in correction of tumor hypoxia (77). Since the secretion of VEGF is stimulated by hypoxia, whether tumors with extensive necrosis (presumably from hypoxia), such as carcinosarcoma, might benefit from an analogous treatment, needs to be tested. A number of tyrosine kinase inhibitors that target VEGF receptors directly, or influence pathways that modulate VEGF or other steps that may be required for vascular integrity (such as pericytes), are other possibilities that target angiogenesis to reduce tumor growth. Drugs such as sorafenib (Nexavar) and SU11248 (sunitinib, Sutent) that inhibit VEGFR2 and PDGFR-β among other kinases (see section below) have been found to be effective against renal cell carcinoma (78). Interestingly, whereas VEGF expression was not correlated with histologic grade in endometrial carcinoma patients, in one study involving 57 patients, VEGF-negative tumors and angiostatin-positive tumors were associated with non-recurrent disease (79). However, both endostatin and VEGF showed a statistically significant elevation in the serum of patients with higher tumor stage (80), which may in part be regulated by estrogen. These studies, although limited, indicate that anti-angiogenic chemo or monoclonal antibody therapy strategies may be useful in preventing malignant progression of endometrial carcinoma.

Epidermal Growth Factor Receptor Inhibitors

Overexpression of erbB2 in approximately 15% of type I (endometrioid) endometrial carcinomas and epidermal growth factor receptor (EGFR) in the majority of endometrial carcinosarcomas (82% in one study), largely in the sarcomatous component (81) has led to interest in trials with trastuzumab, erbB1 and Her2 inhibitors (82–84), EGFR inhibitors, such as erlotinib or gefitinib and/or the monoclonal antibody cetuximab, which have been used in various malignancies including ovarian cancer (85–87). Combinations of these agents with radiation or chemotherapy are likely to be tested in the ensuing years, and are of interest in uterine malignancies.

Other Kinase Inhibitors

The PI3K/Akt signaling pathway, shown to be important in hormone-dependent cancers of the breast, prostate, and endometrium, plays a critical role in regulating proliferation, apoptosis, and mRNA translation of many proteins involved in malignant behavior (88, 89). Constitutive signaling of the PI3k/Akt occurs when PTEN, the master phosphatase and inhibitor of this pathway, is mutated or deleted, as shown in many human cancers (90, 91). Activation of mTOR (mammalian target of rapamycin) by Akt is likely to be important in endometrial cancer and inhibitors of mTOR, such as rapamycin and analogs of this macrolide (used at higher doses for immunosuppresssion following transplantation), are currently in clinical testing and of interest for endometrial carcinoma. In the phase I study of deforolimus, a patient with carcinosarcoma of Müllerian origin achieved a partial response in liver and lung metastases, still ongoing at 22 months (92). Rapamycin has been shown to be inhibitory of growth in endometrial carcinoma cell lines (93) and accordingly, to upregulate p27 in primary cultures of endometrial epithelial cells (Gold et al., unpublished data). As discussed earlier, the loss and/or mutation of PTEN is an early event in endometrial cancer (17–19). Therefore, the use of inhibitors of PI3K/AKT (to reconstitute the growth inhibitory effect of PTEN by blocking Akt or by blocking proteins downstream from this pathway such as mTOR), β-catenin (which regulates transcription of transformation associated genes), and the cyclin-dependent kinase inhibitor, p27, all shown to be aberrantly expressed in endometrial cancer, appear to have potential significance for future clinical trials. Recent data has shown that inhibition of multiple targets results in therapeutic efficacy (e.g. effects of sunitinib or sorafenib in renal cell cancer; effects of lapatinib in breast cancer). The results achieved are an indication of the importance of concurrently inhibiting more than one "activated" pathway. Multitargeted tyrosine kinase (TK) inhibitors of VEGF 1, 2, 3, PDGF α and β, and c-kit will be tested for activity in endometrial cancer (78, 94). To date, sorafenib has also demonstrated antitumor effect against a number of papillary cancers (ovary, thyroid, and kidney) (78).

Proteasome Inhibitors

As discussed previously, another apparent early event in the development of endometrial cancer is the absence and/or cytoplasmic mislocalization of the cyclin dependent kinase inhibitor, p27^{kip1} (p27), which, when in the nucleus, blocks cell cycle progression in late G1 phase by blocking cyclin-dependent kinase activity (Cdk2) and thus, phosphorylation of the retinoblastoma protein (pRb) (95, 96). Gold et al. have further shown that absence of p27 in malignant endometrial glands is due to a high rate of uibiquitin-mediated proteasome degradation (30) and increased levels of the ubiquitin targeting proteins, Cks1 and Skp2 (48, 67, 97). As shown in Fig. 1, whereas TGF-β signaling in normal endometrial epithelial cells induces a marked increase in nuclear p27 to enable growth inhibition, because of lack of TGF-β signaling in endometrial carcinoma cells (46), p27 succumbs to continuous degradation (30). The mechanism of normal induction of p27 by TGF-β signaling, shown to be via Smad2/3 activation, is not at the mRNA level but through preventing its degradation by downregulating Cks1 and Skp2, the rate limiting components of the SCF complex of proteins that ensures the targeting of p27 for proteasomal degradation (48, 67, 96, 97). The importance of p27 as a major cell cycle protein that regulates endometrial cell growth is underscored by the fact that ovarian hormones, estrogen and progesterone, also regulate p27 levels (30) (Fig. 1). Specifically, estrogen induces MAPK-driven proteasomal degradation of p27 in normal endometrial epithelial cells and progesterone causes a marked increase in p27 in primary normal endometrial epithelial cells and most primary endometrial carcinoma cells tested in vitro. These data suggest that TGF-β is unable to exert cell cycle control by preventing the degradation of p27 in the presence of continuous estrogen-driven proteasomal degradation. The mechanisms involved in the hormonal regulation of p27 remain to be determined. It seems apparent that preservation of nuclear p27 levels has emerged as a significant potential target for restoring normal endometrial cell growth. Therefore, a possibility for future therapeutic intervention may be the use of proteasome inhibitors, such as bortezomib (Velcade) or analogs, such as salinosporamide (NPI-0052) (98–100). However, blocking proteasomal degradation of p27, that has already been aberrantly mislocalized to the cytoplasm, could ostensibly have a deleterious effect through its ability to affect the cytoskeleton and mediate metastasis (36, 101). Nonetheless, in other cancers, specifically, multiple myeloma, bortezomib has been shown to be quite effective and its action may also be related to induction of endoplasmic reticulum stress, diminished

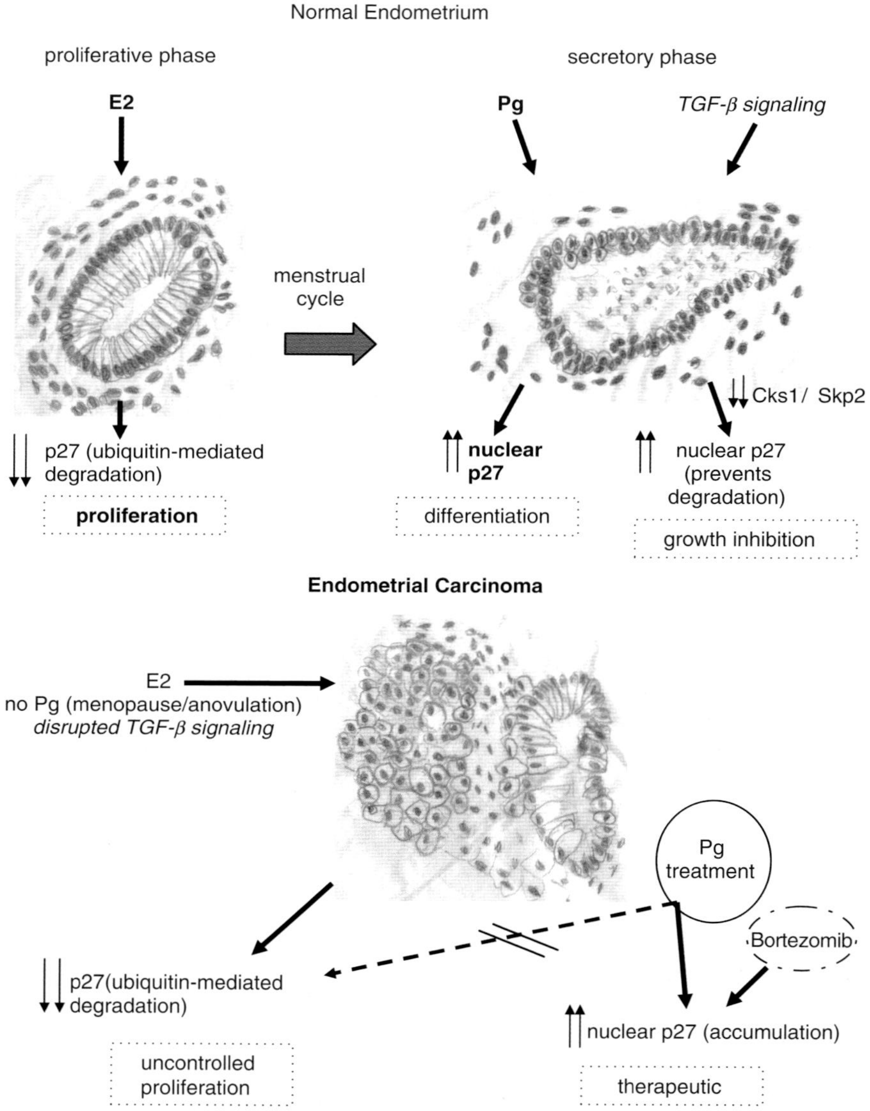

Fig. 1 The cyclin-dependent kinase inhibitor is a major molecular target for growth of normal and malignant endometrium. The model depicts the fate of the cyclin-dependent kinase inhibitor, p27[kip1] (p27) in normal endometrium and in endometrial carcinoma. p27 blocks cyclin-dependent kinase 2 (Cdk2) activity, causing growth arrest in late G_1 phase of the cell cycle (95, 96). In the proliferative phase of the normal menstrual cycle (top), estrogen (E2) induces ubiquitin-mediated degradation of p27 in 26S proteasomes. During the secretory phase, progesterone (Pg) from the corpus luteum increases the levels of p27 in the nucleus of differentiated glandular epithelial cells (30). Similarly, TGF-β/[Smad2/3] signaling induces an accumulation of nuclear p27 in the glandular epithelial cells to promote growth control (30, 46–48, 67). This occurs, at least in part, by preventing p27 degradation through the downregulation of Skp2 [E3-ligase for p27] and Cks1. These proteins are rate-limiting

angiogenesis, or effects on a number of other pathways relying on proteasome degradation of proteins (102).

Future Strategies

The introduction of systemic therapy in the treatment of endometrial cancer is a relatively recent development. The full impact of utilizing systemic therapy in addition to surgery and radiotherapy is difficult to predict at this time. However, clinical trials are providing clear indication of an effect on survival at locally advanced as well as metastatic stages. With better diagnosis and staging, as well as delineation of molecular events accompanying increased risk of distant metastases, systemic treatments will undoubtedly be introduced in earlier stages and in selected patients. Whether postoperative radiation will continue to be part of treatment regimens in stage I with "high-risk features" (e.g. lymphovascular invasion, high grade, focal papillary serous differentiation) will need to be addressed in morbidity-reducing trials.

Future diagnosis and treatment will entail tailoring therapies to the histology of the tumor, the genetic make-up of the individual, and the proteomic profile of the serum (eventually to also include tissue by Laser Capture Microdissection followed by mass spectrometry). Results of such studies may lead to apply combinatorial therapeutic approaches, followed by monitoring the re-expression of certain markers determined proteomically to indicate a return towards normal. Indeed, coupling tumor biology at various stages with developmental therapeutics is the challenge for the future. Endometrial cancer may lend itself particularly well to such target validation due to access to tissue, and the applying of paradigms that have been developed to interrogate mechanisms and pathways involved in endometrial hyperplasia and cancer, as discussed in this chapter.

In other uterine malignancies, because of their relative rarity, the challenge will be to identify less toxic systemic regimens in advanced disease, so that they can be applied widely in clinical trials. Currently, toxicity often inhibits use of chemotherapy for uterine leiomyosarcomas and carcinosarcomas so that chemotherapy is only used when faced with life-threatening advanced and recurrence settings. It is a high priority, therefore, to find more effective and less toxic treatments, based on chemotherapy, radiation, and targeted drugs, at emphasized in Chapter 13.

Fig. 1 (continued) components of the SCF complex that target p27 for ubiquitin-mediated degradation in the proteasome (48, 67). In endometrial carcinoma, both unopposed E2 and loss of TGF-β/Smad2 signaling permit continuous ubiquitin-mediated degradation of p27, leading to uncontrolled proliferation (30, 46–48, 67). Since Pg treatment increases the levels of nuclear p27 in primary cultures of endometrial carcinoma cells, nuclear p27 expression may be a marker of positive response to Pg therapy in vivo (31). In addition, based on in vitro data, proteasome inhibitors, such as bortezomib (98–100, 102), might provide a new therapeutic approach to increase p27 nuclear levels and gain growth control in endometrial carcinoma.

Conclusions

- Future diagnosis and treatments will entail tailoring therapies to the histology of the tumor, the genetic make-up of the individual, and proteomic profiles.
- Coupling tumor biology at various stages with developmental therapeutics is the challenge for the future.
- Endometrial cancer may lend itself to studies of target validation as access to tissues and ability to interrogate mechanisms and pathways at premalignant stages such as endometrial hyperplasia are now available.
- Current therapeutic approaches may also be increasingly guided by ongoing advances in tumor biology.

References

1. Muggia FM, Chia G, Reed LJ, Romney SL. Doxorubicin-cyclophosphamide: effective chemotherapy for advanced endometrial adenocarcinoma. Am J Obstet Gynecol. 1977; 128(3):314–9.
2. Thigpen JT, Blessing JA, DiSaia PJ, Yordan E, Carson LF, Evers C. A randomized comparison of doxorubicin alone versus doxorubicin plus cyclophosphamide in the management of advanced or recurrent endometrial carcinoma: a Gynecologic Oncology Group study. J Clin Oncol. 1994;12(7):1408–14.
3. Thigpen JT, Brady MF, Homesley HD, et al. Phase III trial of doxorubicin with or without cisplatin in advanced endometrial carcinoma: a gynecologic oncology group study. J Clin Oncol. 2004;22(19):3902–8.
4. Fleming GF, Fillaci VL, Bentley RC, et al. Phase III randomized trial of doxorubicin + cisplatin versus doxorubicin + 24-h paclitaxel + filgrastin in endometrial carcinoma: a Gynecologic Oncology Group study. Ann Oncol. 2004;15(8):1173–8.
5. Fleming GF, Brunetto VL, Cella D, et al. Phase III trial of doxorubicin plus cisplatin with or without paclitaxel plus filgrastim in advanced endometrial carcinoma: a Gynecologic Oncology Group study. J Clin Oncol. 2004;22(11):2159–66.
6. Hoskins PJ, Swenerton KD, Pike JA, et al. Paclitaxel and carboplatin, alone or with irradiation, in advanced or recurrent endometrial cancer: a Phase II study. J Clin Oncol. 2001; 19(20):4048–53.
7. Rabdall ME, Brunetto G, Muss H, et al. Whole abdominal radiotherapy versus combination doxorubicin-cisplatin chemotherapy in advance endometrial carcinoma: A randomized Phase III study. J Clin Oncol. 2001;19(20):4048–53.
8. Randall ME, Filiaci VL, Muss H, et al. Randomized phase III trial of whole-abdominal irradiation versus doxorubicin and cisplatin chemotherapy in advanced endometrial carcinoma: a Gynecological Oncology Group Study. J Clin Oncol. 2006;24(1):36–44.
9. Sutton G, Brunetto VL, Kilgore L, et al. A Phase III trial of ifosfamide with or without cisplatin in carcinosarcoma of the uterus: A Gynecologic Oncology Group Study. Gynecol Oncol. 2000;79(2):147–53.
10. Homesley HD, Filiaci VL, Bitterman P, Eaton L, Kilgore LC, Monk BJ. Phase III trial of ifosfamide versus ifosfamide plus paclitaxel as first line treatment of advanced or recurrent uterine carcinosarcoma (mixed mesodermal tumors): a Gynecologic Oncology Group study. SGO. Abstract # 66, 2006.
11. Wolfson AH, Brady MF, Rocereto TF, et al. A Gynecologic Oncology Group randomized trial of whole abdominal irradiation (WAI) vs cisplatin-ifosfamide + mesna (CIM) in surgically cytoreduced stage I-IV carcinosarcoma (CS) of the uterus. Gynecol Oncol. 2007;107:77–85.

12. Yang J, Mani SA, Donaher JL, et al. Twist, a master regulator of morphogenesis, pays an essential role in tumor metastasis. Cell. 2004;117:927–939.
13. Jeon YT, Park IA, Kim YB, et al. Steroid receptor expressions in endometrial cancer: clinical significance and epidemiological implication. Cancer Lett. 2006;239:198–204.
14. Shang Y, Brown M. Molecular determinants for the tissue specificity of SERMs. Science. 2002;295(5564):2465–8.
15. Lupu R and Menendez JA. Targeting fatty acid synthase in breast and endometrial cancer: an alternative to selective estrogen receptor modulators? Endocrinology. 2006;147:4056–66.
16. Barnes KR and Lippard SJ. Cisplatin and related anticancer drugs: recent advances and insight. Met Ions Biol Syst. 2004;42:143–77.
17. Ellenson LH and Wu TC. Focus on endometrial and cervical cancer. Cancer Cell. 2004; 5(6):533–8.
18. Sun H, Enomoto T, Fujta M, et al. Mutational analysis of the PTEN gene in endometrial carcinoma and hyperplasia. Am J Clin Pathol. 2001; 115(1):32–8.
19. Levine RL, Cargile CB, Blazes MS, van Rees B, Kurman RJ, Ellenson LH. PTEN mutations and microsatellite instability in complex atypical hyperplasia, a precursor lesion to uterine endometrioid carcinoma. Cancer Res. 1998;58(15):3254–8.
20. Shedden KA, Kshirsagar MP, Schwartz DR, et al. Histologic type, organ of origin, and Wnt pathway status: effect on gene expression in ovarian and uterine carcinomas. Clin Cancer Res. 2005; 11:2123–2131.
21. Marquez RT, Baggerly KA, Patterson AP, et al. Patterns of gene expression in different histotypes of epithelial ovarian cancer correlate with those in normal fallopian tube, endometrium, and colon. Clin Cancer Res. 2005; 11:6116–26.
22. Kohn EC, Mills GB, Liotta L. Promising directions for the diagnosis and management of gynecological cancers. Int J Gynaecol Obstet. 2003;83:203–209.
23. Souchelnytskyi S. Proteomics of TGF-beta signaling and its impact on breast cancer. Expert Rev Proteomics. 2005;2:925–935.
24. Espina V, Dettloff KA, Cowherd S, Petricoin EF 3rd, Liotta LA. Use of proteomic analysis to monitor responses to biological therapies. Expert Opin Biol Ther. 2004;4:83–93.
25. Wulfkuhle JD, Aquino JA, Calvert VS, et al. Signal pathway profiling of ovarian cancer from human tissue specimens using reverse-phase protein microarrays. Proteomics. 2003;3:2085–2090.
26. Cowherd SM, Espina VA, Petricoin EF 3rd, Liotta LA. Proteomic analysis of human breast cancer tissue with laser-capture microdissection and reverse-phase protein microarrays. Clin Breast Cancer. 2004;5:385–392.
27. Yoshizaki T, Enomoto T, Nakashima R, et al. Altered protein expression in endometrial carcinogenesis. Cancer Lett. 2005;226:101–106.
28. Vilgelm A, Lian Z, Wang H, et al. Akt-mediated phosphorylation and activation of estrogen receptor alpha is required for endometrial neoplastic transformation in Pten + /– mice. Cancer Res. 2006;66(7):3375–80.
29. Zukerberg LR, DeBarnardo RL, Kirley Sd, et al. Loss of cables, a cyclin-dependent kinase regulatory protein, is associated with the development of endometrial hyperplasia and endometrial cancer. Cancer Res. 2004;64:202–208.
30. Lecanda J, Parekh TV, Gama P, et al. Transforming growth factor-beta, estrogen, and progesterone converge on the regulation of p27Kip1 in the normal and malignant endometrium. Cancer Res. 2007;67(3):1007–18.
31. Watanabe J, Watanabe K, Jobo T, et al. Significance of p27 as a predicting marker for medroxyprogresterone acetate therapy against endometrial endometrioid adenocarcinoma. Int J Gynecol Cancer. 2006;16(Suppl 1):452–7.
32. Mutter GL, Lin MC, Fitzgerald JT, et al. Altered PTEN expression as a diagnostic marker for the earliest endometrial precancers. J Natl Cancer Inst. 2000;92:924–930.
33. Podsypanina K, Lee RT, Politis C, Hennessy I, et al. An inhibitor of mTOR reduces neoplasia and normalizes p70/S6 kinase activity in pTen + /- mice. Proc Natl Acad Sci USA. 2001;98(18):10320–5.

34. Stambolic V, Tsao MS, Macpherson D, Suzuki A, Chapman WB, Mak TW. High incidence of breast and endometrial neoplasia resembling human Cowden syndrome in pten + /- mice. Cancer Res. 2000;60:3605–3611.

35. Di Cristofano A, De Acetis M, Koff A, Cordon-Cardo C, Pandolfi PP. Pten and p27KIP1 cooperate in prostate cancer tumor suppression in the mouse. Nat Genet. 2001;27:222–4.

36. Besson A, Gurian-West M, Chen X, Kelly-Spratt KS, Kemp CJ, Roberts JM. A pathway in quiescent cells that controls p27Kip1 stability, subcellular localization, and tumor suppression. Genes Dev. 2006;20:47–64.

37. Payne SR, Kemp CJ. P27(Kip1) (Cdkn1b)-deficient mice are susceptible to chemical carcinogenesis and may be a useful model for carcinogen screening. Toxicol Pathol. 2003;31:355–63.

38. An HJ, Lee YH, Cho NH, et al. Alteration of PTEN expression in endometrial carcinoma is associated with down-regulation of cyclin-dependent kinase inhibitor, p27. Histopathology. 2002;41:437–445.

39. Weng LP, Brown JL, Eng C. PTEN coordinates G(1) arrest by down-regulating cyclin D1 via its protein phosphatase activity and up-regulating p27 via its lipid phosphatase activity in a breast cancer model. Human Mol Genet. 2001;10(6):599–604.

40. Mamillapalli R, Gavrilova N, Mihaylova VT, et al. PTEN regulates the ubiquitin-dependent degradation of the CDK inhibitor p27(KIP1) through the ubiquitin E3 ligase SCF(SKP2). Curr Biol. 2001;11(4):263–267.

41. DeBernardo RL, Littell RD, Luo H, et al. Defining the extent of cables loss in endometrial cancer subtypes and its effectiveness as an inhibitor of cell proliferation in malignant endometrial cells in vitro and in vivo. Cancer Biol Ther. 2005;4:103–107.

42. Zhang H, Duan HO, Kirley SD, Zukerberg LR, Wu CL. Aberrant splicing of cables gene, a CDK regulator, in human cancers. Cancer Biol Ther. 2005;4:1211–1215.

43. Li DM, Sun H. EPT1, encoded by a candidate tumor suppressor locus, is a novel protein tyrosine phosphatase regulated by transforming growth factor beta. Cancer Res. 1997; 57(11):2124–9.

44. Spoelstra NS, Manning NG, Higashi Y, et al. The transcription factor ZRB1 is aberrantly expressed in aggressive uterine cancers. Cancer Res. 2006;66(7):3893–3902.

45. McGrath M, Lee IM, Hankinson SE, et al. Androgen receptor polymorphisms and endometrial cancer risk. Int J Cancer. 2006;118:1261–1268.

46. Parekh TV, Gama P, Wen X, et al. Transforming growth factor beta signaling is disabled early in human endometrial carcinogenesis concomitant with loss of growth inhibition. Cancer Res. 2002;62(10):2778–2790.

47. Gold LI and Parekh TV. Loss of growth regulation by transforming growth factor-beta (TGF-beta) in human cancers: studies on endometrial carcinoma. Semin Reprod Endocrinol. 1999; 17(1):73–92.

48. Gold LI and Lecanda J. Mechanisms of cell cycle regulation by TGF-β dysregulated in cancer. In: Transforming growth factor—β in Cancer Therapy. Vol. 1. Basic and Clinical Biology, Part 1. Basic Concepts of TGF-β signaling in normal physiology and cancer pathobiology, Ed., Sonia Jakowlew, Humana Press, Inc., Totowa, NJ, 2008.

49. Roberts AB and Wakefield LM. The two faces of transforming growth factor beta in carcinogenesis. Proc Natl Acad Sci USA. 2003;100:8621–8623.

50. Muraoka-Cook RS, Dumont N, Arteaga CL. Dual role of transforming growth factor beta in mammary tumorigenesis and metastatic progression. Clin Cancer Res. 2005;11(2 Pt 2): 937s–943s.

51. Dumont N and Arteaga CL. Targeting the TGF beta signaling network in human neoplasia. Cancer Cell. 2003;3(6):531–536.

52. Derynck R, Akhurst RJ, Balmain A. TGF-beta signaling in tumor suppression and cancer progression. Nat Genet. 2001;29(2):117–29.

53. Yingling JM, Blanchard KL, Sawyer JS. Development of TGF-beta signaling inhibitors for cancer therapy. Nat Rev Discov. 2004;3(12):1011–1022.

54. Tsuchida K, Sunada Y, Noji S, Murakami T, Uezumi A, Nakatani M. Inhibitors of the TFG-beta superfamily and their clinical applications. Mini Rev Med Chem. 2006;6(11):1255–1261.

55. Saunier EF, Akhurst RJ. TGF beta inhibition for cancer therapy. Curr Cancer Drug Targets 2006;6(7):565–78.
56. Akhurst RJ. Large- and small-molecule initiators of brainstorming growth factor-beta signaling. Curr Opin Investig Drugs 2006;7(6):513–521.
57. Bierie B and Moses HL. Tumour microenvironment: TGFbeta: the molecular Jekyll and Hyde of cancer. Nat Rev Cancer 2006;6(7):506–520.
58. Bhowmick NA, Neilson EG, Moses HL. Stromal fibroblasts in cancer initiation and progression. Nature. 2004;432(7015):332–337.
59. Orimo A, Tomioka Y, Shimizu Y, et al. Cancer-associated myofibroblasts possess various factors to promote endometrial tumor progression. Clin Cancer Res. 2001;7(10):3097–105.
60. Joyce JA. Therapeutic targeting of the tumor microenvironment. Cancer Cell. 2005; 7:513–520.
61. Radisky DC and Bissell MJ. Cancer. Respect thy neighbor! Science. 2004;303(5659):775–777.
62. Hayward SW, Wang Y, Cao M, et al. Malignant transformation in a nontumorigenic human prostatic epithelial cell line. Cancer Res. 2001;61(22):8135–8142.
63. Ao M, Williams K, Bhowmick NA, Hayward SW. Transforming growth factor-beta promotes invasion in tumorigenic but not in nontumorigenic human prostatic epithelial cells. Cancer Res. 2006;66:8007–16.
64. Ao M, Franco OE, Park D, Raman D, Williams K, Hayward SW. Cross-talk between paracrine-acting cytokine and chemokine pathways promotes malignancy in benign human prostatic epithelium. Cancer Res. 2007;67(9):4244–53.
65. Bhowmick NA, Chytil A, Plieth D, et al. TGF-beta signaling in fibroblasts modulates the oncogenic potential of adjacent epithelia. Science. 2004;303(5659):848–851.
66. Bierie B and Moses HL. Under pressure: stromal fibroblasts change their ways. Cell. 2005; 123(6):985–7.
67. Lecanda J, Ganapathy V, D'Aquino-Ardalan C, et al. TGFbeta prevents proteasomal degradation of the cyclin-dependent kinase inhibitor p27 (Kip1) for cell cycle arrest. Cell Cycle 2009;8(5):742–756.
68. Arnold JT, Kaufman DG, Seppala M, Lessey BA. Endometrial stromal cells regulate epithelial cell growth in vitro: a new co-culture model. Hum Reprod. 2001;16:836–845.
69. Lee GY, Kenny PA, Lee EH, Bissell MJ. Three-dimensional culture models of normal and malignant breast epithelial cells. Nat Methods. 2007;4(4):359–65.
70. Fournier MV, Martin KJ, Kenny PA, et al. Gene expression signature in organized and growth-arrested mammary acini predicts good outcome in breast cancer. Cancer Res. 2006;66(14):7095–102.
71. Thigpen JT, Brady MF, Alvarez RD, et al. Oral medroxyprogesterone acetate in the treatment of advanced or recurrent endometrial carcinoma: a dose-response study by the Gynecologic Oncology Group. J Clin Oncol. 1999;17(6):1736–44.
72. Iwai K, Fukuda K, Hachisuga T, Mori M, Uchiyama M, Iwasaka T, Sugimori H. Prognostic significance of progesterone receptor immunohistochemistry for lymph node metastases in endometrial carcinoma. Gynecol Oncol. 1999;72(3):351–9.
73. Burger RA, Sill MW, Monk BJ, Greer BE, Sorosky JI. Phase II trial of bevacizumab in persistent or recurrent epithelial ovarian cancer or primary peritoneal cancer: a Gynecologic Oncology Group study. J Clin Oncol. 2007;25:5615–71.
74. Kamat AA, Merrit WM, Coffey D, et al. Clinical and biological significance of vascular endothelial growth factor in endometrial cancer. Clin Cancer Res. 2007;13(24):7487–95.
75. Hicklin DJ, Ellis LM. Role of the vascular endothelial growth factor pathway in tumor growth and angiogenesis. J Clin Oncol. 2005;23(5):1011–27.
76. Kamat AA, Merritt WM, Coffey D, et al. Clinical and biological significance of vascular endothelial growth factor in endometrial cancer. Clin Cancer Res. 2007;13(24):7487–95.
77. Willett CG, Boucher Y, diTomaso E, et al. Direct evidence that the VEGF-specific antibody bevacizumab has antivascular effects in human rectal cancer. Nat Med. 2004;10(2):145–147.
78. Motzer RJ, Basch E. Targeted drugs for metastatic renal cell carcinoma. Lancet. 2007; 370(9605):2071–3.

79. Yabushita H, Noguchi M, Kinoshita S, Kishida T, Sawaguchi K, Noguchi M. Angiostatin expression in endometrial cancer. Oncol Rep. 2002;9(6):1193–6.
80. Shaarawy M, El-Sharkawy SA. Biomarkers of intrinsic angiogenic and anti-angiogenic activity in patients with endometrial hyperplasia and endometrial cancer. Acta Oncol. 2001; 40(4):513–8.
81. Livasy CA, Reading FC, Moore DT, Boggess JF, Lininger RA. EGFR expression and Her2/neu overexpression/amplifiction in endometrial carcinosarcoma. Gynec Oncol. 2006;100(1):101–6.
82. Press MF, Lenz HJ. EGFR, HER2 and VEGF pathways: validated targets for cancer treatment. Drugs. 2007;67(14):2045–75.
83. Konecny GE, Venkatesan N, Yang G, et al. Activity of lapatinib a novel HER2 and EGFR dual kinase inhibitor in human endometrial cancer cells. Br J Cancer. 2008;98(6):1076–1084.
84. Ejskjaer K, Sorensen BS, Poulsen SS, Forman A, Nexo E, Mogensen O. Expression of the epidermal growth factor system in endometrioid endometrial cancer. Gynecol Oncol. 2007; 104(1):158–67.
85. Schilder RJ, Sill MW, Chen X, et al. Phase II study of gefitinib in patients with relapsed or persistent ovarian or primary peritoneal carcinoma and evaluation of epidermal growth factor receptor mutations and immunohistochemical expression: a Gynecologic Oncology Group study. Clin Cancer Res. 2005;11(15):5539–48.
86. Gordon AN, Finkler N, Edwards RP, et al. Efficacy and safety of erlotinib HCL, an epidermal growth factor receptor (HER1/EGFR) tyrosine kinase inhibitor, in patients with advanced ovarian carcinoma: results from a phase II multicenter study. Int J Gynecol Cancer. 2005;15:785–792.
87. Secord AA, Blessing JA, Armstrong DK, et al. Phase II trial of cetuximab and carboplatin in relapsed platinum-sensitive ovarian cancer and evaluation of epidermal growth factor receptor expression: a Gynecologic Oncology Group study. Gynecol Oncol. 2008;108(3):493–9.
88. Vivanco I, Sawyers CL. The phosphatidylinositol 3-Kinase AKT pathway in human cancer. Nat Rev Cancer. 2002;2(7):489–501.
89. Wu X, Senechal K, Neshat MS, Whang YE, Sawyers CL. The PTEN/MMAC1 tumor suppressor phosphatase functions as a negative regulator of the phosphoinositide 3-kinase/Akt pathway. Proc Natl Acad Sci U S A. 1998;95(26):15587–91.
90. Ali IU, Schriml LM, Dean M. Mutational spectra of PTEN/MMAC1 gene: a tumor suppressor with lipid phosphatase activity. J Natl Cancer Inst. 1999;91(22):1922–32.
91. Cairns P, Okami K, Halachmi S, et al. Frequent inactivation of PTEN/MMAC1 in primary prostate cancer. Cancer Res. 1997;57(22):4997–5000.
92. Mita MM, Mita AC, Chu QS, et al. Phase I trial of the novel mammalian target of rapamycin inhibitor deforolimus (AP23573; MK-8669) administered intravenously daily for 5 days every 2 weeks to patients with advanced malignancies. J Clin Oncol. 2008;26(3):361–367.
93. Zhou C, Gehrig PA, Whang YE, Boggess JF. Rapamycin inhibits telomerase activity by decreasing the hTERT mRNA level in endometrial cancer cells. Molec Cancer Ther. 2003; 2:789–795.
94. Sonpavde G, Hutson TE. Pazopanib: a novel multitargeted tyrosine kinase inhibitor. Curr Oncol Rep. 2007;9(2):115–9.
95. Slingerland JM, Hengst L, Pan CH, Alexander D, Stampfer MR, Reed SI. A novel inhibitor of cyclin-Cdk activity detected in transforming growth factor beta-arrested epithelial cells. Mol Cell Biol. 1994;14(6):3683–94.
96. Bloom J, Pagano M. Deregulated degradation of the cdk inhibitor p27 and malignant transformation. Semin Cancer Biol. 2003;13(1):41–7.
97. Gold LI, Rahman M, Liarsky V, et al. The downregulation and growth inhibition of endometrial caricinoma cells. Proc Amer Assoc Cancer Res. 2004;910:(Abstract # 3948).
98. Cusack JC Jr, Liu R, Xia L, et al. NPI-0052 enhances tumoricidal response to conventional cancer therapy in a colon cancer model. Clin Cancer Res. 2006;12(22):6758–6764.
99. Mitsiades CS, Mitsiades N, Hideshima T, Richardson PG, Anderson KC. Proteasome inhibitors as therapeutics. Essays Biochem. 2005;41:205–218.
100. Richardson PG, Mitsiades C. Bortezomib: proteasome inhibition as an effective anticancer therapy. Future Oncol. 2005; 1(2):161–171.

101. Denicourt C, Saenz CC, Datnow B, Cui XS, Dowdy SF. Relocalized p27Kip1 tumor suppressor functions as a cytoplasmic metastatic oncogene in melanoma. Cancer Res. 2007; 67(19):9238–43.
102. Richardson PG, Sonneveld P, Schuster MW, et al. Assessment of proteasome inhibition for extending remissions (APEX) investigators. Bortezomib or high-dose dexamethasone for relapsed multiple myeloma. N Engl J Med. 2005;352:2487–2498.

Index

E

EBRT. *See* External beam radiotherapy
EC. *See* Endometrial carcinoma
EGFR. *See* Epidermal growth factor receptor
EMT. *See* Epithelial to mesenchymal
       transition
Endocervical adenocarcinoma, 116
Endocrine therapy, endometrial
       adenocarcinomas and, 217
Endogenous Hormones Breast Cancer
       Collaborative Group, 3
Endometrial adenocarcinoma
   endocrine therapy and, 217
   lymph node sampling of patients with, 164
   subtypes of, 87
   systemic chemotherapy for, 267
Endometrial cancer
   advanced stage, 240–243
   age-specific incidence rates for, 7
   biology of, 260
   Bokhman's type II, 58
   brachytherapy for, low-dose v. high-dose
          rate, 185
   care of, surgical treatment as standard
          of, 143
   chemoprevention of, 9
   chemotherapy in treatment of, 223–230
          combination, 226–227
          single agent, 224–225
   classification of, 161–162
   clinical management guidelines for, 164
   as common, 143, 161, 193
   CT of, 44
   detection
          diagnostic modalities for, 27–28
          early, 46–47
   development of, 275
   diagnosis of, 22, 51
          imaging in, 25–47
          recommendations for, 19
   early-stage type I, 169
          surgical therapy for, 161–170
   early warning signs of, 161
   EBRT treatment of, 186
   epidemiology of, 1–10
   EPT and, 1
   ER expressed by, 269
   estrogen production with development
          of, 243–244
   ET and, 1, 3, 5
   evaluation of, 25
   fertility of patients with, 144, 151, 155
   future directions for treatment of,
          155, 277

   genetic disorders of patients presenting
          with, 145–146
   good prognosis associated with, 237
   high-risk subtypes of, 193
   hormonal agents in disseminated, studies
          of, 218–219
   hormonal therapy treatment for, 219
          follow up after, 153
          method of, 152–153
          studies on, 218–219
   hormonal v. cytotoxic therapy
          responsiveness of, 218
   hormone receptor action in, mechanisms
          of, 153–154
   imaging patients with, protocols for, 35
   increased risk of developing
          BMI increasing associated with, 2, 4
          factors associated with, 14–15
          obesity and, 1, 14–15, 144–146,
                162, 169
          tamoxifen and, 15
          women and, 14
   infertility of presenting patients with, 145
   intraoperative management of, 163
   laparoscopic surgery and, 165–168
          vaginal hysterectomy combined
                with, 166
   management of, conservative, 176–177
   menopausal ET and increased risk of, 1, 3
          lowering, 6
   menstrual irregularity and, 145
   MRI of, 36
   obesity as epidemiologic risk factor for, 1,
          14–15, 144–146, 169
   parity increasing causing decreasing
          risk of, 8
   PET of, 45
   postmenopausal women affected by, 144
   postoperative radiation therapy for,
          241–242
   primary hormonal therapy of, 143–156
   progestins in systemic therapy of, 217
   PR's presence in, 153–154
   PTEN gene and, 92
   quality of life of patients with, 167–168
   radiation therapy for locally recurrent, 237
   recurrent, 46–47
          factors associated with improved
                survival in, 238
          isolated to central pelvis, 230
          risk of, 176
          surgery for stage IV, 239–240
          vaginal, 239
   RT adjuvant therapy for, 175, 178–182

Printed in the United States of America